Maximum Interval Training

John Cissik

Jay Dawes

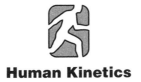

Human Kinetics

Library of Congress Cataloging-in-Publication Data

Cissik, John, 1971-
   Maximum interval training / John Cissik, Jay Dawes.
      pages cm
   Includes bibliographical references.
   1. Physical fitness. I. Dawes, Jay. II. Title.
   GV481.C628 2015
   613.7--dc23

                              2014047772

ISBN: 978-1-4925-0023-0 (print)

This publication is written and published to provide accurate and authoritative information relevant to the subject matter presented. It is published and sold with the understanding that the author and publisher are not engaged in rendering legal, medical, or other professional services by reason of their authorship or publication of this work. If medical or other expert assistance is required, the services of a competent professional person should be sought.

The web addresses cited in this text were current as of January 2015, unless otherwise noted.

Acquisitions Editor: Justin Klug; **Developmental Editor:** Carla Zych; **Managing Editor:** Elizabeth Evans; **Copyeditor:** Bob Replinger; **Permissions Manager:** Martha Gullo; **Graphic Designer:** Kathleen Boudreau-Fuoss; **Cover Designer:** Keith Blomberg; **Photograph (cover):** Jason Allen; **Photographs (interior):** Neil Bernstein; **Visual Production Assistant:** Joyce Brumfield; **Photo Production Manager:** Jason Allen; **Art Manager:** Kelly Hendren; **Associate Art Manager:** Alan L. Wilborn; **Illustrations:** © Human Kinetics, unless otherwise noted; **Printer:** Sheridan Books

We thank D1 Sports Training in Colorado Springs, Colorado, for assistance in providing the location for the photo shoot for this book.

Human Kinetics books are available at special discounts for bulk purchase. Special editions or book excerpts can also be created to specification. For details, contact the Special Sales Manager at Human Kinetics.

Printed in the United States of America   10 9 8 7 6 5 4 3 2 1

The paper in this book is certified under a sustainable forestry program.

Human Kinetics
Web site: www.HumanKinetics.com

United States: Human Kinetics
P.O. Box 5076
Champaign, IL 61825-5076
800-747-4457
e-mail: humank@hkusa.com

Canada: Human Kinetics
475 Devonshire Road Unit 100
Windsor, ON N8Y 2L5
800-465-7301 (in Canada only)
e-mail: info@hkcanada.com

Europe: Human Kinetics
107 Bradford Road
Stanningley
Leeds LS28 6AT, United Kingdom
+44 (0) 113 255 5665
e-mail: hk@hkeurope.com

Australia: Human Kinetics
57A Price Avenue
Lower Mitcham, South Australia 5062
08 8372 0999
e-mail: info@hkaustralia.com

New Zealand: Human Kinetics
P.O. Box 80
Torrens Park, South Australia 5062
0800 222 062
e-mail: info@hknewzealand.com

Fortuna et ira me agunt.
– John Cissik

For my wife, April, and my three wonderful children,
Gabriele, Addison, and Asher.
– Jay Dawes

Contents

Part III
Maximum Interval Program Design

Part IV
Maximum Interval Performance Programs

Exercise Finder

(continued)

Exercise	Muscles worked	Exercise emphasis	Page #
FOUNDATIONAL EXERCISES—*continued*			
Heavy ropes towing	Core; lower body	Strength; stability	85
Heavy ropes pulling	Shoulders; upper back; biceps; core	Strength; stability	86
Heavy ropes tug of war	Total body	Strength; endurance; stability	87
ADVANCED EXERCISES			
Heavy ropes one-handed slam	Total body	Strength; stability; coordination	88
Heavy ropes backpedal slam	Total body	Strength; stability; coordination	90
Heavy ropes shuffle slam	Total body	Strength; stability; coordination	91
Heavy ropes one-legged slam	Total body	Strength; stability; coordination; balance	92
Heavy ropes unstable slam	Total body	Strength; stability; coordination; balance	94
Heavy ropes one-handed wave	Shoulders; chest; upper back; core; lower body	Strength; stability; coordination	95
Heavy ropes one-legged wave	Total body	Strength; stability; coordination; balance	96
Heavy ropes unstable wave	Total body	Strength; stability; coordination; balance	98
Heavy ropes oblique woodchopper	Core	Strength; coordination	100
Heavy ropes one-legged woodchopper	Core; lower body	Strength; coordination; balance	102
CHAPTER 7—SUSPENSION TRAINING			
FOUNDATIONAL EXERCISES			
Suspension chest press	Chest; shoulders; triceps; core	Strength; stability	111
Suspension row	Upper back; shoulders; biceps; core	Strength; stability	112
Suspension biceps curl	Biceps	Strength; stability	113
Suspension triceps extension	Triceps	Strength; stability	114
Suspension squat	Lower body; quadriceps; hamstrings; glutes	Strength; stability	115
Suspension reverse lunge	Quadriceps; hamstrings; glutes	Strength; balance; mobility	116
Suspension hip up	Core	Strength; stability	117
Suspension leg curl	Glutes; hamstrings	Strength	118
Suspension knees to chest	Core	Strength; stability	119
Suspension lying leg raise	Core	Strength; stability	120
ADVANCED EXERCISES			
Suspension push-up	Chest; shoulders; triceps	Strength; stability	121
Suspension fly	Chest; core	Strength; stability	122
Suspension one-armed row	Upper back; shoulder; biceps	Strength; balance; stability	123
Suspension reverse fly	Shoulders; upper back	Strength; stability	124
Suspension one-legged squat	Quadriceps; hamstrings; glutes	Strength; balance; stability	125
Suspension foot-in-trainer one-legged squat	Quadriceps; hamstrings; glutes	Strength; balance; coordination	126

(continued)

Exercise Finder *(continued)*

Exercise	Muscles worked	Exercise emphasis	Page #
FOUNDATIONAL EXERCISES—*continued*			
Sandbag split squat	Lower body	Strength; endurance; balance	165
Sandbag in-place lunge	Lower body	Strength; endurance; balance	166
Sandbag overhead press	Upper body	Strength; endurance	167
Sandbag bent-over row	Upper body	Strength; stability	168
Sandbag upright row	Shoulders; trapezius	Strength; endurance	169
ADVANCED EXERCISES			
Sandbag overhead squat	Total body	Strength; stability; endurance	170
Sandbag farmer's walk	Core	Stability; grip strength	171
Sandbag push-up to overhead press	Total body	Strength; stability; endurance	172
Sandbag Y press	Total body	Strength; stability; endurance	174
Sandbag walkover lunge	Lower body	Strength; balance; stability	175
Sandbag swing and lift	Total body	Mobility; power	176
Sandbag high pull	Shoulders; trapezius	Strength; endurance	177
Sandbag push press	Total body	Strength; coordination	178
Sandbag jerk	Total body	Strength; coordination	178
Sandbag clean	Total body	Strength; coordination	180
Sandbag squat to carry	Total body	Strength; balance; stability	182
CHAPTER 10—ALTERNATIVE TRAINING FORMATS			
HEAVY RESISTANCE BANDS			
Heavy resistance band standing row	Rhomboids; middle trapezius	Endurance	186
Heavy resistance band standing chest press	Chest; shoulders; triceps	Endurance	187
Resistance band push-up	Chest; shoulders; triceps	Strength; endurance	188
Resistance band assisted pull-up	Upper back	Strength	189
Heavy resistance band squat	Lower body	Endurance	190
WATER-FILLED STABILITY BALLS			
Water-filled stability ball lift	Lower body; core	Strength; endurance; stability	192
Water-filled stability ball squat	Lower body; core	Strength; endurance; stability	193
Water-filled stability ball carry	Total body	Strength; stability	194
WEIGHTED TRAINING SLEDS			
Sled push	Total body	Strength; force	195
Sled pull	Upper back; biceps	Strength; endurance	196
Sled drag	Lower body	Strength; endurance	197
HEAVY BOXING BAGS			
Heavy boxing bag jab	Total body	Conditioning	198
Heavy boxing bag cross	Totally body	Conditioning	200
Heavy boxing bag hook	Total body	Conditioning	201
Heavy boxing bag walking lunge	Lower body; core	Strength; stability	202

Preface

The concept of high-intensity interval training has exploded over the last 10 years. It has become popular in our culture through programs like Cross Fit, P90X, and Insanity. In addition to workout videos and social media, these approaches to training also have apparel, television shows, and even fitness certifications associated with them. These programs often advocate the use of many of the newer training tools that have become popular over the last several years. Much of this is accompanied by unsubstantiated marketing claims, unsound exercise techniques, and a lack of understanding of how to integrate everything into a safe and effective training program. *Maximum Interval Training* is intended to give the reader the tools they need to make safe, effective decisions when it comes to conditioning.

To accomplish this, this book is divided into four parts. Part I provides background on maximum interval training to help the reader understand why and how this type of training works the way it does and how to approach training safely. This first part is organized into two chapters. Chapter 1 explains the importance of maximum interval. Chapter 2 covers different equipment options for maximum interval training as well as tips on how to perform these workouts safely.

Part II covers the tools that are used in maximum interval training. It has descriptions of the various tools that are used in modern-day training programs, and it is organized into six chapters. Chapters 3 through 10 detail specific tools—their benefits, drawbacks, and uses—that are used in maximum interval training programs and provide common exercises that are extensively illustrated.

Part III teaches how to design successful metabolic short- and long-term programs. It takes the information that was provided in parts I and II and applies it to designing maximum interval training programs. This part is divided into five chapters. Chapter 11 covers important topics, such the importance of testing. Chapter 12 explains how to assess your fitness, and chapter 13 helps interpret and use the results. Chapters 14 and 15 guide you in designing short-term and long-term programs to achieve your goals.

Part IV provides sample programs that illustrate how to put everything together and apply it to specific situations. Each chapter has an analysis of the conditioning needs of the situation followed by advice on how to integrate maximum interval training into the larger workout. The chapters also have sample workout programs as well as long-term workout programs that help you practice applying maximum interval training.

Maximum interval training is essential for ensuring athletes' success in game situations as well as being able to perform successfully in everyday life. It is important for minimizing the effects of fatigue, helping you to build and maintain muscle mass, increasing your strength, increasing your mobility, and burning calories. *Maximum Interval Training* provides modern tools and approaches to help you achieve your goals!

Key to Muscles

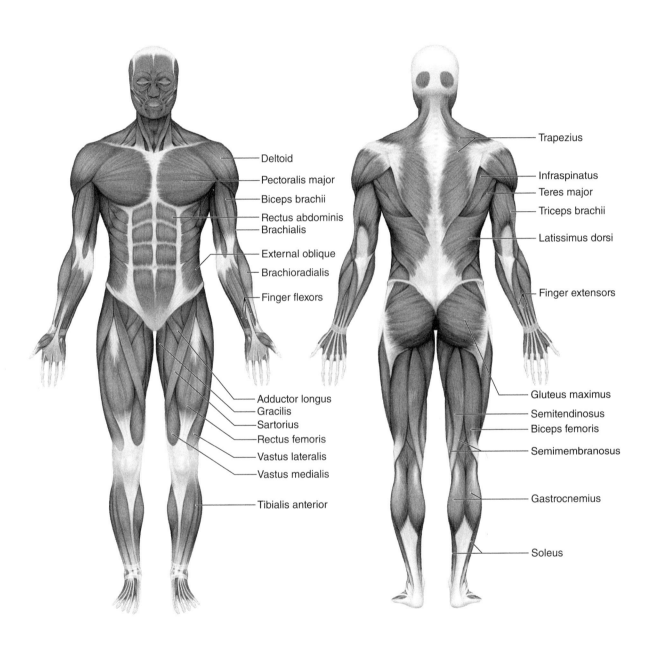

Deltoid

Pectoralis major

Biceps brachii

Rectus abdominis

Brachialis

External oblique

Brachioradialis

Finger flexors

Adductor longus

Gracilis

Sartorius

Rectus femoris

Vastus lateralis

Vastus medialis

Tibialis anterior

Trapezius

Infraspinatus

Teres major

Triceps brachii

Latissimus dorsi

Finger extensors

Gluteus maximus

Semitendinosus

Biceps femoris

Semimembranosus

Gastrocnemius

Soleus

PART I

Maximum Interval Conditioning

CHAPTER 1

Maximum Interval Advantages

In recent years athletes, coaches, and fitness enthusiasts have dramatically increased their use of interval training, especially high-intensity interval training (HIIT). This trend is evidenced by the sheer number of interval-training classes being offered at local gyms and health clubs. Additionally, in the past several years consumers have been bombarded with information about extreme conditioning programs through the Internet, television, and other forms of media. Although these programs may differ in structure, types of exercises and drills, and duration, one thing is relatively consistent: purpose. That purpose is to gain the benefits of aerobic training, anaerobic training, and even strength training in a short, intense period.

The purpose of this book is to help readers develop optimal maximum interval training (MIT) sessions to meet their specific fitness and performance goals in a safe and effective manner. To allow readers to individualize their MIT sessions, a wide variety of modalities and training options are presented so that readers can tailor their training program to their specific needs, preferences, and constraints.

WHAT IS MAXIMUM INTERVAL TRAINING (MIT)?

MIT uses short, intense exercise periods with a variety of exercise modes combined with brief bouts of recovery to improve performance and body image. Typically, exercise bouts are performed at a high intensity level. To allow performance at high intensity, the exercise session has to be brief; otherwise, the person would not be able to maintain the effort. For example, many of the programs in this book have exercise bouts between 20 and 60 seconds in length.

The length of the rest periods is dictated by the intensity of the work bout, meaning that the more intense the work bout is, the greater the amount of recovery is needed before the next work bout begins. In simple terms, intensity and volume are inversely related. If one of these training variables increases, the other must decrease and vice versa. The selected duration and intensity depend on the primary energy system being emphasized, the mode of training being used, and the adaptational responses desired.

MIT differs dramatically from traditional steady-state, cardiorespiratory training, in which a relatively constant intensity at or below the lactate threshold is maintained for the duration of the exercise session.

BENEFITS OF MAXIMUM INTERVAL TRAINING

Although athletes have used interval training for over a century, it is now becoming a mainstream concept for developing overall fitness. You only have to turn on the TV or go on to social media to see examples of these programs. This model is in contrast to the old view of fitness, which held that long-term aerobic exercise was required to work the heart, lungs, and circulatory system. But many of the cardiorespiratory benefits produced by traditional aerobic training methods are also provided by interval training. These benefits include improved ability to consume oxygen, greater ability to transport oxygen to exercising muscles, and an increase in mitochondrial size and density, allowing greater production of energy.

Besides improving cardiorespiratory performance, MIT may serve as an effective tool for weight loss and weight management. The old thinking was that to burn fat, people needed to exercise at a low intensity. The problem with this line of thinking is that low-intensity exercise doesn't burn as much fat! Although low- to moderate-intensity, steady-state cardio burns a greater percentage of fat during a workout, the total amount of fat burned and the total caloric expenditure are significantly greater when using a HIIT training program (Tremblay, Simoneau, and Bouchard 1994; Boutcher 2011). Thus, for those attempting to lose weight or maintain a healthy weight, performing MIT may be more beneficial than doing traditional steady-state aerobic training.

Energy system development (ESD) for explosive and intermittent-style sports is another benefit associated with MIT. We ultimately use a substance called ATP, or adenosine triphosphate, to fuel movement. When we want to exercise or perform in sport, we break down the ATP to release energy. We rely on three primary energy pathways to create ATP—two anaerobic pathways (the ATP–PCr system and the fast-glycolytic system) and one aerobic pathway (the oxidative system). The ATP–PCr system provides energy for explosive activities that last approximately 7 to 15 seconds, which would include activities such as the 40-yard dash, pro-agility, or vertical jump. For moderate- to high-intensity activities of longer duration, such as a 400- or 800-meter run, we start to rely more on the fast-glycolytic energy system to provide energy through glycolysis. Finally, for activities performed at a lower intensity for greater than 2 or 3 minutes, we start to rely on the aerobic energy system for ATP production. Although each of these energy systems are working to some degree at any given time, the one that dominates in ATP production is dictated by the intensity and duration of the activity as well as our ability to use oxygen (Baechle and Earle 2008).

During intermittent, or discontinuous, team and court sports, such as basketball, hockey, and tennis, the anaerobic energy pathways are called on to provide energy to sustain performance. Thus, to yield the greatest carryover to performance, the training method selected must reflect the metabolic demands of the sport and challenge the energy systems that supply athletes with fuel during competition. The athlete should engage in training that requires intermittent bouts of high intensity performed over short durations and allows brief recovery bouts using active or complete rest. This form of training also stimulates aerobic adaptations because the athlete will have an increase in oxygen consumption in an attempt to recover from the stressors between work bouts (Brewer 2008). The athlete would have a similar experience during a game or match: high-intensity bouts (acceleration and deceleration, rapid changes of direction, jumping, and so on) followed by lower-intensity bouts (jogging, time-outs, waiting for the next play, and so on) that rely heavily on the oxidative system for recovery.

MIT stimulates an increase in anaerobic enzymes, allowing greater anaerobic energy turnover and more efficient use of lactate as a fuel source during exercise. Athletes can thus work at a higher intensity for a longer time, which provides them with a distinct advantage over their competition. From a physiological standpoint, higher-intensity bouts of training also provide greater stimulation to explosive muscle fibers (Type II) than traditional steady-state aerobic training does. Athletes are thus able to preserve a greater amount of lean muscle mass tissue, allowing greater force production. Those attempting to manage their weight may benefit as well because this method promotes the preservation of lean mass while stimulating fat loss.

MIT can be done using a variety of training modalities and equipment, such as calisthenics, repeat sprints, and kettlebells. Many of these options are discussed in greater detail in chapter 2. Users have many training options; they are not limited to long, slow distance training or whatever cardio equipment is available at the local gym or health club. Having more options helps combat the boredom that many people experience when performing continuous-style cardiorespiratory training; the various alternatives may increase exercise adherence, self-efficacy, self-esteem, and enjoyment.

Finally, MIT is a time-efficient method of training. In general, MIT sessions last approximately 10 to 20 minutes (including rest periods). For example, 15 minutes of intense exercise, performed in as few as six sessions over a 2-week period, has been shown to have a positive effect on oxidative capacity during aerobic-based exercise (Gibala and McGee 2008). Furthermore, performing seven HIIT sessions over 2 weeks has been shown to produce a significant improvement in fatty acid oxidation during exercise (Talanian et al. 2007). Also, because MIT does not necessarily require a lot of expensive equipment, a session can be performed practically anywhere, so not having time to get to the gym is no longer a barrier. Therefore, MIT may provide the perfect solution for those with limited time to work out.

CHAPTER 2

Equipment Options and Safety Considerations

Maximum interval training is a fun and effective way to train. It can stand alone or supplement other training. This type of training uses a variety of training tools. This chapter provides an overview of the equipment used in maximum interval training and helps you select the right equipment. A major section of the chapter focuses on ensuring that the maximum interval-training experience is a safe one.

EQUIPMENT OPTIONS FOR MAXIMUM INTERVAL TRAINING

When we think of strength training many of us think of barbells and dumbbells. When we think about getting in shape, we normally think of some type of cardiovascular exercise done at low intensity over a long duration. Maximum interval training uses different tools, techniques, and training approaches to achieve the benefits described in the previous chapter. Maximum interval training uses body weight, medicine balls, heavy ropes, suspension training, kettlebells, sandbags, and some unusual training devices to achieve our goals. These tools are described in detail in chapters 3 through 10.

Body weight is a great training tool to a point. A notable advantage is that special equipment is not needed to perform the exercises. Bodyweight exercises include things like squats, lunges, push-ups, pull-ups, dips, and mobility drills. The challenge with bodyweight training is that it is hard to make the exercises more difficult as fitness increases.

Medicine balls are heavy balls that come in various weights. They can be carried, pressed, pulled, rowed, thrown, swung, and caught. Although medicine balls are a fun way to train, a lot of space may be required, especially if you are going to throw the balls.

Heavy ropes are extra-thick ropes 60 to 100 feet (18 to 30 m) long that are used for unique total-body exercises. Most of the exercises done with heavy ropes are a variation of lifting the rope up and slamming it to the ground. Exercising with heavy ropes can be enjoyable, but it is hard to make these exercises more difficult and this tool requires a great deal of space.

Suspension training involves performing bodyweight exercises while part of the body (the feet or the hands) is suspended off the ground. Suspension training develops balance, coordination, and stabilizing muscles. But it has some of the same challenges as bodyweight exercises and requires space to connect the suspension trainer and perform the exercises.

Kettlebells are weighted balls with handles. Their unique shape allows many exercises to be performed, thus permitting a great deal of exercise variety. Their main challenge is the initial difficulty of learning to perform the exercises.

Sandbags are just what the name implies. Adding sand adds weight, which can make the exercise more difficult. In addition, the sand shifts while the exercise is being performed, which increases the challenge. Many free-weight exercises are performed with sandbags. The biggest challenge is the potential mess and finding a facility that is OK with that possibility.

Many other training tools are used with maximum interval training. Traditional strong-man implements include heavy tires, sledgehammers, and logs. These tools provide variety but can be difficult to acquire and are not included in this book.

Sprinting is frequently used either as a conditioning tool or as a component of a workout that uses other tools. Sprinting is extremely sport specific, highly technical, and unforgiving of technique mistakes. Poor instruction in sprinting can cause people to run slowly with bad technique, which is obviously not desirable in sport.

You can use many tools with maximum interval training. The wonderful thing is that you can focus on one tool (for example, on a given day you might do all your training with kettlebells) or incorporate several tools into each workout. Having a variety of options can make figuring out what to do a daunting prospect. To simplify the process, use the following criteria to assess which tools are most appropriate for you:

- Access
- Advantages and disadvantages
- Likes and dislikes

Access to equipment will be a major limiting factor in your choices. If you are training in your home, what equipment do you have and what can you afford to purchase? If you are training in a facility, what equipment does it have? Another factor that determines access is your comfort level with the technical aspect of the various training tools.

Every type of exercise equipment has advantages and disadvantages, which are described in detail in the appropriate chapters. This aspect must be factored in when it comes to selecting a training tool. Why are you training? If your training goals align with the advantages of a given tool, then it is probably a good match for you.

Finally, your individual likes and dislikes are important when it comes to selecting training tools. For example, if you find bodyweight training to be incredibly boring, then it probably should not be a key component of your conditioning program. Using tools that you strongly dislike will not result in a rewarding training experience and may discourage you from exercising. On the other hand, if you occasionally incorporate a type of training that you only mildly dislike, you may develop an appreciation for it over time.

SAFETY CONSIDERATIONS

With any kind of exercise program, numerous factors may contribute to accidents or injuries. When it comes to training safely, each of the following areas should be carefully evaluated: environment, preparation, attire, technique, and progression.

Environment

Most injuries associated with exercise relate to the workout environment. The temperature and condition of the workout space can have a significant effect on your well-being.

A hot or humid environment, combined with intense exercise, is a recipe for health problems. If you are going to exercise in this kind of environment, drink water frequently.

Drink before, during, and after exercise. To prevent becoming dehydrated, you should begin drinking water several hours before exercise. To get a sense of how much water you need to be drinking during a workout, weigh yourself before and after the workout. According to the American College of Sports Medicine's Position Stand on Exercise and Fluid Replacement, you should drink enough water during exercise so that you do not lose more than 2 percent of your body weight from sweating. After exercise, you should drink approximately 1.5 liters of water per kilogram of body weight lost during the exercise session (Bergeron, Hargreaves, Haymes, et al. 2007).

Get acclimatized to warm temperatures gradually. Becoming acclimatized to heat takes time. When beginning an exercise program in a hot environment, you should give yourself several days of gradually increasing the intensity and duration to give your body a chance to get used to the heat.

Recognize the symptoms of heat illness and stop exercising if they occur. This recommendation is tough to follow because extreme heat affects our ability to think. Symptoms include cramps, fatigue, nausea and vomiting, dizziness, and drenching sweat accompanied by cold, clammy skin. When heat illness becomes life threatening, signs and symptoms include hot, flushed, dry skin; shortness of breath; decreased sweating; confusion; and even convulsions. When these symptoms begin, immediately seek medical attention.

Cold environments can also be problematic. More than a few people train in unheated garages during the winter, and some even train outside! In cold environments, drinking water is still important, although it's more difficult to judge the need for water because of the cold. Dressing appropriately is important. In cold environments, shivering, lack of coordination, and drowsiness are signs of possible hypothermia. Don't ignore these symptoms. You should also be aware of possible frostbite, which can begin as a painful, itching sensation and progress to a cold or burning feeling and numbness.

Crowding and clutter are common sources of injuries during exercise. When fixed equipment in a facility is too close together or when equipment or personal belongings are left lying on the floor, the stage is set for accidents related to tripping and collisions. For those reasons, you need to be aware of your surroundings and put smaller equipment items back where they belong when you are finished with them. Choose a public space where others observe the same good habits.

Preparation

Many people overestimate their activity levels and abilities or fail to pay attention to symptoms that could be serious. Before taking up an aggressive exercise program involving maximum interval training, you must realistically evaluate your status; if you don't, the consequences could be serious. You should visit with a physician and be sure that you are healthy enough to participate in an intense exercise program.

Always warm up at the start of an exercise session. The warm-up prepares the body for work by gradually increasing heart rate, moving blood into the tissues that will be exercised, developing psychological focus, and allowing practice of the movements that will be done later at higher intensity. In other words, the warm-up prevents injury and improves performance.

When it comes to maximum interval training, an effective warm-up involves several steps. First, perform some type of low-intensity cardiovascular exercise for 3 to 5 minutes, just enough to increase heart rate and get a light sweat going. For example, jog 400 yards. Second, perform 5 to 10 minutes of total-body mobility exercises. These movements work the entire body and force the muscles to work through their full range of motion. Finally, start the actual workout light and easy and progress in difficulty.

Table 2.1 Multistep Warm-Up and Workout Example

Warm-up step 1	Warm-up step 2	Warm-up step 3	Workout
Jog 400 yards (meters)	Perform each exercise for 30 seconds or 10 yards: Leg swing, front and back Leg swing, side to side March High-knee walk Walk on toes Arm circle Bear crawl Jump rope for 3 to 5 minutes	Perform each exercise for 30 seconds: Squat Lunge Push-up Pull-up	Perform each exercise for 30 seconds. Rest for 10 seconds after each exercise. Repeat 2 ×: Kettlebell swing Kettlebell snatch (right hand) Kettlebell snatch (left hand) Kettlebell clean (right hand) Kettlebell clean (left hand) Kettlebell push-up Kettlebell press

Table 2.1 shows a sample warm-up and workout. It begins with a light jog (step 1) to raise the heart rate and get a sweat going. Step 2 has mobility exercises that focus on most of the muscles and joints of the body. Step 3 has simple exercises that continue to prepare the body for the workout, although this step uses exercises that are at a higher intensity than the previous ones. Finally, the workout (step 4) is a total-body kettlebell conditioning workout.

Attire

Dressing appropriately for exercise is more than a fashion statement; it's a safety issue. For example, wearing shoes that have closed toes is important, for several reasons. First, you would be surprised how often something is dropped on the feet in this environment. Although a shoe won't cushion the foot from a dropped 45-pound (20.4 kg) plate, it will help prevent a nail from being ripped off. Second, an amazing number of viruses and bacteria grow on the floors in exercise facilities. Wearing shoes greatly reduces the risk of contracting those. Finally, wearing shoes means that you are less likely to slip on the floor.

Jewelry and overly baggy clothing should be avoided when performing maximum interval training. Necklaces, bracelets, watches, earrings, and rings can interfere with your ability to grasp or manipulate equipment properly. They can catch on hard surfaces or become enmeshed in soft surfaces, causing mishaps and injuries. They collect and transmit germs, and they can be scratched and banged up from coming into contact with the equipment.

In hot environments, wear light-colored clothing that breathes. Light-colored clothing reflects heat, whereas dark-colored clothing absorbs it. Therefore, light-colored clothing is preferable when exercising in hot environments. You should also wear either somewhat loose-fitting clothing or clothing that is made to breathe so that sweat has a chance to evaporate rather than become trapped. In cold environments, clothing should be layered so that it can be added to or removed as conditions dictate.

Technique

A lot of space in this book is devoted to descriptions and photos of how to perform the exercises included in the workout programs. This emphasis reflects the importance of correct technique. Correct technique ensures appropriate loading of the joints and prevents injuries. Correct technique also ensures that the muscles being trained are the ones that will produce the desired training effect.

For example, let's say that we are performing a Romanian deadlift. Ideally, we keep the chest out and the shoulders pulled back throughout. This technique evenly distributes the stress of the exercise across the lumbar vertebrae. It also ensures that when we are leaning forward, we are targeting the hamstring muscles. But if we allow the shoulders to slump forward, several things happen. First, the weight is loading the front of the vertebrae, which increases the chances of a disc injury. Second, because the shoulders are slumped forward, we'll perform the movement by bending from the trunk, which will emphasize the lower back muscles instead of the hamstrings. As you can see, one subtle technique change can have major ramifications.

Progression

Wanting to jump straight into the advanced exercises and advanced workout programs is perfectly natural. The problem with doing this is that it prevents two things from happening. First, it does not allow us to develop the physical foundation that we need to be safe and successful with our training experience. Second, it means that we have not mastered the fundamental techniques of how to perform these exercises safely. Injuries become more likely to occur.

Use the right amount of weight and don't try to advance too quickly. As mentioned earlier, technique is extremely important both to ensure safety and to ensure that the exercise is training what we want it to. Eight of the chapters in this book cover various exercises that can be used for maximum interval training. These chapters are divided into foundational exercises and advanced exercises. The intent of the foundational exercises is to teach techniques that you will use with the advanced exercises and to develop the physical foundation that you will need for success with the advanced exercises. In addition, advanced athletes still use many of the fundamental exercises. Each advanced exercise has prerequisites. You should master these prerequisites before attempting the advanced exercises. If you have mastered the prerequisites, you have the technical and physical foundation to perform the advanced exercises safely and effectively.

The final six chapters in this book cover interval-training programs. Each of the maximum interval programs covered is meant to support the type of training that is the focus of the chapter. For example, in the strength and power chapter, the maximum interval-training program is meant to support someone who is focusing on strength and power training. Each workout chapter has a foundational program and an advanced one. The foundational programs should be mastered first. The foundational programs include foundational exercises. The advanced programs have foundational exercises but also include advanced exercises, that is, exercises that have prerequisites. This means that you need to master the prerequisites before attempting an advanced program.

Maximum Interval Exercises

Bodyweight Training

Of all the exercise equipment you could ever own, your own body may be the best! It is always with you, so you don't need to buy any equipment or go to the gym to use it. Bodyweight exercises can develop strength, power, and stamina, as well as improve your body's ability to move with skill and efficiency. Additionally, you need to master many of these exercises before you perform the advanced drills and progressions found in this book that use various pieces of equipment to overload the muscles.

GETTING STARTED

Many of the exercises in this section may be classified as either strength or endurance exercises, depending on your initial strength level. As a rule, if you can perform no more than 10 repetitions of a given exercise, such as dips or pull-ups, the exercise would place a greater emphasis on strength than endurance. In comparison, if you are able to perform significantly more than 10 repetitions of a particular bodyweight exercise, you are emphasizing endurance. Both strength and endurance exercises may be selected when performing interval training, but exercises that require more strength will require more rest before you can perform subsequent sets of the same exercise. Therefore, using a superset approach that combines two or more exercises that work opposing muscle groups may be a good strategy for keeping the metabolic demands high throughout the training session while allowing adequate recovery between muscle groups to perform your best on each exercise. Table 3.1 includes examples of exercises that can be performed as supersets.

Table 3.1 Superset Examples

Perform one set of each exercise in the superset without resting. Repeat in the same order for the desired number of supersets

Superset 1	Push-up → Pull-up → Squat
Superset 2	Split squat → Dip → Walking plank

FOUNDATIONAL EXERCISES

The foundational bodyweight exercises in this section are essential for learning good movement technique, as well as reducing your risk of injury. You should master each of these fundamental exercises before you progress to the more advanced exercises in this section or add resistance (dumbbells, medicine balls, sandbags, and so on). These drills are the cornerstone for more advanced training options and higher levels of performance in the future.

Bodyweight Jumping Jacks

Intended Uses

This exercise develops basic coordination and cardiorespiratory fitness and prepares the body for more complex forms of training (such as plyometrics).

Prerequisites

- Absence of lower-extremity or shoulder injuries.

Steps

- Start with the feet together and hands down to the sides.
- Jump the feet to the sides while simultaneously lifting the hands up overhead.
- Return to the starting position and repeat this movement.
- Repeat for the desired number of repetitions or the desired time.

Variations

- Move the feet forward and backward in a scissor-like fashion.

Key Points

- Maintain a good rhythm between upper- and lower-body movements.

Bodyweight Crab Kick

Intended Uses

This drill helps develop shoulder mobility and stability, as well as hip stability of the support leg.

Prerequisites

- Good shoulder stability and mobility.
- No previous shoulder injuries.

Steps

- While sitting on the floor, place your palms flat on the ground behind your back and then bend the knees.
- Lift the hips off the ground.
- Extend your left leg out (*a*).
- Simultaneously kick the right leg out while pulling the left leg back to the starting position in a scissor-like fashion (*b*).
- Repeat this drill for a set number of repetitions or for a specified time.

Key Points

- Do not allow the hips to drop throughout the duration of the exercise.

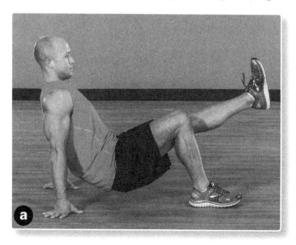
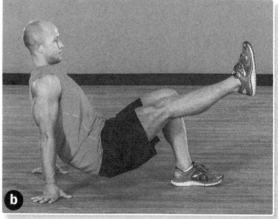

Bodyweight Inchworm

Intended Uses

This exercise is excellent for improving shoulder and trunk stability. It is also a great exercise for improving hamstring flexibility, strength, and endurance.

Prerequisites

- Good hamstring flexibility.
- Good shoulder and trunk stability.

Steps

- Begin in a push-up position with the arms straight (*a*).
- While keeping the legs straight, walk the feet up (*b*) until they are at or close to the hands (*c*).
- After doing this, walk the hands out to return to the push-up position.
- Perform this drill for the desired distance.

Key Points

- Keep the legs as straight as possible without hyperextending the knee.
- Maintain a rigid torso.

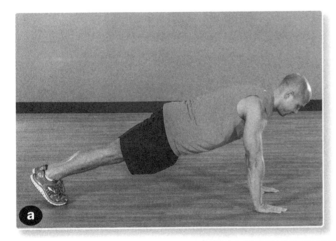

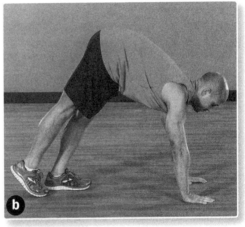

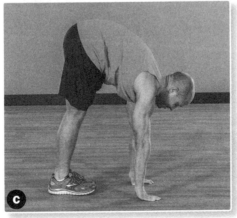

Bodyweight Bear Crawl

Intended Uses

This drill can be used to help improve upper- and lower-body coordination, as well as trunk stability.

Prerequisites

- No shoulder pain or injuries.
- Good trunk strength and endurance.

Steps

- Begin in a push-up position with the arms straight.
- Bend the ankles, knees, and hips until the knees are directly under the hips and you are on the balls of your feet.
- From this position, walk forward on all fours by alternating the right arm and left leg and then the left arm and right leg (a-b).
- Perform this drill for the desired distance.
- This drill can be performed forward, backward, and laterally.

Key Points

- Maintain a rigid torso.

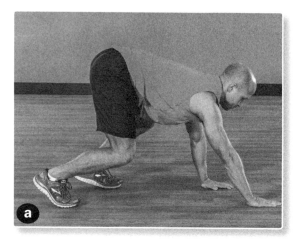 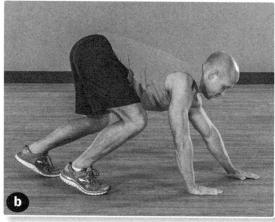

Bodyweight Mountain Climber

Intended Uses

This drill increases cardiorespiratory fitness and emphasizes dynamic core engagement and stability.

Prerequisites

- Ability to perform a plank and stabilize the trunk.

Steps

- Assume a plank position with the arms fully extended and palms in contact with the ground.
- While maintaining a neutral spine, drive the right knee toward the chest (*a*).
- Simultaneously straighten the right leg while driving the left knee toward the chest (*b*).
- Continue alternating legs for a set time or for the desired number of repetitions.

Key Points

- Lock the hips and maintain a neutral spine throughout the duration of the exercise.
- Keep the neck in a neutral position.

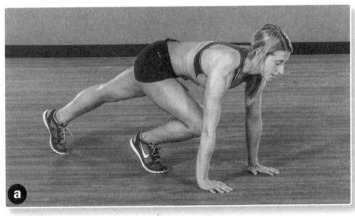

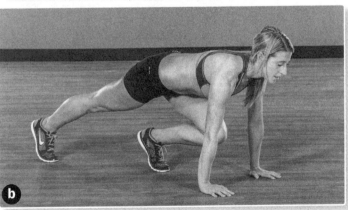

Bodyweight Groiner

Intended Uses

This drill provides a great dynamic warm-up for the hips and adductors. Additionally, when you become proficient at this movement, it can be extremely challenging from a metabolic standpoint.

Prerequisites

- Good hip mobility and hamstring flexibility.
- Good trunk strength and endurance.

Steps

- Begin in a push-up position with the arms straight.
- While maintaining a rigid spine, move the right leg out, drive the knee forward, and plant your right heel at, or slightly past, your right shoulder.
- Straighten the right leg to return it to its starting position and then repeat this motion on the left side.
- Continue this pattern, alternating between sides for a set time or the desired number of repetitions.

Key Points

- Do not allow the back to arch while performing this exercise.

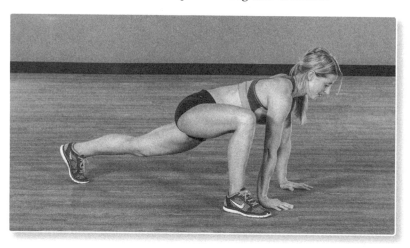

Bodyweight Scissors

Intended Uses

This drill can be used to develop quick feet and change-of-direction speed.

Prerequisites

■ No lower-body injuries.

Steps

■ Stand on an imaginary line.
■ Begin with the right foot in front of the line and the left foot behind the line.
■ Bend the arms at 90 degrees and, using a reciprocating opposite arm and leg action, alternate the feet back and forth in a rapid scissor-like manner (*a-b*).
■ Perform this exercise for the desired number of repetitions or the desired time.

Key Points

■ Maintain an opposite arm and leg movement pattern to ensure balance and coordination.
■ Keep the chest up, shoulders back, and torso rigid.

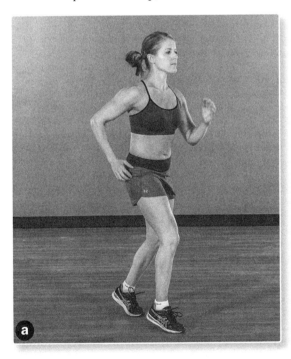
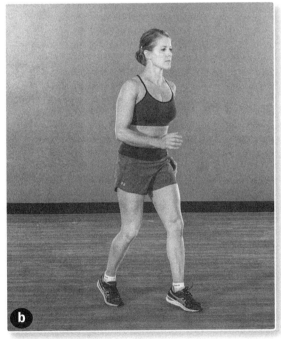

Bodyweight Pull-Up

Intended Uses

This drill improves local muscular endurance in the back, biceps, and shoulders. It develops the strength of the upper back, shoulders, and biceps and enhances shoulder stability.

Prerequisites

- Upper-body strength.

Steps

- With the arms fully extended, grab the bar using an overhand grip (*a*).
- Bend the elbows and pull the body upward until the chin is over the bar (*b*).
- Lower the body in a controlled manner back to the starting position.

Variations

- To reduce the intensity of this exercise, position a barbell in a squat rack so that when you grab the bar and lean back, your torso is at an angle approximately 45 degrees to the ground.
- With the ankles "cast," that is, rigid with the toes up, and the heels in contact with the floor, pull the body up toward the bar until the chest touches the bar.
- Perform this exercise for the desired number of repetitions.

Key Points

- Visualize pulling the bar to your chest.
- Do not swing the torso, or "kip," during the exercise.

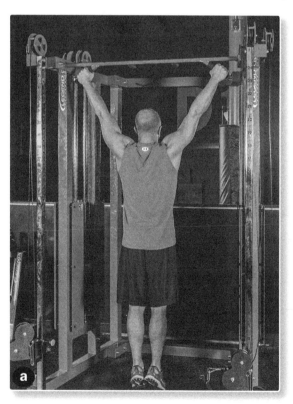 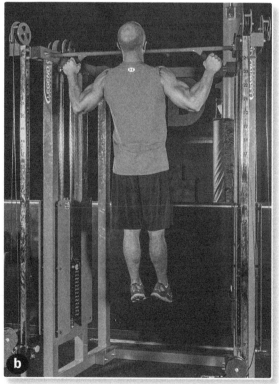

Bodyweight Push-Up

Intended Uses

This exercise develops the muscles of the chest, shoulders, and triceps and improves upper-body muscular endurance.

Prerequisites

- Ability to perform a plank.
- No preexisting pain or shoulder injuries.

Steps

- Assume a plank position with the arms fully extended and palms in contact with the ground (*a*).
- While maintaining a rigid torso, lower the chest, hips, and trunk toward the ground by bending the elbows until the upper portion of the arms is parallel to the ground (*b*).
- Perform this exercise for the desired number of repetitions or the desired time.

Variations

- The intensity of this drill can be reduced by placing the hands on a bench or putting the knees on the ground.
- The intensity of this exercise can be increased by elevating the feet on a bench or stability ball.
- The intensity of this exercise can also be increased by changing limb positions with the lower body (e.g., hip abduction, lift knee toward shoulder).

Key Points

- Do not allow the hips to drop or elevate throughout the duration of this movement.

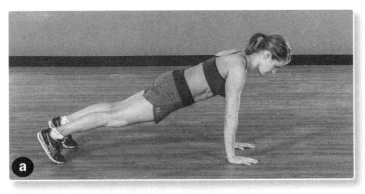

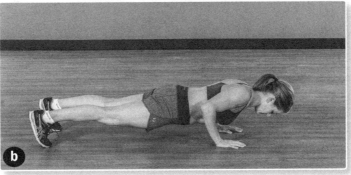

Bodyweight Dip

Intended Uses

This exercise develops the muscles of the chest, shoulders, and triceps and improves upper-body pushing strength and muscular endurance.

Prerequisites

- No shoulder injuries.

Steps

- Position yourself between two dip bars.
- With your palms facing your body, place a hand on each bar.
- Push yourself up by extending the elbows so that the hands are directly beneath the shoulders. Bend the knees so that the shins are parallel to the ground (*a*).
- Then, in a controlled manner, lower your body by allowing the elbows to bend until the upper arms are approximately parallel to the ground (*b*).
- Extend the elbows and use the chest and shoulders to press the body back to the starting position.
- Perform this exercise for the desired number of repetitions.

Variations

- The intensity of this drill can be reduced by performing this exercise between two benches (heels on one bench and palms of hands on the other).

Key Points

- Perform this exercise in a smooth and controlled manner.
- Avoid any bobbing or jerking movements.

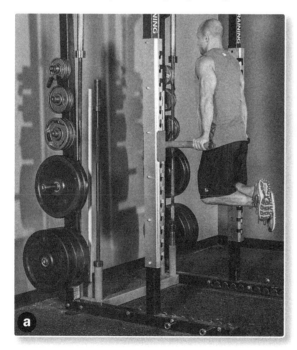 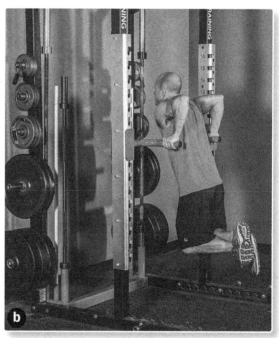

ADVANCED EXERCISES

You should perform the advanced exercises described in this chapter only after you master the foundational exercises. Many of these exercises have a technical or fitness foundation that you must acquire to ensure your safety. In addition, if you perform these exercises incorrectly, they will not produce the desired results.

Bodyweight Traveling Plank

Intended Uses

This exercise is excellent for engaging the core and developing trunk stability. This progression of the static plank significantly increases the metabolic demands of the exercise.

Prerequisites

- Ability to perform a static prone plank for a minimum of 30 seconds.
- No previous history of shoulder injury.

Steps

- Begin by lying on your belly and forearms.
- Pull the toes back toward your shins and in one continuous movement lift your hips and torso until your elbows are directly under your shoulders and your upper arms are perpendicular to the ground (*a*).
- While maintaining a rigid torso and flat back, lift the right forearm and left foot and move them forward.
- Pull the body forward by pressing down and back with the right elbow (*b*). Repeat this action, walking the left forearm and right foot forward.
- Continue alternating until you cover the desired distance.

Variations

- Perform this drill traveling backward and laterally.

Key Points

- Do not allow the hips to rotate as you move forward.
- Keep the torso stiff throughout the duration of the exercise.
- Lateral traveling planks increase the demands placed on the adductors of the lead leg and the chest muscles as the body is pulled laterally.

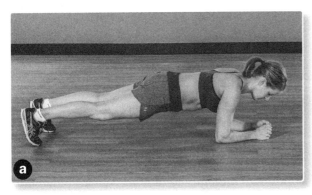
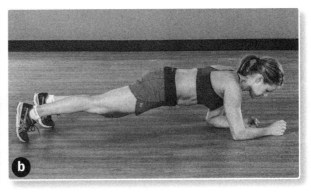

Bodyweight Walking Plank

Intended Uses

This advanced variation of the plank is great for developing shoulder and trunk stability, coordination, and cardiorespiratory fitness.

Prerequisites

- Ability to perform a static prone plank for a minimum of 30 seconds.
- No previous history of shoulder injury.

Steps

- Begin by lying on your belly and forearms.
- Pull the toes back toward your shins and in one continuous movement lift your hips and torso until your elbows are directly under your shoulders and your upper arms are perpendicular to the ground.
- Shift your weight to your right elbow (*a*) and then to the left elbow (*b*).
- Extend the left arm and place the left palm down. Then extend the right arm and place the right palm down until you are in a push-up position (*c*).
- After attaining this position, place the left forearm down, followed by the right forearm.
- Repeat this process, alternating in a clockwise and counterclockwise fashion for the desired number of repetitions.

Key Points

- Keep the torso stiff throughout the duration of the exercise.
- Maintain a rhythmic cadence: 1 = left palm down, 2 = right palm down, 3 = left forearm down, 4 = right forearm down.

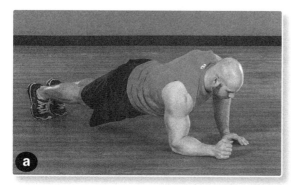
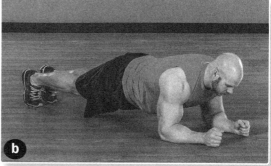
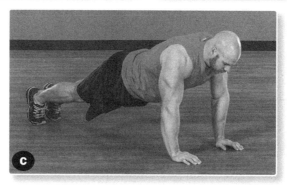

Bodyweight Frog Hop

Intended Uses

Aside from enhancing cardiorespiratory fitness and building muscular endurance, this drill can be used to improve hip mobility and improve squat depth.

Prerequisites

- Ability to squat below parallel with good, consistent technique.
- Ability to perform a minimum of 20 bodyweight squats.
- Ability to maintain good postural alignment throughout the duration of the exercise.

Steps

- Begin in a plank position.
- Simultaneously jump both feet forward and land in a deep squat position with the palms and feet in full contact with the ground (*a*).
- From this position, jump up as high as possible (*b*).
- Go back to the starting position and repeat for the desired number of repetitions.

Key Points

- Maintain a rigid trunk and a neutral posture.
- When in the squat position, focus on keeping the chest up.

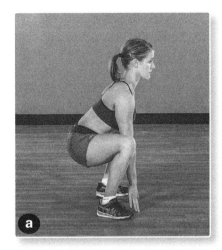

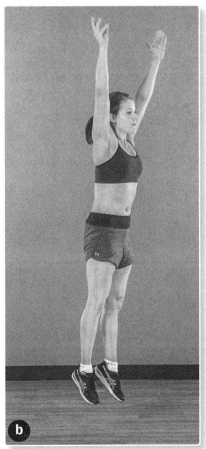

Bodyweight Line Jump

Intended Uses

This drill can be used to develop quick feet and change-of-direction speed.

Prerequisites

- No lower-body pain or injuries.

Steps

- While standing and facing a taped line on the floor, jump forward (*a*) over the line and back (*b*) as quickly as possible.

Variations

- Perform this drill jumping side to side.

Key Points

- Keep your center of mass over the line so that you can transition quickly between jumps.
- Keep the chest up, shoulders back, and torso rigid.

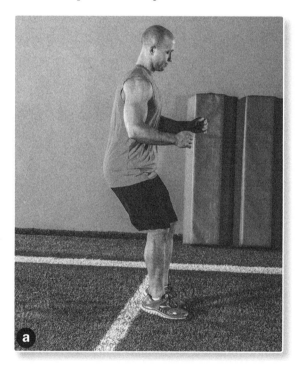
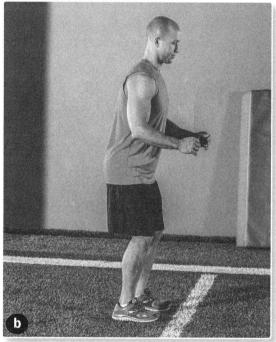

Bodyweight Staggered Push-Up

Intended Uses

This variation of the push-up increases core engagement and develops unilateral strength in the upper body. It is also a good exercise for enhancing shoulder stability.

Prerequisites

- Ability to perform push-ups with good, consistent technique.
- Ability to perform a minimum of 10 push-ups.
- No preexisting shoulder pain or injuries.

Steps

- Assume a plank position, with the arms fully extended and palms in contact with the ground.
- Position the left hand forward just above the head and place the right hand directly below the chest (*a*).
- While maintaining a rigid torso, lower the chest, hips, and trunk toward the ground by bending the elbows until the upper portion of the arms is parallel to the ground (*b*).
- From that position, extend your arms until you are back in the starting position.
- Bring the right hand forward and the left hand back. Then perform another push-up.
- Continue alternating hand positions and performing push-ups for the desired number of repetitions or a set time.

Key Points

- Do not allow the hips to drop or elevate throughout the duration of this movement.

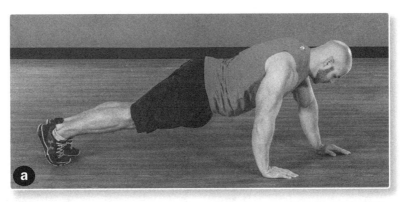

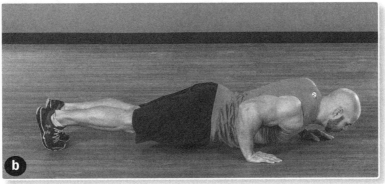

Bodyweight Speed Squats

Intended Uses

This drill can be used as a foundational progression into plyometric exercises. It also helps train your lower body to be more explosive.

Prerequisites

- Good mobility in the ankles, knees, and hips.
- Ability to perform the squat exercise with consistent, good form.
- Ability to perform at least 20 bodyweight squats.

Steps

- While keeping the trunk braced, chest up, and shoulder blades together, sit back at the hips, allowing the hips, knees, and ankles to flex.
- When the tops of the thighs are parallel to the ground (*a*), extend the hips, knees, and ankles and return to the starting position (*b*).
- Perform as quickly as possible while maintaining good form and technique. Try to jump from the squat position without leaving the ground.

Key Points

- When you do the movement correctly, you will almost lose ground contact because of the explosive force generated as you return to the starting position.
- Make certain that the knees do not pass the toes and stay aligned with the second toe.

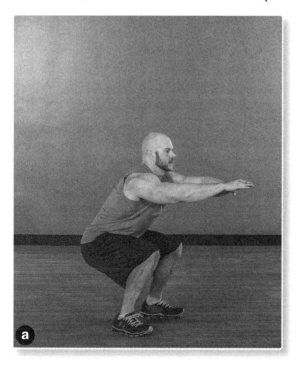
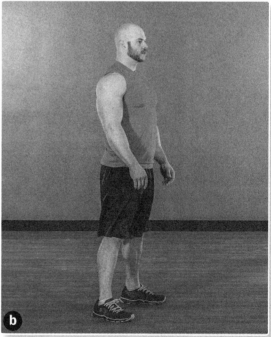

Bodyweight Speed Split Squat

Intended Uses

This variation of the squat increases the load placed on a single leg and requires greater balance laterally than the traditional squat does.

Prerequisites

- Good balance and coordination.
- No ankle, knee, or hip pain or injuries.

Steps

- Without rotating the hips, step back with one foot and assume a staggered stance (*a*).
- While keeping the trunk braced, chest up, and shoulder blades together, allow the hips, knees, and ankles to flex until the knee of the back leg almost touches the ground (*b*).
- When the top of the front (working) leg thigh is parallel to the ground, extend the hips, knees, and ankles and explode back up to the starting position.
- Perform for the desired number of repetitions and then switch legs.

Variations

- This drill can be progressed by elevating the rear foot on a bench or chair.

Key Points

- Perform the same number of repetitions on each leg.
- When you do the movement correctly, you will almost lose ground contact because of the explosive force generated as you return to the starting position.
- Make certain that the knee does not pass the toes of the lead leg and stays aligned with the second toe.

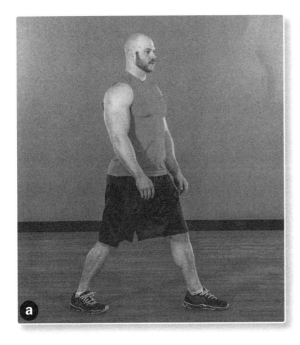
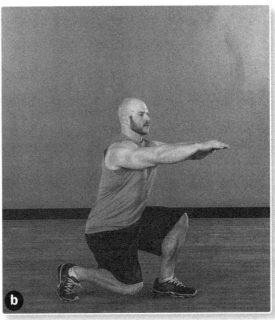

Bodyweight Squat Hold

Intended Uses

This drill develops isometric strength of the lower body.

Prerequisites

- Ability to perform the squat exercise with consistent, good form.
- Ability to perform at least 20 bodyweight squats.

Steps

- Placing the hands on the hips or keeping them at your sides, perform a squat until the tops of the thighs are parallel to the ground.
- Hold this position for the desired time.

Variations

- Lift the hands overhead and extend the arms, simultaneously pulling the shoulder blades down and together. Descend into the squat and attempt to hold this position for the desired time.

Key Points

- Maintain proper knee, hip, and postural alignment throughout the duration of the exercise.
- Maintain a rigid torso, keeping the chest up and shoulders back.
- Push the elbows back and stick the chest out and up.

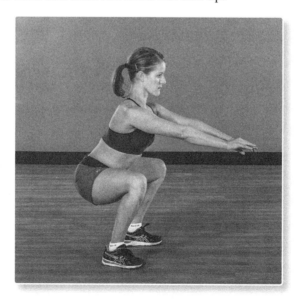

Bodyweight Lateral Squat

Intended Uses

This drill can be used to improve lower-body stability and balance while you shift your weight from side to side. It also assists with developing groin and hip strength and flexibility.

Prerequisites

- Good balance and stability.
- No lower-body pain or injuries.

Steps

- Extend the arms and raise them to shoulder level.
- Stand with the feet just wider than shoulder-width apart.
- Bend the ankle, knee, and hip of the left leg and sit back while simultaneously shifting your center of mass to the left (a). Repeat by shifting your center of mass to the right (b).
- The arms should remain extended at shoulder level throughout the duration of the exercise to provide counterbalance.

Key Points

- Make certain that the knee does not pass the toes of the lead leg and stays aligned with the second toe.

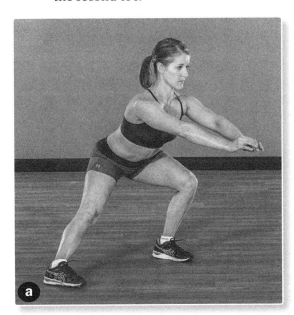
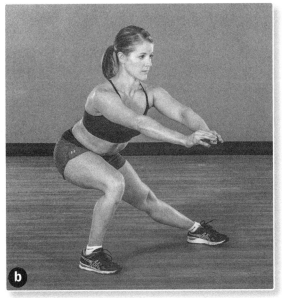

Bodyweight 180-Degree Squat Turn

Intended Uses

This exercise is good for improving lower-body muscular endurance, coordination, and body awareness.

Prerequisites

- Balance, stability, and coordination.
- No lower-body pain or injuries.

Steps

- Perform a squat (*a*).
- As you ascend, lift the left foot, pivot on the right foot, and turn to the left until you are facing the opposite direction (*b*).
- Immediately perform another squat and then repeat this process, pivoting off the left foot and turning to the right.
- Continue alternating until you have performed the desired number of repetitions.

Key Points

- Make certain that the knees do not pass the toes.

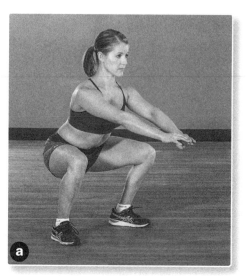

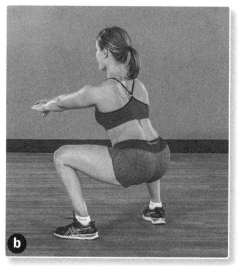

Bodyweight Reverse Lunge

Intended Uses

This drill improves lower-body muscular endurance and coordination and develops unilateral strength and endurance.

Prerequisites

- Good balance and coordination.
- No lower-body pain or injuries.
- Ability to perform a forward lunge with good, consistent technique.

Steps

- While maintaining a rigid torso, step back with the right foot as far as possible.
- Simultaneously allow the left leg, ankle, knee, and hip to bend until the top of the thigh is parallel to the ground (*a*).
- Extend the left leg and move the right foot forward until you are back in the starting position (*b*).
- Repeat this action, stepping back with the left foot and allowing the right leg to take the lead.
- Continue alternating until you have performed the desired number of repetitions.

Variations

- After extending the lead leg and moving the trail leg back to the starting position, immediately perform a high knee drive with the leg that trailed and add a front kick. Return the kicking leg to the starting position and repeat this sequence for the desired number of repetitions. Repeat this action on the opposite side.

Key Points

- Make certain that the lead leg knee stays aligned with the second toe of the same-side foot.

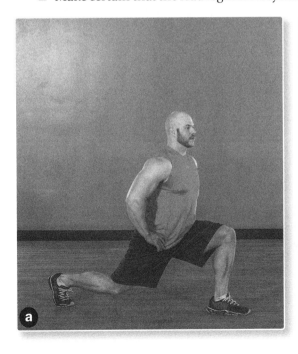
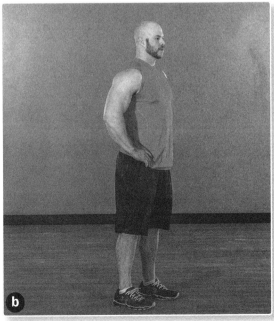

Bodyweight Walking Lunge

Intended Uses

This drill improves lower-body muscular endurance, balance, and coordination. It also develops unilateral strength and endurance.

Prerequisites

- Good balance, stability, and coordination.
- No lower-body injuries.
- Ability to perform a forward lunge with good, consistent technique.

Steps

- Begin in a standing position.
- Set your back.
- Take an exaggerated step forward with the right foot (*a*).
- Allow the right ankle, knee, and hip to bend until the thigh is parallel to the ground (*b*).
- Perform the lunge with the left leg.
- Continue alternating until you have covered the desired distance.

Variations

- This drill can also be performed moving laterally.
- Hockey lunges are performed in the same manner as the walking lunge, but the exaggerated step forward should be at a 45-degree angle rather than straight ahead.

Key Points

- Keep the lead leg knee aligned with the second toe of the same-side foot.
- Focus on driving the knee toward the chest, stepping over the lead leg.

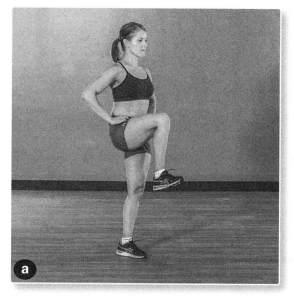
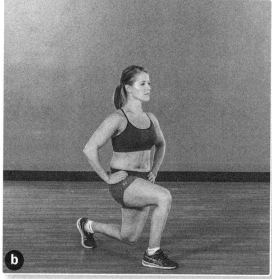

Bodyweight Alternating Step-Up

Intended Uses

This drill improves lower-body muscular endurance, balance, and hip stability. It also develops unilateral strength and endurance.

Prerequisites

- Good balance and hip stability.
- No lower-body pain or injuries.

Steps

- Stand facing a 12- to 16-inch (30 to 40 cm) box.
- Lift the knee and place the left foot completely flat on top of the box (*a*).
- Push off with the left leg and lift the right foot. Place the right foot on top of the box (*b*).
- Step back with the right foot first, placing it completely on the ground. Then step back with the left foot.
- Repeat this exercise, leading with the right leg.
- Continue alternating sides for the desired number of repetitions.

Variations

- Perform the desired number of repetitions on one leg and then switch and perform the same number of repetitions on the opposite leg.
- Lateral and rotational step-ups may be used to add variety and incorporate different movement planes.

Key Points

- Make certain that the foot is flat on the ground or box.
- Keep the knees aligned with the second toe and do not allow the hips to rotate.

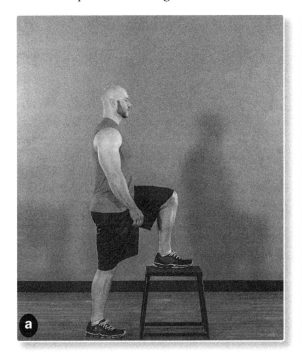
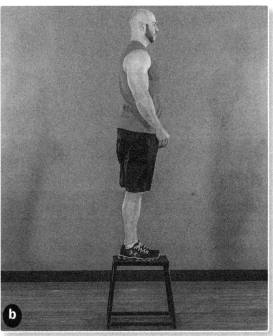

Bodyweight Burpee

Intended Uses

This drill can be used for total-body agility and power. It is also an excellent total-body conditioning exercise.

Prerequisites

- Good trunk stability.
- Ability to perform a deep squat with good form and technique.
- No lower- or upper-body pain or injuries.

Steps

- Begin in a standing position. Then drop down into a push-up, or plank, position by placing both palms on the ground and jumping the feet back (*a*).
- Explosively thrust the feet forward toward the chest (*b*). When both feet are in full contact with the ground, jump up as high as possible (*c*).
- Repeat for a set time or the desired number of repetitions.

Variations

- After thrusting the feet forward, simply stand up rather than jump. This less-stressful version of the exercise can be used to continue challenging the metabolic system when you cannot achieve or maintain proper form while jumping.

Key Points

- Keep the arms bent at 90 degrees.
- Maintain a rigid torso with a slight lean forward (10 degrees) at the hips.
- With each skip, visualize pushing the ground away from you.
- Minimize your vertical movement (or bobbing and bouncing up and down) as much as possible while performing the skip.

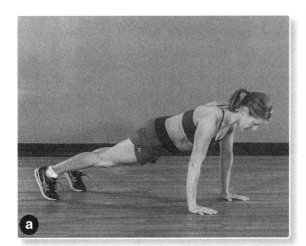

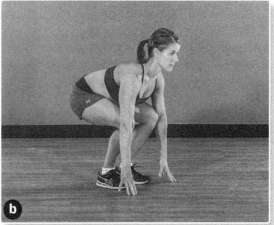

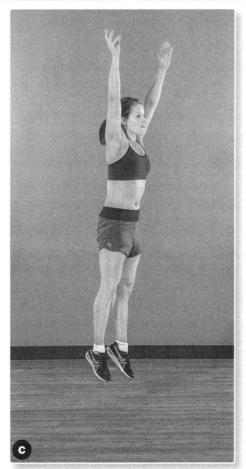

Bodyweight Quick Feet on Box

Intended Uses

This drill can be used for coordination, balance, single-leg stability, and foot quickness.

Prerequisites

- Ability to stabilize and maintain balance on one leg.
- No lower-body pain or injuries.

Steps

- Bend the arms at the elbows until they reach a 90-degree angle. Place the tips of the finger of the left hand at eye level and place the right hand at the same level as the back hip pocket.
- Lift the right foot and place just the toes on a 6- to 12-inch (15 to 30 cm) box (*a*).
- Lean slightly forward from the hips and rapidly alternate the arms and feet in a running-like manner until the right hand is at the right cheek, the left hand is by the back left hip pocket, the left foot is on the box, and the right foot is on the ground (*b*).
- Continue this pattern for the desired time or number of repetitions.

Key Points

- Use opposite arm and leg action.
- Keep the torso rigid.
- Lean slightly forward (10 degrees) at the hips.
- Tap the top of the box with the toes of the lead leg.

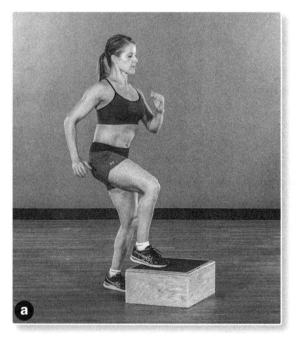
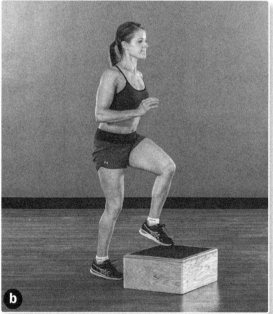

INTRODUCTORY PROGRAM

If you have never exercised regularly, knowing where to start can be challenging. Table 3.2 presents a four-week program that will help you get comfortable with bodyweight exercises. You should perform this program twice a week for four weeks. Do the exercises in the order listed. Each exercise should be performed for 20 seconds. Do not rest between exercises. After you have been through the entire list of exercises, rest for 2 minutes and repeat. Perform the entire list of exercise three times in each workout session.

Table 3.2 Introductory Bodyweight Training Program

Day 1	Day 2
Bodyweight jumping jacks, p. 13	Bodyweight jumping jacks, p. 13
Bodyweight crab kick, 14	Bodyweight push-up, p 21
Bodyweight inchworm, p 15	Bodyweight crab kick, p 14
Bodyweight bear crawl, p 16	Bodyweight dip, p 22
Bodyweight climber, p 17	Bodyweight inchworm, p 15
Bodyweight groiner, p 18	Bodyweight pull-up (modified, if necessary), p 20
Bodyweight scissors, p 19	Bodyweight mountain climber, p 17
Bodyweight push-up, p 21	Bodyweight scissors, p 19
Bodyweight dip, p 22	Bodyweight groiner, p 18
Bodyweight pull-up, p 20	Bodyweight bear crawl, p 16

CHAPTER 4

Sprinting

Sprinting, or running at a high rate of speed, is extremely important in many sports. Athletes are often required to execute multiple sprints over varying distances during a match or competition. Because they need to run quickly over short distances even when tired, sprinting is a frequently used training tool in sport conditioning programs.

Performing sprints for conditioning has advantages and disadvantages. A major advantage of using sprints is that they are an effective method of maximum interval training. Sprinting at high speeds is intense. Additionally, because most athletes have to sprint to be successful in their sports, it is a sport-specific form of interval training. For this reason, using sprints provides high potential for direct transfer to improved sport performance.

On the other hand, sprinting is a highly technical motion. Speed is highly dependent on running mechanics, stride length (the length of each stride), stride frequency (how quickly you take strides), strength, and mobility. Good sprinting technique requires moving the limbs quickly with skill and efficiency to maximize the amount of force being exerted against the ground and to prevent injuries, particularly to the hamstrings and shins. If sprinting is performed in a fatigued state, a breakdown in form and technique often results, which increases the risk of injury. Also, when technique breaks down, the pace slows. In other words, if sprint training for conditioning is done improperly, sloppy rather than ideal sprint mechanics are emphasized. Poor movement mechanics hinder speed development—a chain of events that we want athletes to avoid at all costs!

With that in mind, this chapter focuses on identifying and performing each component of good sprinting mechanics to help you understand what the movement should look like. Drills that you can use to learn proper running form and technique are presented (these drills also make good conditioning exercises in their own right). Finally, advanced approaches to employing sprinting as conditioning are discussed.

GETTING STARTED

Depending on distance, a sprint can have up to three distinct phases. The first phase is called acceleration. During the acceleration phase, we are starting to build up speed. The second phase is maximum velocity. In this phase of the sprint, we achieve the fastest speed possible. The final phase is speed endurance, in which we attempt to maintain maximum velocity for as long as possible.

Distinguishing between phases is important because acceleration and maximum velocity sprinting have subtly different techniques. In addition, specific phases may apply to some sports but not others. For example, baseball requires players to accelerate over relatively short distances. Therefore, a baseball player rarely is able to build up enough speed to reach maximal velocity. In contrast, an athlete running the 400-meters event in track and field must progress through all three phases.

Maximum Velocity

When discussing sprinting technique, running at maximum velocity is typically addressed first. Achieving maximum velocity is always the goal, whether taking a single step or running 200 meters.

When running at maximum velocity, the foot lifts off the ground. As the foot breaks contact with the ground, it should be brought up behind your body to your hip (figure 4.1). The goal is to touch your gluteal muscles (glutes) with your heel. To understand the path of the leg and foot, picture yourself sliding your right foot up a wall behind you. From this position, swing the leg forward to the point where the thigh is roughly parallel to the ground, allowing your lower leg to unfold as you do so. From this position, drive the foot toward the ground using the hip. The ball of the foot should contact the ground slightly in front of the body. As the right foot strikes the ground, bring the left foot up toward your glutes. Pull yourself forward until your body passes over your foot and then repeat.

Whenever you are sprinting, your feet and ankles should be rigid. Sometimes this position is referred to as being "cast." When sprinting with the feet and ankles cast, the toes should not point down. One strategy to help you keep them in the correct position is to think about lifting the big toe of each foot up while sprinting.

Posture is also important when sprinting. You should stay tall when the foot strikes the ground and not allow yourself to slump forward. Staying tall maximizes your ability to exert force against the ground, whereas slumping hinders the amount of force that you can produce.

Good arm mechanics are also critical for sprinting. Your arms should be bent and held at a natural angle. Your hands can be open or closed depending on what is comfortable for you, but you should not clinch your hands into fists because this increases tension in the upper body. Additionally, the arms should move straight forward and backward; they should never cross in front of the body. Crossing the body creates rotation, which negatively affects sprinting speed (figure 4.2).

Acceleration

For a sprinter, the acceleration phase has two subphases: pure acceleration and transition. During pure acceleration, the sprinting technique is slightly different than when running at maximum velocity. During transition, the technique is almost identical to that used for maximum velocity, although the velocity is not maximal.

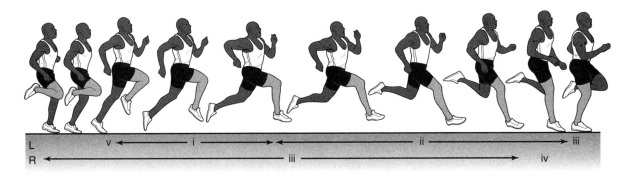

Figure 4.1 Path of the legs and feet during the maximum velocity phase of sprinting: heel to glutes, leg swing forward, and footstrike.

Adapted, by permission, from G. Schmolinsky, 2000, *The East German textbook of athletes* (Toronto: Sport Books).

Pure acceleration relies on frontside mechanics, in which the leg action takes place in front of the body. When accelerating, you pick your right foot off the ground. As you do this, you lift your right knee up in front of the body. Then, using your glutes, you drive your right foot down into the ground so that you land on the ball of your foot. As you drive the right foot down, you lift the left foot, and then you continue to alternate.

Most people reach the transition phase after about 10 to 15 meters of acceleration. At this point you begin incorporating backside mechanics into the sprint, and the technique is identical to that used for maximum velocity sprinting.

When accelerating, as when sprinting at maximum velocity, you swing your arms forward and backward and maintain a good, straight body posture (although you may be leaning forward slightly as your velocity increases). Your feet and ankles should still be rigid, or cast.

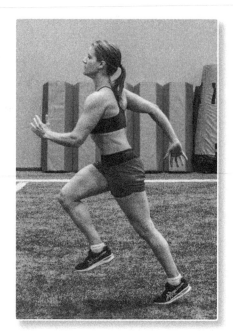

Figure 4.2 Proper form for sprinting at maximum velocity: Feet and ankles are cast, posture is upright, and loosely bent arms move forward and back without crossing.

Speed Endurance

Speed endurance is the ability to maintain maximum velocity. Except for track and field athletes, there's not a lot of need to worry about speed endurance. Few sporting situations allow an athlete to run in a perfectly straight line and accelerate continuously long enough for this quality to come into play. Occasionally, however, speed endurance may be required, especially if a critical mistake or several mistakes are made. In this case, realize that the running mechanics are identical to those used for running at maximum velocity. The challenge is that maximum velocity can be maintained only for a few seconds. So at this stage we are simply trying to slow down as little as possible.

Although speed endurance is not as critical except in track and field, repeated sprint ability is essential for sports that require intermittent bursts of speed, such as soccer, lacrosse, and rugby. Integrating sprint conditioning work into the training programs for these sports can pay huge dividends on the playing field, especially during the latter stages of a competition. Players who are better conditioned are able to generate bursts of speed throughout a match. In many cases, this training allows an athlete to beat the opponent to the ball, get enough separation to make a catch, or outlast the competition in a dead heat. Speed endurance can literally be the difference between winning and losing.

FOUNDATIONAL EXERCISES

When it comes to using sprinting as a maximum interval-training tool, technique is critical for preventing injury and ensuring both the effectiveness and the transferability of the exercises. With that in mind, the foundational exercises are meant to break this complicated skill down into parts that can be easily mastered. After these skills have been mastered, these foundational exercises make great warm-up drills and can still be used for conditioning workouts.

Sprinting Footstrike

Intended Uses

This drill teaches how to lift the foot off the ground, how to plant the foot on the ground, and which part of the foot should make contact while sprinting. This is also a valuable exercise for developing sprint-specific shin and foot strength. It can be done slowly (as described) or as a low-intensity plyometric exercise.

Prerequisites

- Ability to "cast" the foot.
- Understanding which part of the foot to strike the ground with.

Steps

- Begin by facing the course.
- Keeping the leg straight, swing the left leg forward from the hip (*a*).
- As you swing the leg forward, cast the foot as it breaks contact with the ground.
- Swing the leg forward so that the left foot touches the ground just ahead of your hips (*b*).
- Your foot should land so that the ball of the foot contacts the ground.
- Pull your body forward with the left leg as you swing the right leg forward.
- Continue alternating until you have covered the desired distance.

Key Points

- The foot should be cast as soon as it leaves the ground.
- Keep the legs straight and move forward from the hips.
- Land on the ball of the foot.

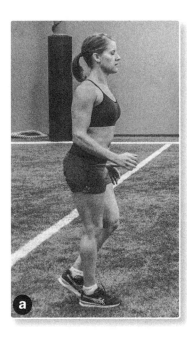
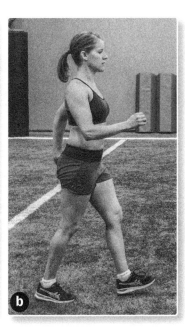

Sprinting Lift the Foot

Intended Uses

This drill reinforces the skills developed by the previous drill while teaching backside mechanics. This drill teaches you how to lift your foot up to your hips during the sprinting motion. After you have mastered this technique, the drill is a useful warm-up and conditioning drill in its own right.

Prerequisites

- Ability to cast the foot.
- Understanding which part of the foot to strike the ground with.
- Ability to perform the footstrike drill with consistent, good technique.

Steps

- Begin by facing the course.
- Lift the right foot off the ground and cast the foot as you lift it (*a*).
- Lift the right foot behind the body, as if sliding it up a wall (*b*).
- Lift the right foot up until it touches the right buttock or as close as you can comfortably get.
- Keeping the foot cast, step forward with the right foot, landing on the ball of the foot.
- Repeat using the left leg.
- Continue alternating until you have covered the desired distance.

Key Points

- The foot should be cast as soon as it leaves the ground.
- Slide the cast foot behind you until it touches your buttock.
- Land on the ball of the foot.

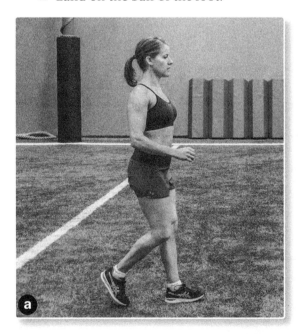
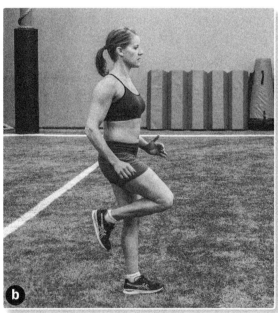

Sprinting Swing the Leg

Intended Uses

This drill reinforces the need to keep the foot cast and to land on the ball of the foot. This drill teaches frontside mechanics and teaches you how to drive the foot toward the ground using your hips. After you have mastered it, this is another drill that makes a great warm-up and conditioning exercise.

Prerequisites

- Ability to cast the foot.
- Understanding which part of the foot to strike the ground with.
- Ability to maintain good posture during the drill.

Steps

- Begin by facing the course.
- Lift the right knee in front of the body.
- As the right foot leaves the ground, cast the foot.
- Lift the right knee until the thigh is parallel to the ground.
- Keeping the foot cast, step forward with the right foot, landing on the ball of the foot.
- Repeat using the left leg.
- Continue alternating until you cover the desired distance.

Key Points

- The foot should be cast as soon as it leaves the ground.
- Land on the ball of the foot.
- Stay tall while performing this exercise; keep the chest out and shoulders back.

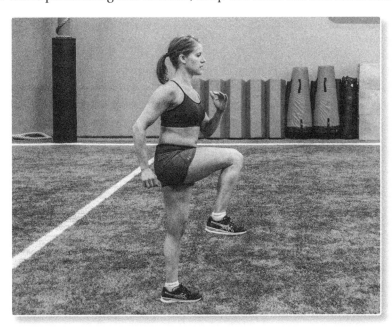

Intended Uses

This drill combines all the previous drills and simulates running at maximum velocity. It reinforces each of the skills that have been taught to this point while requiring you to put everything together. It is also an effective warm-up drill and can be used to help condition the hamstrings in a sprinting-specific manner.

Prerequisites

- Ability to cast the foot.
- Understanding which part of the foot to strike the ground with.
- Understanding of backside mechanics.
- Understanding of frontside mechanics.
- Ability to maintain good posture during the drill.

Steps

- Begin by facing the course.
- Lift the right foot off the ground, casting the foot as you lift it.
- Lift the right foot behind the body; picture it sliding up a wall.
- Lift the right foot up until it touches the right buttock or as close as you can comfortably get.
- Swing the right leg forward so that the right thigh ends up parallel to the ground.
- As you swing the right leg forward, the foot should uncouple, or separate, from the buttock.
- Using the hip, drive the right foot down toward the ground in front of the body.
- The right foot should contact the ground on the ball of the foot.
- As the right foot strikes, repeat the movement with the left leg.
- Continue alternating for the desired distance.

Key Points

- The foot should be cast as soon as it leaves the ground.
- Land on the ball of the foot.
- Stay tall while performing this exercise; in other words, hold the chest out and shoulders back.
- Use the glutes to drive the foot toward the ground.

ADVANCED EXERCISES

The foundational exercises are important because they teach and refine aspects of sprinting, which is a more complicated movement skill than many people believe. The foundational exercises also serve as useful conditioning exercises, especially when incorporated with other exercise modes. Having said all that, they are not a substitute for sprinting. The advanced exercises described in this chapter represent ways to use sprinting as a stand-alone tool for maximum interval training. Table 4.1 outlines suggested distances, times, and rest periods for the advanced sprinting exercises.

Table 4.1 Distances, Times, and Rest Periods for Advanced Sprinting Exercises

Constant distance sprinting (time in seconds, rest period in seconds)	Stepwise sprinting (time in seconds, rest period in seconds)	Finite time sprinting (total sprint and rest time)
10 × 100 meters (25 sec, 50 sec)	1 × 20 meters (10 sec, 20 sec) 1 × 40 meters (15 sec, 30 sec) 1 × 60 meters (20 sec, 40 sec) 1 × 80 meters (25 sec, 50 sec) 1 × 100 meters (30 sec, 60 sec) 1 × 80 meters (25 sec, 50 sec) 1 × 60 meters (20 sec, 40 sec) 1 × 40 meters (15 sec, 30 sec) 1 × 20 meters	1 × 40 meters (20 sec) 1 × 100 meters (30 sec) 2 × 80 meters (25 sec each) 2 × 60 meters (20 sec each) 3 × 40 meters (20 sec each) 1 × 100 meters

Stepwise Sprinting

Intended Uses

This exercise is more sport specific than constant distance sprinting. It replicates athletics in the sense that it provides a variety of sprinting distances and recovery intervals. The downside is that this exercise can be predictable, unlike sprinting in sport.

Prerequisites

- Understanding of correct sprinting mechanics.
- Sufficient endurance to sprint the desired distance using correct technique.

Steps

- Line up at the start line and face the course.
- On the start command, run the desired distance.
- In this approach to sprinting, you run a specific distance on the first sprint. Distance increases on subsequent sprints; alternatively, it could decrease on subsequent sprints or increase first and then decrease as the sprints progress (see table 4.1 for an example).

Key Points

- Correct technique has to be emphasized.
- For safety reasons, when technique breaks down, the exercise should be stopped.
- Recovery between sprints should be active; do not sit down or lie down because inactivity will encourage fatigue and cramping. You should walk around or even perform a slow jog between sprints.

Constant Distance Sprinting

Intended Uses

This approach is a simple way to program sprinting as a maximum interval-training tool. Many sports, because of the playing field or tradition, use this approach for their conditioning. For example, an American football field is 100 yards long, which makes running 100 sprints logical. The downside is that athletes tend to save themselves for the last few sprints, which defeats the purpose of the exercise.

Prerequisites

- Understanding of correct sprinting mechanics.
- Sufficient endurance to sprint the desired distance using correct technique.

Steps

- Line up at the start line and face the course.
- On the start command, run the desired distance.
- In this approach to sprinting, you run a specific number of sprints at a predetermined distance; for example, you run 10 sprints of 100 yards.
- This drill is most effective when there is a standard for running the sprints and a standard for recovery times. For example, 100-yard sprints could be run in 20 seconds with 60 seconds of recovery. If you take less than 20 seconds to run the sprint, you have more time to rest; if you take longer than 20 seconds, you have less time to rest. See table 4.1 for an example.

Key Points

- Correct technique must be emphasized.
- For safety reasons, when technique breaks down, the exercise should be stopped.
- Recovery between sprints should be active; do not sit down or lie down because inactivity will encourage fatigue and cramping. You should walk around or even perform a slow jog between sprints.

Finite Time Sprinting

Intended Uses

This sprinting exercise is the most advanced one in the book. It is random, and it is unforgiving of those who are slow or tired. For these reasons, it resembles what happens in sport. The challenge with this exercise is that you need someone to inflict it on you to keep it random and unpredictable.

Prerequisites

- Understanding of correct sprinting mechanics.
- Sufficient endurance to sprint the desired distance using correct technique.

Steps

- Line up at the start line and face the course.
- On the start command, run the desired distance.
- For this approach to sprinting, you run a specific distance. You are told that distance right before starting the sprint. This distance is random and changes from sprint to sprint.
- You have a specific time to run the sprint and recover from it, but that time is never communicated to you. When the time is up, it's time to run the next sprint. See table 4.1 for an example.

Key Points

- Correct technique has to be emphasized.
- For safety reasons, when technique breaks down, the exercise should be stopped.
- Recovery between sprints should be active. Do not sit down or lie down because inactivity will encourage fatigue and cramping. You should walk around or even perform a slow jog between sprints.
- Total volume should be kept to no more than 500 to 750 yards (450 to 700 m).
- The times to complete each sprint should be realistic for you to run the sprint and recover before the next one. Remember that correct technique and speed are critical to sprints!

INTRODUCTORY PROGRAM

The following three-day-a-week workout program will help you become proficient with sprinting technique and build your foundation so that you can effectively use sprinting in maximum interval training. This program is meant to be done for four weeks. The first day focuses on technique drills and maximum velocity, so the distances are long enough that you have a chance to reach top speed. The second day focuses on technique drills and acceleration, which means that the sprints are shorter and the focus is on frontside mechanics. The final day focuses on technique speed endurance, which means that the sprints are longer and full recovery occurs after each sprint. After completing this program, you should be proficient with technique and have a fitness base that allows you to use the more advanced exercises. This program is detailed in table 4.2.

Table 4.2 Introductory Sprinting Program

Monday	Wednesday	Friday
Warm-up: 400-meter jog	Warm-up: 400-meter jog	Warm-up: 400-meter jog
Sprinting footstrike, 2 × 20 meters, p. 43	Sprinting footstrike, 2 × 20 meters, p. 43	Sprinting footstrike, 1 × 20 meters, jog back, p. 43
Sprinting lift the foot, 2 × 20 meters, p. 44	Sprinting lift the foot, 2 × 20 meters, p. 44	Sprinting lift the foot, 1 × 20 meters, jog back, p. 44
Sprinting swing the leg, 2 × 20 meters, p. 45	Sprinting swing the leg, 2 × 20 meters, p. 45	Sprinting swing the leg, 1 × 20 meters, jog back, p. 45
Sprinting put it all together, 2 × 20 meters, p. 46	Sprinting put it all together, 2 × 20 meters, p. 46	Sprinting put it all together drill, 1 × 20 meters, jog back, p. 46
3–5 × 40 meters, full recovery	3 × 5 meters, full recovery	2 × 5 meters, full recovery
	3 × 20 meters, full recovery	2 × 20 meters, full recovery
		5 × 150 meters, full recovery

CHAPTER 5

Medicine Balls

Medicine balls have been around for centuries. According to Thomas (2002), although the medicine ball may date back to the ancient Egyptians, the Greek physician Claudius Galen (ca. AD 130–200) is thought to be the first to prescribe the use of balls for therapeutic purposes. In the 16th century Girolamo Mercuriale promoted the use of light balls filled with air or feathers and heavy balls filled with sand to prevent and heal illness. The medicine ball was also used by the United States Military Academy in the late 1800s and early 1900s and by the United States Army as a reconditioning tool during World War II.

Medicine balls are not only an extremely versatile training tool but are also relatively inexpensive when compared with other forms of traditional gym equipment. They come in various weights, sizes, and types, allowing the use of a wide variety of training styles and the development of various physical attributes. Any local sporting goods store will offer traditional leather-bound balls, sand-filled medicine balls, rubberized medicine balls designed to bounce, and even balls with handles. Furthermore, you can make your own medicine ball by simply taking an old basketball or soccer ball and adding water. In addition to versatility, medicine balls have one major benefit not available with other training devices: They can be released and thrown! This attribute allows users to accelerate the ball throughout the entire range of motion, which maximizes the amount of power that they can generate. This occurs because the muscles responsible for decelerating the weight are not activated during the end range of the movement to slow down the implement.

Creating a Medicine Ball With Water

Step 1: Remove the plug from an old soccer or basketball (needle-nosed pliers may be necessary for removal).
Step 2: Use a garden hose to fill the ball with water.
Step 3: Reinsert the plug.
Step 4: Use an inflation needle and air pump to pressurize the ball.

Adapted from Chandler and Reuter, 1994.

GETTING STARTED

There are currently no standard recommendations for selecting medicine ball weight. In fact, the weight of the ball selected depends on several factors, such as the type of exercise being performed and the desired training outcome. In general, you should select a weight that allows you to perform the desired number of repetitions with good form and technique. By using a load that is too heavy, you may develop poor movement patterns. Breaking these poor habits later is difficult. Furthermore, using an excessive load may lead to injury. If the training load selected is too light, the user may see no performance gains. When aiming to train for muscular endurance or speed, select a load that can be performed for a minimum of 15 to 20 repetitions with good form and technique. If the training goal is strength or power, heavier loads that allow the user to maintain good form and technique for 10 to 12 repetitions may be more beneficial. If you are still uncertain about what size of medicine ball to use, start with the following guideline:

$$\text{Medicine ball weight} = (\text{Body weight} \setminus 2) \times .1$$

$$\text{Example: 8 pounds} = (160 \setminus 2) \times .1, \text{ or } 3.6 \text{ kg} = (72 \setminus 2) \times .1$$

The following exercises and drills focus on a wide range of health and skill-related fitness objectives such as muscular strength and endurance, cardiorespiratory fitness, mobility, balance, coordination, speed, and power. Although an almost infinite number of exercises can be performed with medicine balls, we have tried to narrow them down to the ones that we believe will allow you to maximize your training efforts and hit the broadest range of physical attributes per exercise. Remember, however, that to get the best results from your training program, you should select the exercises and drills that match your desired training outcome.

FOUNDATIONAL EXERCISES

The exercises described in this section are great for developing the core, total-body strength, and power. These exercises not only teach foundational techniques but also are valuable to athletes at all stages of development.

Medicine Ball Chop

Intended Uses

This drill develops upper-body endurance as well as endurance of the core muscles.

Prerequisites

- No pain or history of shoulder injury.
- Ability to plank.

Steps

- Stand with the feet approximately shoulder-width apart while holding a medicine ball overhead (*a*).
- Keep the arms straight and extend the shoulders, moving the ball downward toward the hips (*b*).
- While keeping the arms straight, flex the shoulders and return the ball back overhead.

Key Points

- Maintain a rigid torso throughout.
- Do not allow the arms to bend.
- Go as fast as you can while maintaining proper form and technique.

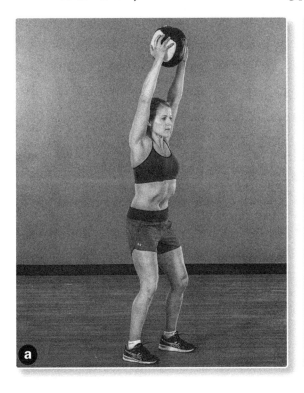
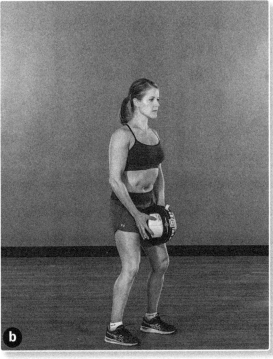

Medicine Ball Alphabet

Intended Uses

This drill primarily develops upper-body endurance. It also requires an athlete to stabilize the core while performing it.

Prerequisites

- No history of shoulder injury.
- Ability to plank.

Steps

- Stand with the feet approximately shoulder-width apart holding the medicine ball at shoulder or chest level (*a*).
- While keeping the arms straight, write the alphabet using the medicine ball (*b-c*).
- Perform this drill for a predetermined time, or to a certain letter. Then repeat the process writing the letters backward (mirror image) for the second set.

Key Points

- Maintain a rigid torso throughout.
- Do not allow the arms to bend.
- Go as fast as you can while maintaining proper form and technique.

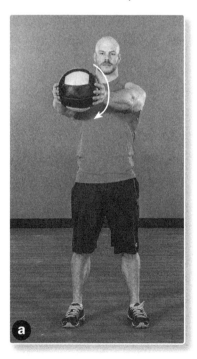
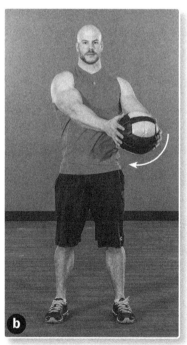
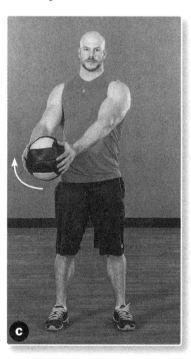

Medicine Ball Thruster

Intended Uses

This drill increases the cardiopulmonary demands of the traditional squat and is a total-body conditioning drill.

Prerequisites

- No shoulder, back, or lower-body injury.
- Ability to perform a squat properly.

Steps

- Assume an athletic position while holding the medicine ball at chest level.
- Perform a squat (*a*).
- While ascending from the squat, press the medicine ball overhead (*b*) and then return to the starting position.
- Perform for a set duration or specified number of repetitions.

Key Points

- Maintain a rigid torso throughout the exercise.
- Press the ball overhead until the upper arms are parallel to the ears.

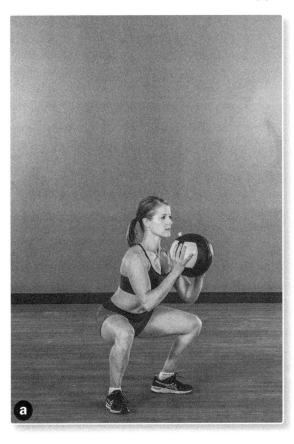 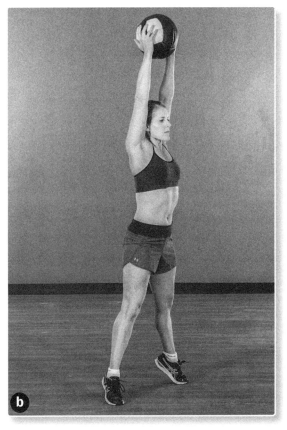

Medicine Ball Bulgarian Squat

Intended Uses

This exercise is excellent for improving single-leg balance and developing hip strength and stability.

Prerequisites

- Ability to squat using proper form and technique.
- Good trunk stability.

Steps

- While holding a medicine ball either overhead or directly in front of the body, assume a split stance, elevating the rear foot on a bench or chair (*a*).
- Allow the ankle, knee, and hip to flex until the top of the thigh is approximately parallel to the ground (*b*).
- Extend the ankle, knee, and hip to return to the starting position.
- Perform for the desired number of repetitions and then repeat using the opposite leg.

Key Points

- Do not allow the knee on the working leg to fall or collapse inward.

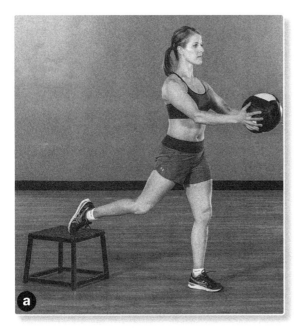
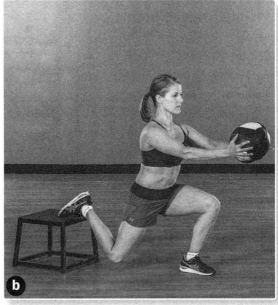

Medicine Ball Wall Ball

Intended Uses

This drill improves total-body power or power endurance.

Prerequisites

- No shoulder or back injuries.
- Ability to perform a squat properly.

Steps

- Begin by facing a cinderblock wall.
- Assume an athletic position while holding the medicine ball at chest level.
- Perform a squat (*a*).
- Ascend from the squat explosively and release the ball at the top of the movement (*b*).
- After the ball has hit the wall overhead, catch it and in one smooth motion return to the squat position to prepare for the next throw.

Key Points

- Keep your eye on the ball and receive it with soft hands, as you would catch a basketball.

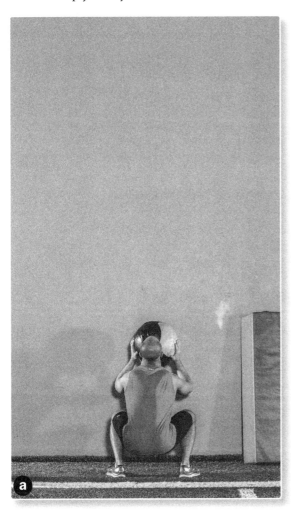

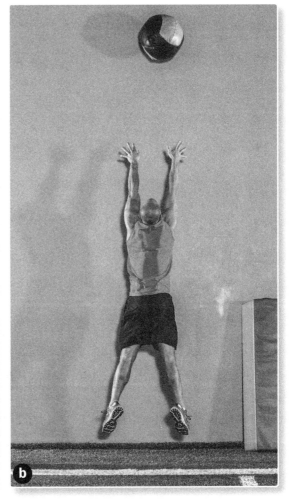

Medicine Ball Touch and Jump

Intended Uses

This drill is used primarily to improve power endurance.

Prerequisites

- Ability to perform a squat with good form and technique.

Steps

- While holding a medicine ball in front of the chest, assume an athletic stance.
- Perform a squat and touch the medicine ball to the ground between the feet (*a*).
- Jump upward explosively, while lifting the medicine ball off the floor and pressing it overhead (*b*).

Key Points

- Allow the ankle, knee, and hip to flex until the top of the thigh is approximately parallel to the ground.
- Do not allow the knees to fall or collapse inward during this drill.

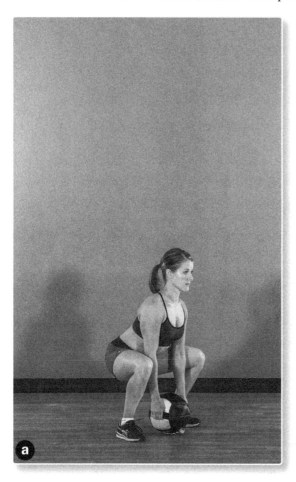
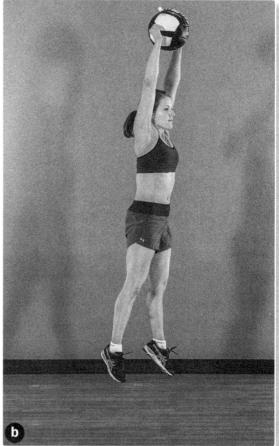

Medicine Ball Slam

Intended Uses

This drill develops upper-body power and power endurance.

Prerequisites

- Ability to maintain a rigid torso.
- No shoulder or back injuries.

Steps

- Assume an athletic stance while extending the arms and holding a medicine ball directly overhead (*a*).
- Forcefully chop the arms downward and slam the ball into the ground just in in front of and between the feet (*b*).
- If you are using a medicine ball that bounces, receive the ball and repeat for the desired number for petitions. If the ball does not bounce, pick it up and repeat this action for the desired time or number of repetitions.

Key Points

- Slam the ball as hard as possible for each repetition.
- Keep your eye on the ball and use soft hands to receive.

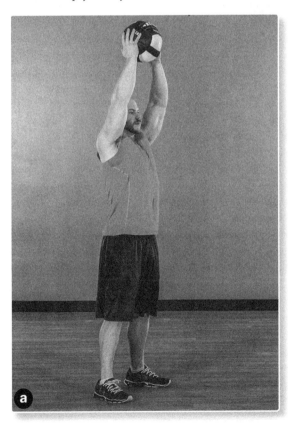
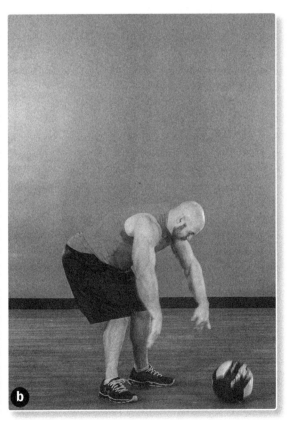

Medicine Ball Chest Pass

Intended Uses

This drill improves upper-body power endurance.

Prerequisites

- No lower-body injuries.

Steps

- Assume an athletic stance in front of a cinderblock wall, rebounder, or with a partner while holding the medicine ball against the chest (a).
- Pass the ball as quickly as possible against the wall or rebounder for a set time or number of repetitions (b).

Key Points

- Get rid of the ball quickly, as if it were on fire.

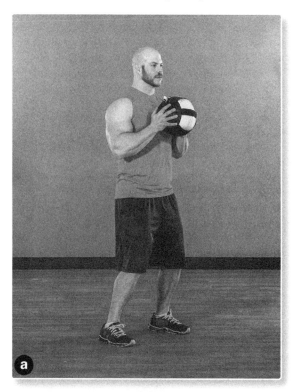

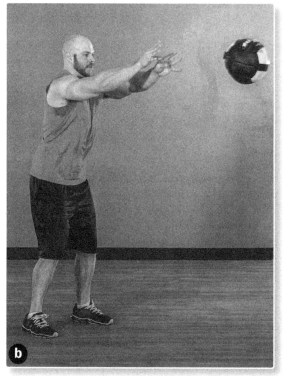

Medicine Ball Seated Twist

Intended Uses

This drill improves core endurance and thoracic spine mobility.

Prerequisites

- No history of back injury.
- Good isometric strength in the trunk.

Steps

- While holding a medicine ball, sit on the ground with the knees slightly bent and heels in contact with the ground.
- Lean back at the hips until your torso is at about a 45-degree angle and rotate the medicine ball back and forth from one hip to the other (*a-b*).

Key Points

- Maintain a rigid torso.
- Go as fast as possible while maintaining good form and technique.

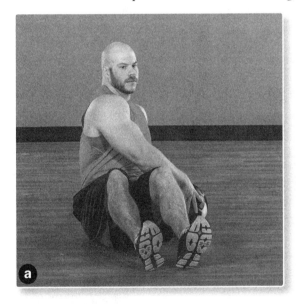
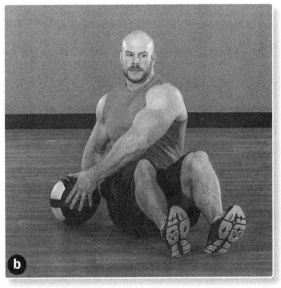

Sit-Up With Medicine Ball Lift

Intended Uses

This drill is excellent for improving trunk and shoulder stability and endurance, flexibility through the lats, and hip flexor strength.

Prerequisites

- Ability to perform a proper sit-up.
- Adequate shoulder mobility and upper-body flexibility.

Steps

- Lie on your back with the knees bent and feet flat on the ground.
- While holding a medicine ball, fully extend your arms and position the ball against the thighs (*a*).
- Perform a sit-up while simultaneously lifting the medicine ball up and back until it is overhead and your torso is perpendicular to the ground (*b*).

Key Points

- Keep your trunk braced and arms fully extended throughout the duration of the exercise.
- Lower your torso in a controlled manner and do not allow your back to slam against the ground.

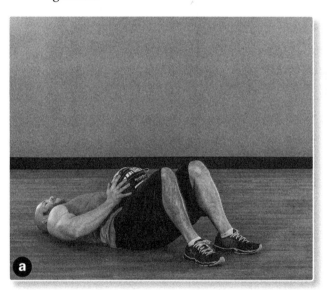
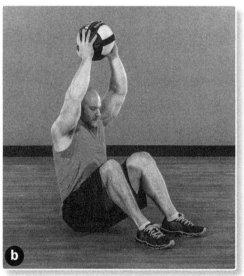

Medicine Ball Modified Pike

Intended Uses

This drill increases core muscular endurance and hamstring flexibility.

Prerequisites

- Ability to perform a proper sit-up.

Steps

- Lie on your back with the right knee bent and right foot flat on the ground (*a*).
- Keep the left leg straight and the left foot pulled back toward the shin.
- While holding a medicine ball, fully extend your arms overhead until the ball is contact with the ground.
- While keeping the left ankle casted, lift the left leg up while simultaneously performing a sit-up and chopping the medicine ball toward the left foot (*b*).
- Switch sides. Continue alternating for the desired number of repetitions.

Key Points

- Keep your trunk braced and arms fully extended throughout the duration of the exercise.
- Lower your torso in a controlled manner and do not allow your back to slam against the ground.
- Keep the arms straight throughout the exercise.

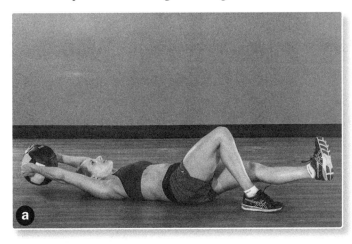
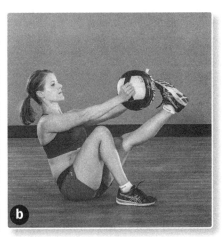

ADVANCED EXERCISES

The advanced medicine ball exercises are a little more complicated, are performed a little faster, or call for better balance than the foundational exercises do. You should master the foundational exercises before attempting these advanced exercises. Athletes should spend two to three months getting comfortable with the foundational exercises before attempting the following exercises.

Medicine Ball Chop With Knee Punch

Intended Uses
This drill improves balance, coordination, and mobility and builds endurance through a dynamic movement pattern.

Prerequisites
- Ability to balance on one leg.
- Ability to perform a plank.

Steps
- Assume a staggered stance with the right foot forward and left foot back.
- Extend the arms so that you are holding the medicine ball directly overhead in front of you (a).
- Simultaneously chop the medicine ball downward toward the back of the left hip and lift the left knee upward toward the right shoulder (b).
- After performing the desired number of repetitions, switch sides.

Key Points
- Punch the knee toward the shoulder.
- Chop the ball to the back hip pocket.

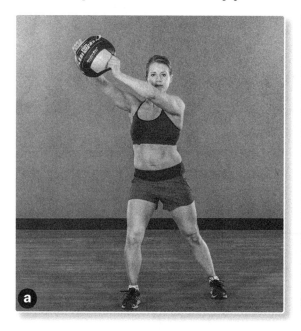 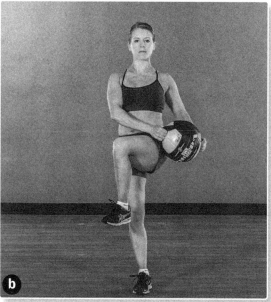

Medicine Ball Speed Squat With Push

Intended Uses

This exercise improves lower-body endurance and trunk and shoulder stability.

Prerequisites

- No lower-back or shoulder injury.
- Ability to squat properly.

Steps

- Assume an athletic stance while holding the medicine ball across the chest (*a*).
- Squat downward while simultaneously extending the arms and pushing the medicine ball away from the body (*b*).
- Pull the medicine ball back toward the chest while returning to the starting position.
- Repeat this action as quickly as possible using good form and technique.

Key Points

- Maintain a rigid trunk.
- Keep the hands at shoulder or chest level while pushing and pulling.
- Sit the hips back, or straight down, to perform the squat.

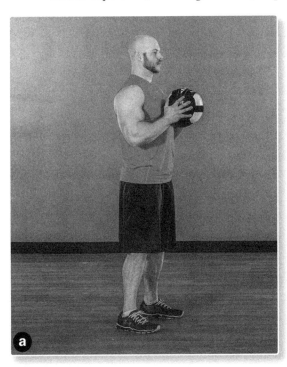
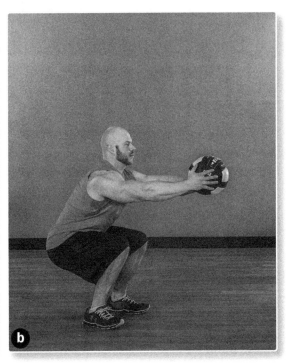

Medicine Ball Multiplanar Squat

Intended Uses

This drill improves lower-body endurance, trunk stability, and mobility using an off-center load.

Prerequisites

- Ability to perform the speed squat with push drill.

Steps

- Assume an athletic stance while holding the medicine ball against the chest (*a*).
- Squat downward while extending the arms and pushing the medicine ball away from the body until it is directly over the left knee (*b*).
- Pull the medicine ball back toward the chest while returning to the starting position.
- Repeat this action, pushing the ball outward over the right knee.

Key Points

- Maintain a rigid trunk.
- Keep the hands at shoulder or chest level while pushing and pulling.
- Sit the hips back, or straight down, to perform the squat.

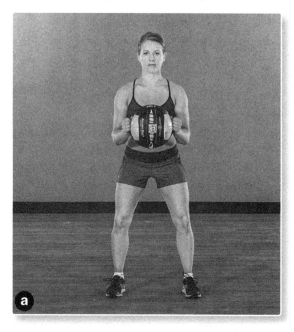
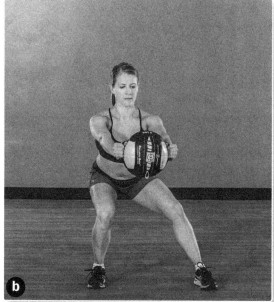

Medicine Ball Step-Box Change

Intended Uses

- This drill is good for improving lower-body footwork and coordination and developing upper- and lower-body muscular endurance.

Prerequisites

- Good balance and coordination.

Steps

- Place the right foot on top of a 4- to 12-inch (10 to 30 cm) aerobic step or plyometric box while holding a medicine ball at chest level (*a*).
- Shift the feet to the right (*b*), so that the left foot is on top of the box and the right foot is on the ground (*c*).
- Shift the feet back to the left, so that the right foot is on the box and the left foot is on the ground.
- Repeat this process, traversing the box for the desired time or number of repetitions.

Key Points

- Focus on good footwork and mechanics.
- Try to look forward rather than downward because looking down will change your body position.

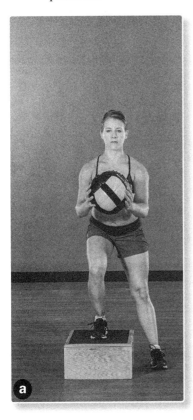
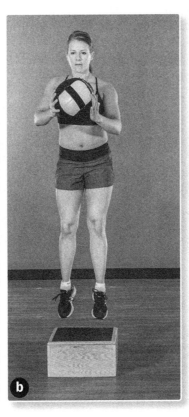
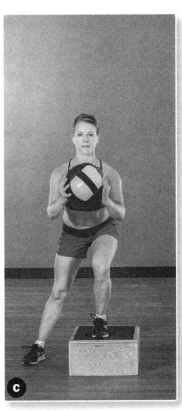

Medicine Ball Single-Leg Squat

Intended Uses

This drill improves leg and hip stability, strength, and endurance.

Prerequisites

- Good balance.
- Ability to perform a squat with proper form and technique.

Steps

- While sitting in a chair and holding a medicine ball in front of you, lift the left foot off the ground (*a*).
- Using only your right leg, stand up (*b*).
- Repeat for the desired number of repetitions and then switch legs.

Key Points

- If it is difficult to maintain your balance, pressing the medicine ball outward on the ascent may help you better counterbalance your body.
- Do not allow the knee on the working leg to fall or collapse inward.

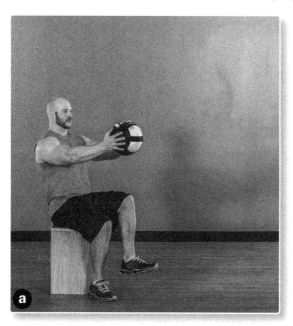 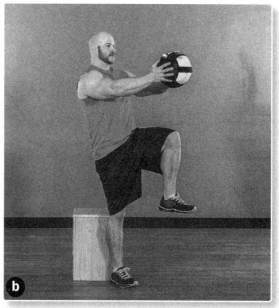

Medicine Ball 90-Degree Jump-Squat and Push

Intended Uses

This drill is good for improving total-body agility and power.

Prerequisites

- Ability to perform a squat with good form and technique.

Steps

- While holding a medicine ball in front of the chest, assume an athletic stance.
- Perform a squat (*a*) and then jump upward and rotate the body toward the left so that the feet are pointing approximately 90 degrees from the starting position (*b*).
- While jumping, push the medicine ball outward so that when landing the arms are fully extended and the ball is at chest height (*c*).
- Pull the medicine ball back toward the chest, jumping and rotating the body so that you are back to the starting position. Repeat this process, only this time jumping to the right.
- Continue alternating between jumps to the left and the right until you have completed the desired number of repetitions.

Key Points

- Allow the ankle, knee, and hip to flex until the top of the thigh is approximately parallel to the ground.
- Do not allow the knees to fall or collapse inward during this drill.

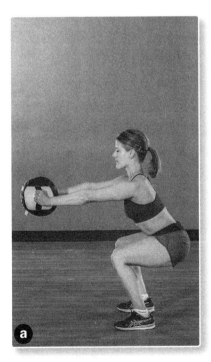
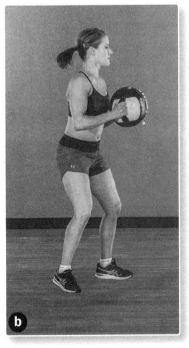
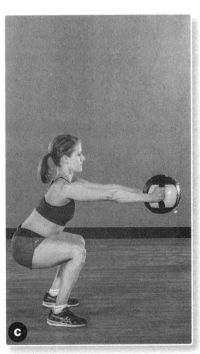

Medicine Ball Rotational Slam

Intended Uses

This drill can be used to improve upper-body power and coordination.

Prerequisites

- Ability to perform slams properly.

Steps

- This drill is performed in the same manner as the medicine ball slam, except that you rotate the torso to the left by pivoting on the right foot.
- Keep the right foot pointed straight ahead (*a*).
- Slam the ball to the outside of the left foot (*b-c*).
- Receive the ball and then repeat in the opposite direction.

Key Points

- Slam the ball as hard as possible for each repetition.
- Keep your eye on the ball and use soft hands to receive.

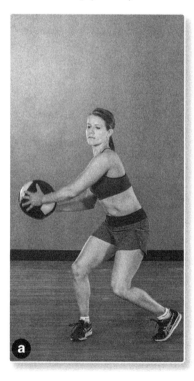 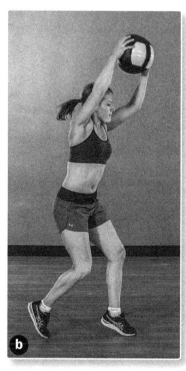 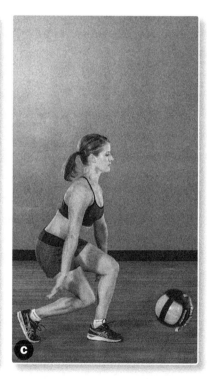

Medicine Ball Bomb Toss to Sprint

Intended Uses

This drill improves total-body power and acceleration.

Prerequisites

- Ability to land properly from a jump (knees aligned with toes, chest up, and shoulders back).
- No previous shoulder injuries.

Steps

- While holding a medicine ball at hip level, assume an athletic stance.
- Perform a vertical jump while explosively throwing the medicine ball overhead and backward (*a*).
- Immediately turn 180 degrees and sprint to the ball (*b*). Then perform another toss in the opposite direction.
- Repeat this drill for four to six repetitions.

Key Points

- Explode upward and throw the ball behind you as far as possible.

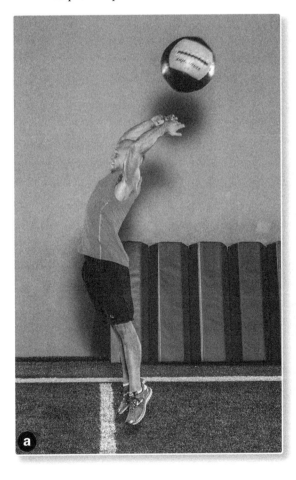
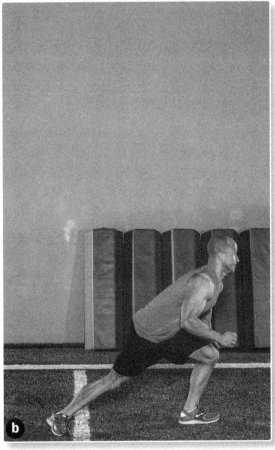

Medicine Ball Off-Centered Plyo Push-Up

Intended Uses

This drill is used primarily to increase upper-body muscular endurance, but it also may enhance shoulder and trunk stability. Additionally, this variation on the push-up increases the load demands on the side that has the hand in contact with the ground.

Prerequisites

- Good shoulder strength and stability.
- No previous shoulder injuries.
- Good trunk stability.

Steps

- Assume a push-up position with one hand on a medicine ball and the other on the ground.
- Perform a push-up (*a*) and then explode upward while shifting the upper body toward the medicine ball and transitioning the hand that was on the ground to the medicine ball and vice versa (*b*).

Key Points

- Most of your weight should be shifted toward the hand on the ground, never the medicine ball.
- Maintain a rigid trunk throughout the duration of the exercise.

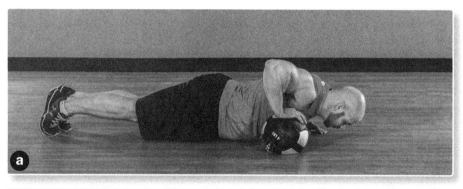

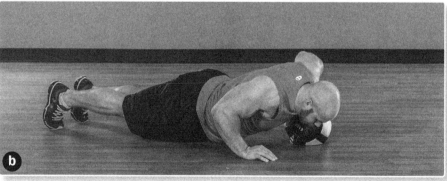

INTRODUCTORY PROGRAM

The program shown in table 5.1 is a four-week program to help you get comfortable with medicine ball exercises. This program also makes a good warm-up for a more advanced athlete. The intent is to train twice a week, circuit style, for four weeks. Perform the exercises in the order listed. Each exercise should be performed for 30 seconds with as little rest as possible. After the circuit has been completed, it can be repeated as many times as desired.

Table 5.1 Four-Week Introductory Medicine Ball Circuit Training Program

Day 1	Day 2
Circuit: 　Medicine ball chop, p. 53 　Medicine ball thruster, p. 55 　Medicine ball touch and jump, p. 58 　Sit-up with medicine ball lift, p. 62 　Medicine ball chest pass, p. 60 　Medicine ball alphabet, p. 54	Circuit: 　Medicine ball slam, p. 59 　Medicine ball Bulgarian squat, p. 56 　Medicine ball touch and jump, p. 58 　Medicine ball modified pike, p. 63 　Medicine ball seated twist, p. 61 　Medicine ball wall ball, p. 57

CHAPTER **6**

Heavy Ropes

Heavy ropes are long, extra-thick ropes that are used for a variety of exercises. Heavy ropes are typically between 50 and 100 feet (15.2 and 30.5 m) long and may be as much as 2 inches (51 mm) in diameter. These tools are used for a number of total-body and core exercises. Every heavy rope exercise has the potential to be rhythmic in nature, which means that heavy ropes are ideal for maximum interval training. These exercises are performed standing up, they use most of the muscles of the body, and they require a great deal of core involvement. All of this combined suggests that heavy ropes have excellent transfer to athletics and real-life situations. In addition, ropes provide a form of dynamic and active resistance that mimics many sport-specific scenarios, such as grappling.

Heavy ropes exercises have some drawbacks that you should be aware of. After a person becomes fit, it is challenging to make heavy ropes exercises more difficult. The ropes are a specific length and weight, so you cannot add weight to the rope when the exercise becomes easier. The only options here are to exercise for a longer duration, rest less, integrate other exercises with the heavy ropes, or use a rope with a larger length or diameter (see table 6.1). These options, while valid, may cause you to train the wrong qualities if you are using this tool for sport performance. Another drawback is that the range of exercises is more limited than it is with other tools. Finally, heavy ropes take up a lot of space. A 50-foot (15.2 m) heavy rope will need 20 to 25 feet (6 to 8 m) of space for most exercises, and space requirements will only increase as the length of the rope increases. Table 6.1 lists size and diameter recommendations by training level.

Table 6.1 Heavy Rope Sizing Options

Training level	Diameter	Length
Beginner	1.25 in. (32 mm)	50–60 ft (15.2–18.3 m)
Beginner–intermediate	1.5 in. (38 mm)	50–60 ft (15.2–18.3 m)
Intermediate	1.5 in. (38 mm)	60 ft (18.3 m)
Advanced	2 in. (51 mm)	50–60 ft (15.2–18.3 m)
Expert	>2 in. (51 mm)	40–60 ft (12.2–18.3 m)

GETTING STARTED

Most heavy rope exercises involve your holding one end of the rope in each hand. This means that the heavy ropes need to be secured to perform most of these exercises. This is normally done by wrapping the rope around a hook or pole or by using something like a heavy kettlebell to secure the rope. Keeping the rope anchored is important; if it is not anchored it tends to move around so much that the exercise becomes ineffective.

Besides anchoring the rope properly, you need to understand the grip types used with heavy rope exercises. These are the one-handed grip, the two-handed grip, and the double grip.

One-Handed Grip

The one-handed grip (figure 6.1) is used for most heavy rope exercises. When an exercise is performed using the one-handed grip, the middle of the rope is anchored. One end of the rope is on your right side and one end is on your left side. You grip one end of the rope with your right hand, palm facing down, and grip the other end your left hand (palm also facing down). Alternatively, you can use an underhand grip. When gripping the rope, your palm should wrap around it.

Two-Handed Grip

The two-handed grip (figure 6.2) is used on exercises that primarily target the core. When using a two-handed grip, the rope should be anchored. Use both hands and hold both ends of the rope together in your hands. Wrap your thumbs around the rope.

Double Grip

This grip is similar to the one-handed grip, but you fold the rope in half to increase the challenge to grip strength (figure 6.3).

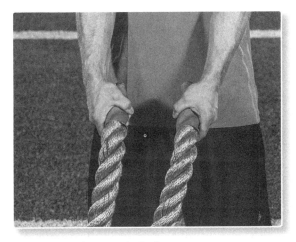

Figure 6.1 One-handed grip.

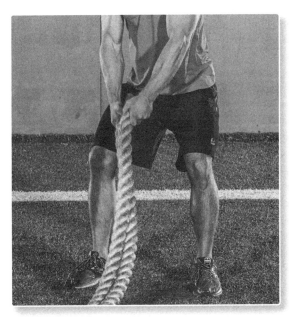

Figure 6.2 Two-handed grip.

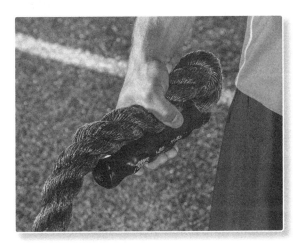

Figure 6.3 Double grip.

FOUNDATIONAL EXERCISES

The foundational exercises for heavy ropes are extremely important. They teach fundamental techniques that you must master before you move on to the advanced exercises. Each of these exercises is appropriate for all levels of development and does an excellent job of conditioning the muscles and energy pathways.

Heavy Ropes Jumping Jacks

Intended Uses

This exercise can be used as a warm-up and conditioning exercise. It is a rhythmic exercise that involves most of the muscles of the body, so it can be performed for a defined number of repetitions or a preset time. It is also a relatively low-skill exercise, so it is conducive to all skill levels.

Prerequisites

- Ability to perform jumping jacks without heavy ropes.
- Understanding how to use the one-handed grip on the heavy ropes.

Steps

- Secure the heavy rope and take a one-handed grip on each end of the rope.
- Stand so that you are holding the ends of the rope at the sides (a).
- Set the back.
- Keep the weight on the balls of the feet.
- Jump so that the feet move out to the sides, about hip-width apart.
- As you move the feet to the sides, raise the hands (and rope) to the sides so that they end up higher than the shoulders (b).
- Lower and repeat for the desired time.

Key Points

- Keep the back set throughout the exercise.
- Keep your weight on the balls of your feet throughout.
- Keep the rope at the sides. Allowing the handles to drift too far forward may cause you to lose balance.

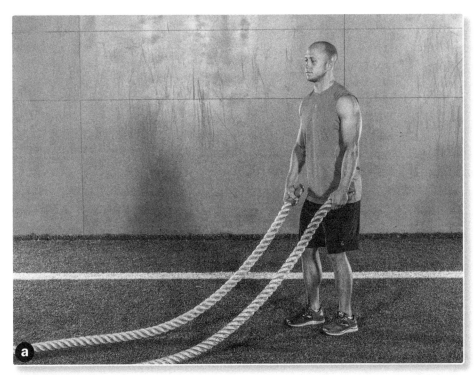

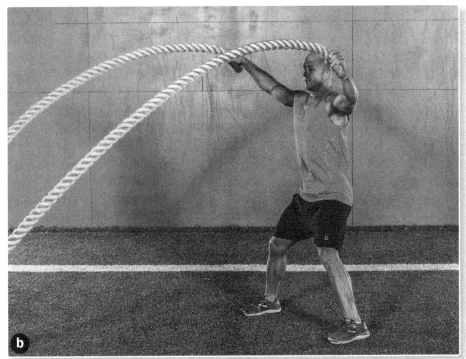

Heavy Ropes Two-Handed Slam

Intended Uses

This exercise is probably one of the most used foundational exercise for heavy ropes. It can be used as a warm-up exercise. It is rhythmic in nature and involves most of the muscles of the body, so it makes a great conditioning exercise. It also involves the muscles of the core.

Prerequisites

- Ability to perform squats.
- Sufficient strength to lift the rope with straight arms.
- Understanding how to use the one-handed grip on the heavy ropes.

Steps

- Secure the heavy rope and take a one-handed grip on each end of the rope.
- Stand so that you are holding the ends of the rope at the sides.
- Set the back.
- Keep the weight on the heels.
- Pushing the hips back, quickly move into a quarter squat.
- Reverse directions and stand up. As you are doing this, move the arms and ropes up until the arms are about parallel to the floor (*a*).
- Without pausing at the top, squat back down, driving the ropes toward the ground (*b*).
- Repeat for the desired time.

Key Points

- Keep the back set throughout the exercise.
- Keep your weight on your heels throughout.
- The squats should be fast and continuous when you are performing the exercise.

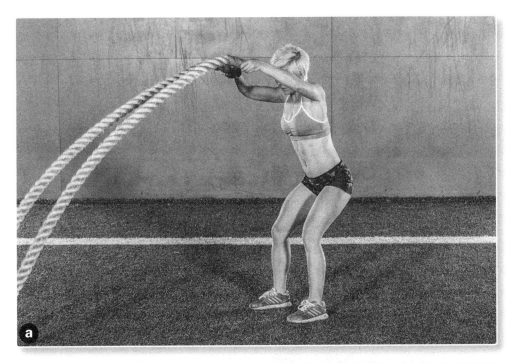

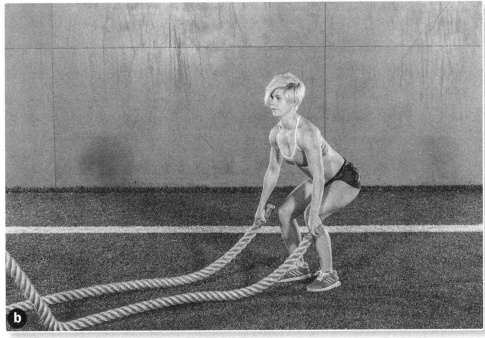

Heavy Ropes Wave

Intended Uses

This rhythmic exercise can be used in a conditioning program. It works the muscles of the shoulders, chest, and upper back. It also requires the lower body and core to stabilize the body during the performance of the exercise.

Prerequisites

- Ability to maintain a quarter squat during the performance of the exercise.
- Sufficient strength to lift the rope with straight arms.
- Understanding how to use the one-handed grip on the heavy ropes.

Steps

- Secure the heavy rope and take a one-handed grip on each end of the rope.
- Stand so that you are holding the ends of the rope at the sides.
- Set the back.
- Keep the weight on the heels.
- Pushing the hips back, move into a quarter squat.
- While maintaining the quarter squat, lift the arms and ropes up until the arms are parallel to the floor.
- Maintaining the squat, lift one arm up and drive the other arm down toward the floor (*a*). Reverse directions (*b*).
- Continue alternating for the desired time.

Key Points

- Keep the back set throughout the exercise.
- Keep your weight on your heels throughout.

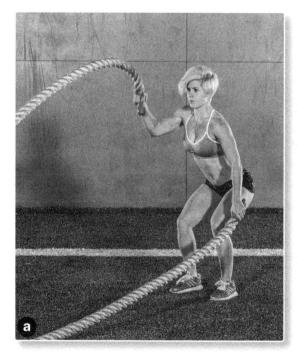 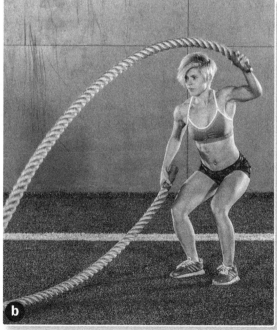

Heavy Ropes Woodchopper

Intended Uses

This exercise primarily trains the muscles of the core. It is rhythmical in nature, so it is appropriate for conditioning. Like the other heavy ropes exercises, it is performed standing up and involves the coordinated movement of both the upper body and the lower body.

Prerequisites

- Ability to perform a quarter squat.
- Sufficient strength to lift the rope on straight arms.
- Understanding how to use the two-handed grip on the heavy ropes.

Steps

- Secure the heavy rope and take a two-handed grip on the rope.
- Stand so that you are holding the ends of the rope at waist level.
- Set the back.
- Keep the weight on the heels.
- Pushing the hips back, quickly move into a quarter squat.
- Reverse directions and stand up quickly. As you are doing this, lift the arms and rope above your head.
- Without pausing at the top, reverse directions and squat back down. As you are squatting, drive the rope into the ground in front of you.
- Reverse directions and repeat for the desired time.

Key Points

- Keep the back set throughout the exercise.
- Keep your weight on your heels throughout.
- Perform the squats quickly and rhythmically for the desired time.

Heavy Ropes Twist

Intended Uses

This exercise is primarily meant to train the muscles of the core, especially the obliques. The exercise is rhythmical in nature, so it is appropriate for conditioning. It is performed standing up and involves stabilization of the lower body.

Prerequisites

- Ability to perform a quarter squat.
- Sufficient strength to lift the rope with straight arms.
- Understanding how to use the two-handed grip on the heavy ropes.

Steps

- Secure the heavy rope and take a two-handed grip on the rope.
- Stand so that you are holding the ends of the rope at waist level.
- Set the back.
- Keep the weight on the heels.
- Pushing the hips back, move into a quarter squat.
- From this position, lift the arms until they are about parallel to the floor (*a*).
- While keeping the arms up, quickly turn the shoulders to the left (*b*).
- Without pausing, turn the shoulders to the right.
- Continue repeating for the desired time.

Key Points

- Keep the back set throughout the exercise.
- Keep your weight on your heels throughout.

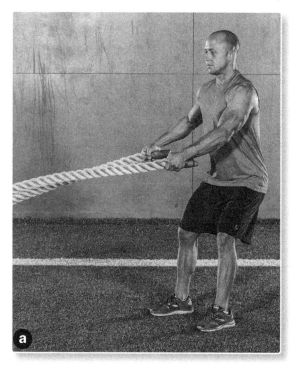 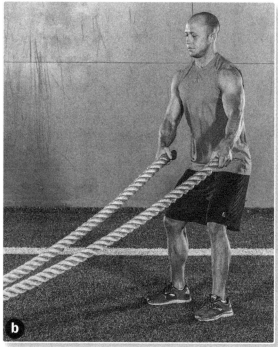

Heavy Ropes Clockwise Arm Circle

Intended Uses

This exercise focuses primarily on the shoulders, upper back, and chest muscles. It is rhythmic in nature, so it is appropriate for conditioning. In addition, performing the exercise requires you to use your core and lower body in a stabilizing role.

Prerequisites

- Ability to perform a quarter squat.
- Sufficient strength to lift the rope on straight arms.
- Understanding how to use the one-handed grip on the heavy ropes.

Steps

- Secure the heavy rope and take a one-handed grip on the rope.
- Stand so that you are holding the ends of the rope at the sides.
- Set the back.
- Keep the weight on the heels.
- Pushing the hips back, move into a quarter squat.
- From this position, lift the arms out to the sides until they are parallel to the floor (*a*).
- While keeping the arms parallel to the floor, make large clockwise circles with the arms for the desired time (*b*).

Key Points

- Keep the back set throughout the exercise.
- Keep your weight on your heels throughout.
- Keep the arms parallel to the floor.

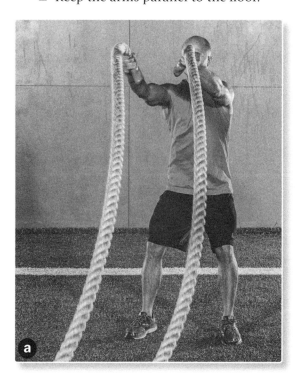
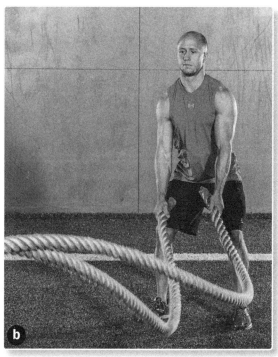

Heavy Ropes Counterclockwise Arm Circle

Intended Uses

This exercise focuses primarily on the shoulders, upper back, and chest muscles. It is rhythmic in nature, so it is appropriate for conditioning. In addition, performing the exercise requires you to use your core and lower body in a stabilizing role.

Prerequisites

- Ability to perform a quarter squat.
- Sufficient strength to lift the rope on straight arms.
- Understanding how to use the one-handed grip on the heavy ropes.

Steps

- Secure the heavy rope and take a one-handed grip on the rope.
- Stand so that you are holding the ends of the rope at the sides.
- Set the back.
- Keep the weight on the heels.
- Pushing the hips back, move into a quarter squat.
- From this position, lift the arms out to the sides until they are parallel to the floor.
- While keeping the arms parallel to the floor, make large counterclockwise circles with the arms for the desired time (a-b).

Key Points

- Keep the back set throughout the exercise.
- Keep your weight on your heels throughout.
- Keep the arms parallel to the floor.

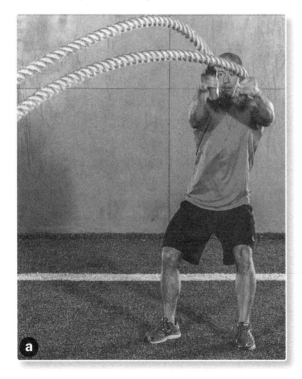 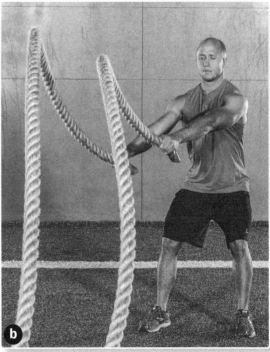

Heavy Ropes Towing

Intended Uses

Towing is an exercise that you can do for distance. It is appropriate for a conditioning workout and for a workout aimed at increasing strength. It challenges the muscles of the lower body and requires the core to stabilize the trunk.

Prerequisites

- Ability to perform a quarter squat.
- Sufficient strength to lift the rope over the shoulder.
- Understanding how to use the two-handed grip on the heavy ropes.

Steps

- Secure one end of the rope around the object that is to be towed.
- Face away from the object.
- Sling one end of the rope over each shoulder and grip the ends.
- Set your back.
- Move into a quarter squat and lean forward.
- Walk forward, dragging the object behind you, for the desired distance (a-b).

Key Points

- Keep the back set throughout the exercise.

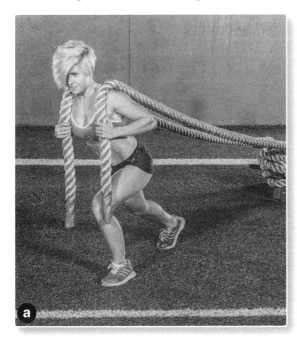
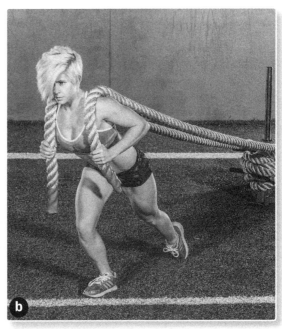

Heavy Ropes Pulling

Intended Uses

Pulling is another exercise that can be done for distance. It is appropriate for a conditioning workout and for a workout aimed at increasing strength. It focuses on the muscles of the shoulders, upper back, and biceps and requires the core to stabilize the trunk.

Prerequisites

- Sufficient strength to lift the rope.

Steps

- Secure one end of the heavy rope to the object that is to be pulled.
- Sit down an appropriate distance away from the object.
- Sit up tall and set the back.
- Grip the end of the rope closer to you with an overhand grip.
- Pull the object toward you with the right hand (*a*).
- Pull the object toward you with the left hand.
- Continue alternating hands until the object has traveled the desired distance (*b*).

Key Points

- For this exercise, wearing gloves might be a good idea to keep the hands from blistering.
- Sit up tall and keep the back set.
- Avoid swinging the upper body to help pull the object toward you.

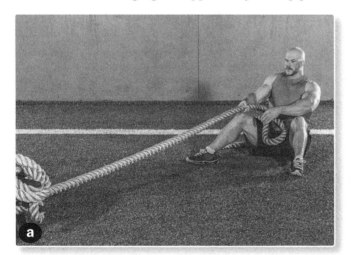
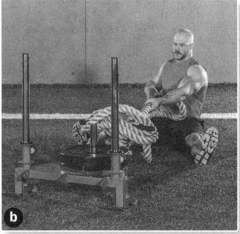

Heavy Ropes Tug of War

Intended Uses

This total-body exercise develops strength, endurance, and trunk and lower-body stabilization. In addition, it is fun and introduces some competition into training.

Prerequisites

- A partner of similar size to yourself.
- Ability to move into a quarter squat.
- Ability to hold the rope.

Steps

- Stretch the heavy rope out on the ground.
- Partners stand at opposite ends of the rope, facing each other.
- Grasp the rope with a two-handed grip and stand up.
- On command, attempt to back up or pull the rope toward you. The idea is to move the other person forward without being moved yourself.

Key Points

- For this exercise, wearing gloves might be a good idea to keep the hands from blistering.

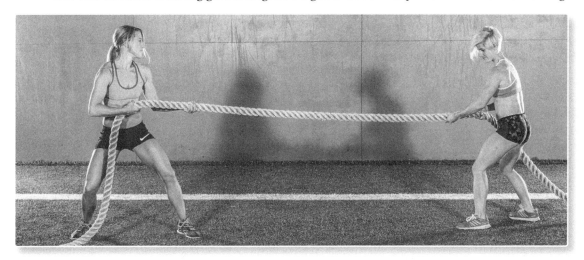

ADVANCED EXERCISES

The advanced exercises described in this chapter build on the foundational exercise techniques. Many of them also require a fitness base. You should master the prerequisites before attempting the advanced exercises; failure to do so may render the exercises harmful or ineffective.

Heavy Ropes One-Handed Slam

Intended Uses

The one-handed slam requires you to squat and stand up, just as you did for the two-handed slam. The exercise requires the muscles of the core to stabilize the trunk. The difference is that only one arm is working at a time. For that reason, the exercise develops a little more coordination than the two-handed variation and is a little more fatiguing. This is a good conditioning exercise because it is rhythmic in nature.

Prerequisites

- Consistent, good technique on the two-handed slam exercise.
- Performance of two-handed slams for a minimum of three months.

Steps

- Secure the heavy rope and take a one-handed grip on each end of the rope.
- Stand so that you are holding the ends of the rope at the sides.
- Set the back.
- Keep the weight on the heels.
- Pushing the hips back, quickly move into a quarter squat (*a*).
- Reverse directions and stand up. As you are doing this, move the right arm and rope up until the arm is parallel to the floor or above the shoulder (*b*).
- Without pausing at the top, squat back down and drive the rope toward the ground.
- Repeat with the left arm.
- Continue alternating between arms for the desired time.

Key Points

- Keep the back set throughout the exercise.
- Keep your weight on your heels throughout.
- The squats should be fast and continuous when you are performing the exercise.

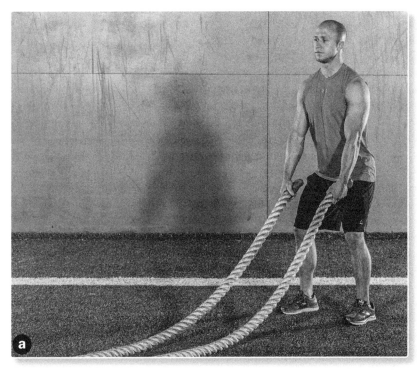

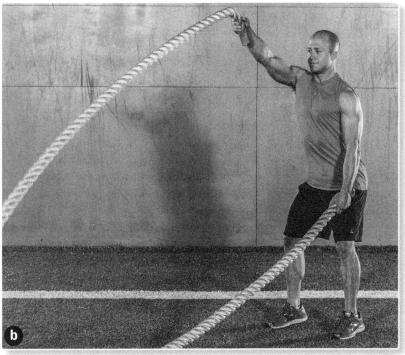

Heavy Ropes Backpedal Slam

Intended Uses

This exercise adds a layer of complexity and variety to the two-handed slam exercise, requiring more coordination. This total-body exercise is appropriate for a conditioning workout.

Prerequisites

- Consistent, good technique on the two-handed slam exercise.
- Performance of two-handed slams for a minimum of three months.
- Sufficient agility to perform a backpedal.

Steps

- Secure the heavy rope and take a one-handed grip on each end of the rope.
- Stand so that you are holding the ends of the rope at the sides.
- Stand close to where the rope is secured so that you have room to move backward.
- Set the back.
- Pushing the hips back, quickly move into a quarter squat.
- Keeping both arms straight, quickly lift your arms and the ropes up until your arms are parallel to the floor (*a*).
- Slam the ropes down toward the ground (*b*).
- As you are lifting and slamming the ropes, perform a backpedal.

Key Points

- Keep the back set throughout the exercise.
- When backpedaling, your weight is on the balls of your feet.
- Maintain the quarter-squat position for balance.

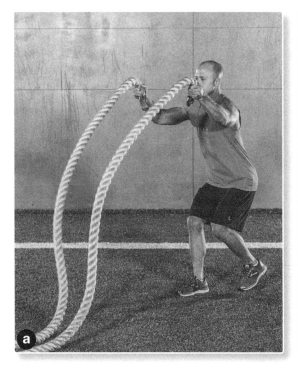 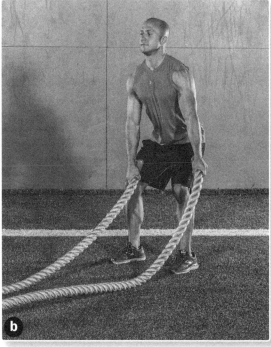

Heavy Ropes Shuffle Slam

Intended Uses

This exercise adds a layer of complexity and variety to the two-handed slam exercise, requiring more coordination. Besides providing the benefits of the slam, this total-body exercise is appropriate for a conditioning workout.

Prerequisites

- Consistent, good technique on the two-handed slam exercise.
- Performance of two-handed slams for a minimum of three months.
- Sufficient agility to perform a backpedal.

Steps

- Secure the heavy rope and take a one-handed grip on each end of the rope.
- Stand so that you are holding the ends of the rope at the sides.
- Stand close to where the rope is secure so that you have room to move backward.
- Set the back.
- Pushing the hips back, quickly move into a quarter squat.
- Keeping both arms straight, quickly lift your arms and the ropes up until your arms are parallel to the floor (a).
- Slam the ropes down toward the ground (b).
- As you are lifting and slamming the ropes, perform a shuffle to the right or left.
- Continue shuffling for the desired time, making sure to spend the same amount of time shuffling in each direction.

Key Points

- Keep the back set throughout the exercise.
- With shuffles, your weight is on the balls of your feet.
- Do not cross the feet during shuffling.
- Maintain the quarter-squat position for balance.

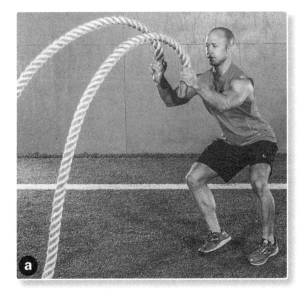
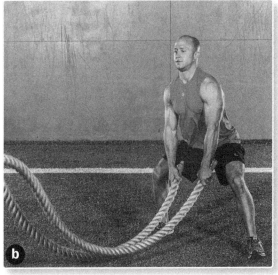

Heavy Ropes One-Legged Slam

Intended Uses

Besides providing the benefits of the slam, this variation requires you to develop balance to perform the exercise. This variation also develops the muscles of the ankle, foot, and shin, which will have to work hard to keep you standing. With practice, this is an appropriate conditioning exercise.

Prerequisites

- Consistent, good technique on the two-handed slam exercise.
- Performance of two-handed slams for a minimum of three months.
- Ability to stand on one foot for at least 60 seconds.

Steps

- Secure the heavy rope and take a one-handed grip on each end of the rope.
- Stand so that you are holding the ends of the rope at the sides.
- Set the back.
- Keep the weight on the heels.
- Lift one foot off the ground and keep it off the ground.
- Pushing the hips back, quickly move into a quarter squat.
- Reverse directions and stand up. As you are doing this, move the arms and ropes up until the arms are parallel to the floor (a).
- Without pausing at the top, squat back down and drive the ropes toward the ground (b).
- Repeat for the desired time and then switch the foot that is off the ground.

Key Points

- Keep the back set throughout the exercise.
- Make sure that you are balanced before attempting to perform the slam.
- Keep your weight on your heel throughout.
- The squats should be fast and continuous when you are performing the exercise.

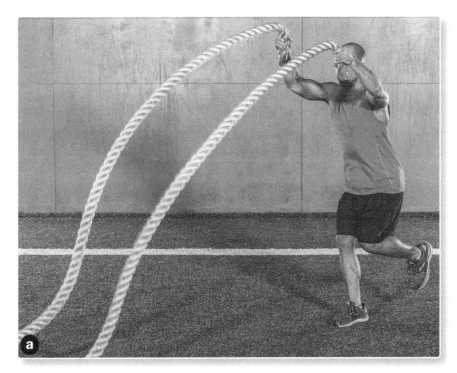

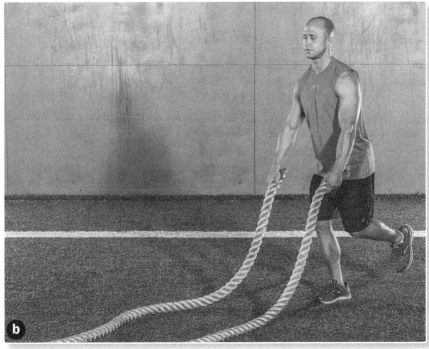

Heavy Ropes Unstable Slam

Intended Uses

Besides providing the normal benefits of the slam, this variation requires you to develop balance to perform the exercise. This variation also develops the muscles of the ankle, foot, and shin, which will have to work hard to keep you standing. With practice, this is an appropriate conditioning exercise.

Prerequisites

- Consistent, good technique on the two-handed slam exercise.
- Performance of two-handed slams for a minimum of three months.
- Ability to perform one-legged slams with consistent, good technique.

Steps

- Secure the heavy rope and take a one-handed grip on each end of the rope.
- Stand so that you are holding the ends of the rope at the sides.
- Set the back.
- Step onto the unstable surface.
- Pushing the hips back, quickly move into a quarter squat.
- Reverse directions and stand up. As you are doing this, move the arms and ropes up until the arms are parallel to the floor (*a*).
- Without pausing at the top, squat back down and drive the ropes toward the ground (*b*).
- Repeat for the desired time and then switch the foot that is on the unstable surface.

Key Points

- Keep the back set throughout the exercise.
- Make sure that you are balanced before attempting to perform the slam.
- Keep your weight on your heel throughout.
- The squats should be fast and continuous when you are performing the exercise.

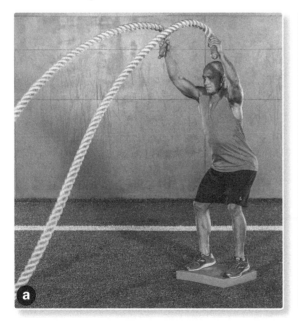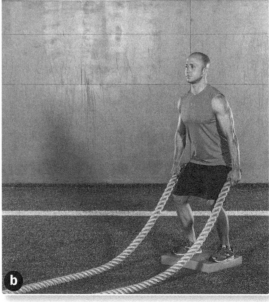

Heavy Ropes One-Handed Wave

Intended Uses

Like the two-handed wave, the one-handed wave requires the muscles of the core to stabilize the trunk. The difference is that only one arm is working at a time. The exercise thus develops more coordination than the two-handed variation does and is a little more fatiguing. This is a good conditioning exercise because it is rhythmic in nature.

Prerequisites

- Consistent, good technique on the two-handed wave exercise.
- Performance of the two-handed wave for a minimum of three months.

Steps

- Secure the heavy rope and take a one-handed grip on each end of the rope.
- Stand so that you are holding the ends of the rope at the sides.
- Set the back.
- Keep the weight on the heels.
- Pushing the hips back, move into a quarter squat.
- While maintaining the quarter squat, lift the right arm and rope up until the arm is parallel to the floor (*a*).
- Maintaining the squat, drive the right arm down toward the floor (*b*). Reverse directions.
- Continue alternating for the desired time and then switch arms.

Key Points

- Keep the back set throughout the exercise.
- Keep your weight on your heels throughout.

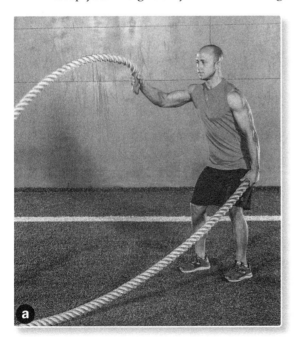
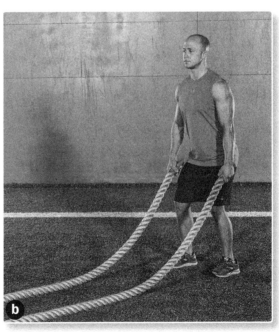

Heavy Ropes One-Legged Wave

Intended Uses

Besides offering the normal benefits of the wave, this variation requires you to develop balance to perform the exercise. This variation also develops the muscles of the ankle, foot, and shin, which will have to work hard to keep you standing. With practice, this is an appropriate conditioning exercise.

Prerequisites

- Consistent, good technique on the two-handed wave exercise.
- Performance of the two-handed wave for a minimum of three months.
- Ability to stand on one foot for at least 60 seconds.

Steps

- Secure the heavy rope and take a one-handed grip on each end of the rope.
- Stand so that you are holding the ends of the rope at the sides.
- Set the back.
- Lift one foot off the ground and keep it off the ground.
- Keep the weight on the heel.
- Pushing the hips back, move into a quarter squat.
- While maintaining the quarter squat, lift the arms and ropes up until the arms are parallel to the floor (*a*).
- Maintaining the squat, drive the other arm down toward the floor immediately followed by the other arm (*b*).
- Continue alternating for the desired time and then switch legs.

Key Points

- Keep the back set throughout the exercise.
- Get your balance before performing the wave.
- Keep your weight on your heel throughout.

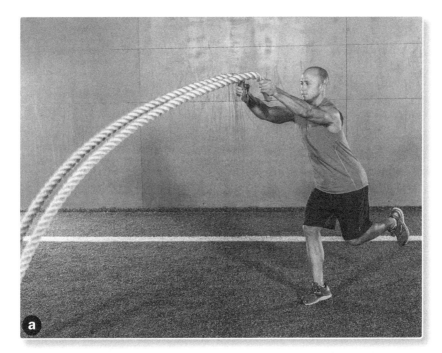

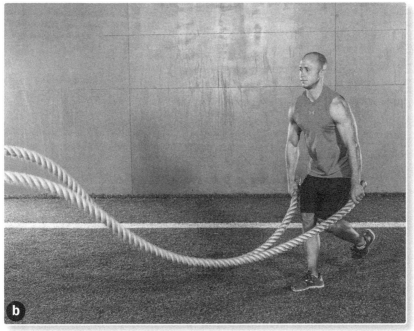

Heavy Ropes Unstable Wave

Intended Uses

Besides offering the normal benefits of the wave, this variation requires you to develop balance to perform the exercise. This variation also develops the muscles of the ankle, foot, and shin, which will have to work hard to keep you standing. With practice, this is an appropriate conditioning exercise.

Prerequisites

- Have consistent, good technique on the two-handed wave exercise.
- Performance of the two-handed wave for a minimum of three months.
- Ability to perform the one-legged wave with consistent, good technique.

Steps

- Secure the heavy rope and take a one-handed grip on each end of the rope.
- Stand so that you are holding the ends of the rope at the sides.
- Set the back.
- Step onto the unstable surface.
- Pushing the hips back, move into a quarter squat.
- While maintaining the quarter squat, lift the arms and ropes up until the arms are parallel to the floor.
- Maintaining the squat, lift one arm up and drive the other arm down toward the floor. Reverse directions (a-b).
- Continue alternating for the desired time and then switch legs.

Key Points

- Keep the back set throughout the exercise.
- Get your balance before performing the wave.
- Keep your weight on your heel throughout.

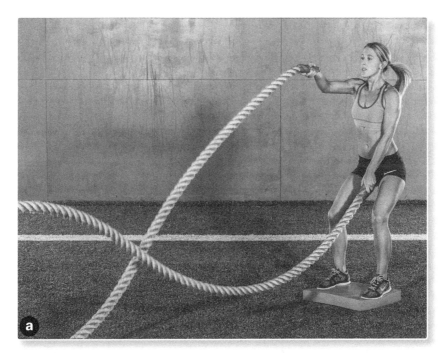

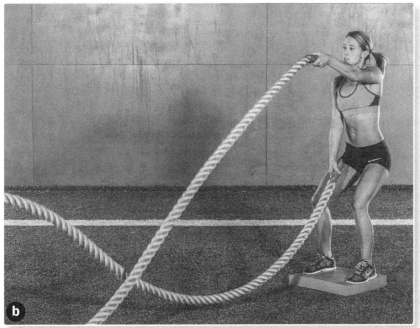

Heavy Ropes Oblique Woodchopper

Intended Uses

Woodchoppers are primarily meant to train the muscles of the core. This exercise is rhythmical in nature, so it is appropriate for conditioning. Like the other heavy ropes exercises, it is performed standing up and involves the coordinated movement of both the upper body and the lower body. This variation targets the muscles of the obliques.

Prerequisites

- Consistent, good technique on the woodchopper exercise.
- Performance of woodchoppers for a minimum of three months.

Steps

- Secure the heavy rope and take a one-handed grip on the rope.
- Stand so that you are holding the ends of the rope at waist level.
- Set the back.
- Keep the weight on the heels.
- Pushing the hips back, quickly move into a quarter squat.
- Reverse directions and stand up quickly. As you are doing this, lift the arms and rope above your head (*a*).
- Without pausing at the top, reverse directions and squat back down. As you are squatting, drive the rope into the ground on your left side (*b*).
- Stand back up from the quarter squat quickly and lift the rope overhead, reverse directions, and drive the rope into the ground on your right side.
- Continue alternating for the desired time.

Key Points

- Keep the back set throughout the exercise.
- Keep your weight on your heels throughout.
- Perform the squats quickly and rhythmically for the desired time.

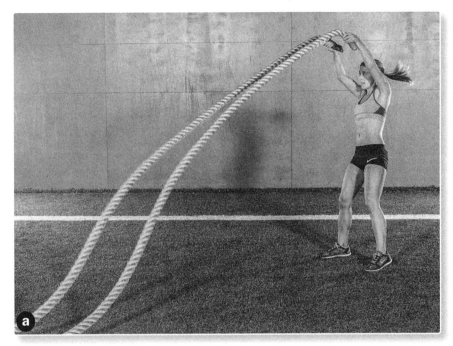

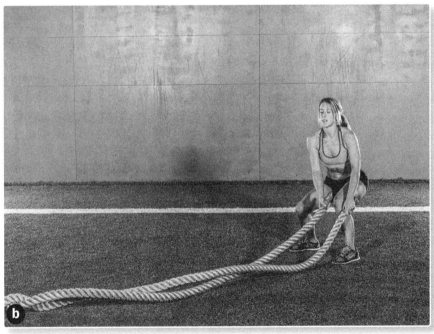

Heavy Ropes One-Legged Woodchopper

Intended Uses

This advanced version of the woodchopper trains the muscles of the core, but its one-legged nature requires the development of balance. It also trains the muscles of the ankle, foot, and shin to support the body while standing on one leg.

Prerequisites

- Consistent, good technique on the woodchopper exercise.
- Performance of woodchoppers for a minimum of three months.
- Ability to stand on one foot for a minimum of 60 seconds.

Steps

- Secure the heavy rope and take a one-handed grip on the rope.
- Stand so that you are holding the ends of the rope at waist level.
- Set the back.
- Stand on one foot.
- Keep the weight on the heel.
- Pushing the hips back, quickly move into a quarter squat.
- Reverse directions and stand up quickly. As you are doing this, lift the arms and rope above your head (a).
- Without pausing at the top, reverse directions and squat back down. As you are squatting, drive the rope into the ground in front of you (b).
- Reverse directions and repeat for the desired time. Then switch legs.

Key Points

- Keep the back set throughout the exercise.
- Get your balance before performing the woodchoppers.
- Keep your weight on your heels throughout.
- Perform the squats quickly and rhythmically for the desired time.

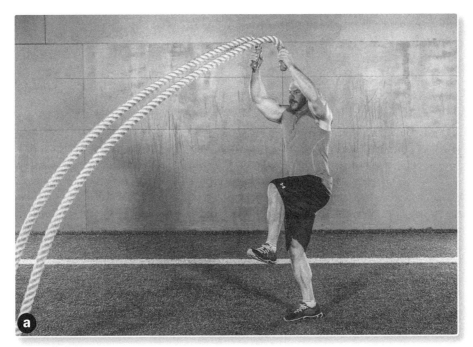

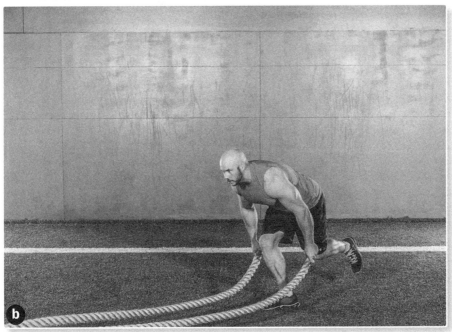

INTRODUCTORY PROGRAM

The introductory program will familiarize you with heavy rope exercises if you have never done them before. It will teach the fundamental movement skills and develop a conditioning foundation that can be applied to more advanced exercises and workouts in the future. This program should be performed two times per week. Because it is a circuit program, each exercise is performed for a set period. After you complete one exercise, you perform the next immediately, without rest. Table 6.2 outlines the program. In this example, you perform the exercises for 30 seconds each. After you have performed all the exercises, rest for 2 minutes and perform the circuit again.

Table 6.2 Introductory Heavy Ropes Training Program

Day 1	Day 2
Circuit:	Circuit:
Heavy ropes two-handed slam, p. 78	Heavy ropes wave, p. 80
Heavy ropes clockwise arm circle, p. 83	Heavy ropes woodchopper, p. 81
Heavy ropes wave, p. 80	Heavy ropes jumping jacks, p. 76
Heavy ropes counterclockwise arm circle, p. 84	Heavy ropes clockwise arm circle, p. 83
Heavy ropes jumping jacks, p. 76	Heavy ropes twist, p. 82
Heavy ropes woodchopper, p. 81	Heavy ropes counterclockwise arm circle, p. 84
Heavy ropes twist, p. 82	Heavy ropes two-handed slam, p. 78

CHAPTER 7

Suspension Training

The use of the suspension trainer has exploded in the fitness industry over the last 10 years. For the most part, suspension-training exercises are variations of bodyweight exercises (bodyweight push-up, squat, lunge, and so forth) with part of the body suspended in the air by the trainer. The suspension trainer is not fixed; all of its parts move in space while the exercise is being performed. For that reason, you must recruit more muscles to perform the movement and stabilize yourself. Using a suspension trainer increases the involvement of the muscles of the core, shoulders, and glutes to perform this stabilizing movement. A tremendous variety of exercises can be performed with the suspension trainer, which helps to keep workouts interesting. The suspension trainer is easily portable, so it's ideal for workouts for those who are on vacation or deployed to remote areas.

Suspension training does have drawbacks. First, these exercises are difficult to learn. They require so much balance and stabilization that even simple exercises like a push-up take time to master. Second, because all the parts of the suspension trainer move in space, safety is a concern. For example, if you are performing a push-up and your hands are in the trainer, allowing one of the hands to move suddenly could be a recipe for a shoulder injury. Third, suspension-training units tend to be expensive, costing upward of $200 each. Finally, suspension training has built-in overload challenges. After you have finished learning and have developed your fitness base, making the exercises more challenging is difficult. You can always perform the exercises for longer periods, but in the case of athletics, you may be training the wrong energy systems and qualities. Because of that, suspension training is frequently integrated with other modes of exercise for an advanced person's program (see table 7.1).

Table 7.1 Sample of Suspension Training Integrated With Other Forms of Training

Kettlebell two-handed swing (30 sec), p. 135	Kettlebell two-handed swing (30 sec), p. 135
Heavy ropes two-handed slam (30 sec), p. 78	Heavy ropes two-handed slam (30 sec), p. 78
Suspension row (30 sec), p. 112	Suspension squat (30 sec), p. 115
Kettlebell two-handed swing (30 sec), p. 135	Kettlebell two-handed swing (30 sec), p. 135
Heavy ropes two-handed slam (30 sec), p. 78	Heavy ropes two-handed slam (30 sec), p. 78
Suspension chest press (30 sec), p. 111	Suspension reverse lunge (30 sec), p. 116

GETTING STARTED

Suspension training involves a little more in terms of setup, adjustment, and basic positions than the other exercise modes covered in this book. Recognizing this requirement helps ensure a safe, successful experience. With that in mind, this part of the chapter covers how to secure and adjust the suspension trainer, the basic grips that are used, and the basic positions used in the exercises.

Securing and Adjusting

The suspension trainer needs to be secured to an object. The object that it is secured to should be able to handle your body's weight without moving or breaking. For example, a tree limb may be tall enough, but if the limb isn't big enough it will break when you try to perform a chest press or push-up. A pull-up bar or a set of monkey bars is ideal for securing a suspension trainer, but a door or small tree limb is not because it may not be able to handle the weight of your body.

Suspension trainers generally have a strap with some sort of carabiner. The carabiner is on one end of the strap, and the rest of the suspension trainer is attached to the other end. The carabiner and strap are looped around the object that the trainer is to be attached to, and the carabiner is then attached to the strap (figure 7.1).

If you want the suspension trainer to be farther off the ground, the strap can be looped around the object it is being attached to multiple times to draw up the suspension trainer. If you want the suspension trainer to be closer to the ground, the strap can be looped around the object that it is being attached to fewer times, which will result in the trainer being lower to the ground. Some exercises should have the trainer higher, some are better if the trainer is lower, and several are best when the trainer is in between. The positioning depends on the exercise and the desired difficulty level.

The handles on most suspension trainers also adjust up or down. Generally, this is done with a buckle that unlocks the strap attached to the handle. After the buckle is released, the handle can be adjusted upward or downward (figure 7.2). This mechanism provides another way to make the trainer closer to the ground or farther from it.

Grips

Four basic grip types are used for suspension trainer exercises. For each grip, the thumb and fingers should be wrapped around the handles. The first grip type is the prone grip, sometimes referred to as an overhand grip (figure 7.3). For the prone grip, the palm faces away from the body or down. So a push-up or a chest press is an example of a prone grip. The second grip type is the supine grip, sometimes called an underhand grip (figure 7.4). For the supine grip, the palms face up or toward the body. An example of this is a biceps curl. The third grip type is the neutral grip (figure 7.5), in which the palms face in toward the body (and toward each other).

The fourth grip type is used for one-handed exercises. A one-handed exercise may use a supine, prone, or neutral grip. The big difference here is that the suspension trainer has to be set up to perform a one-handed exercise. To perform a one-handed exercise, one of the handles is drawn through the other handle (see figure 7.6). After the handle is drawn through, it is used to perform the exercises.

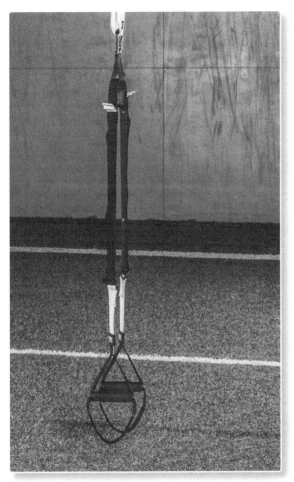

Figure 7.1 Suspension trainer with strap and carabiner.

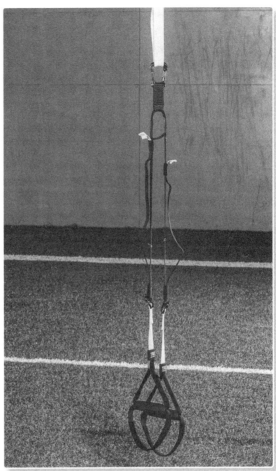

Figure 7.2 Suspension trainer with adjustable handle.

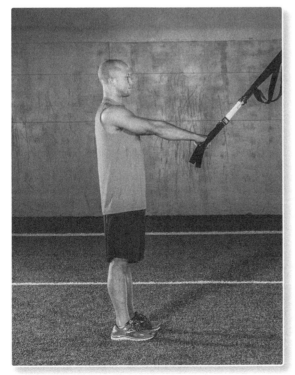

Figure 7.3 Prone grip (overhand).

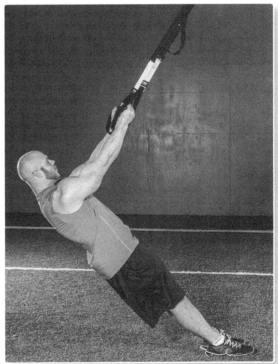

Figure 7.4 Supine grip (underhand).

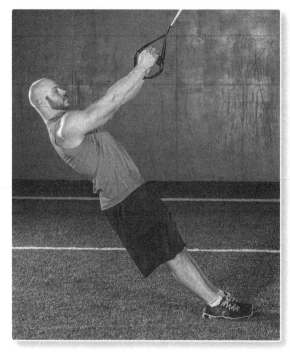

Figure 7.5 Neutral grip (palms toward body).

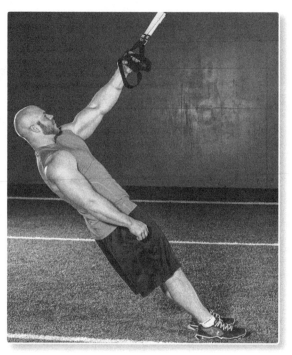

Figure 7.6 One-handed grip (one handle is drawn through the other).

Positions

This book shows five basic body positions for suspension-training exercises. A huge number of exercises and variations are possible using these five positions. The five are supine standing position, supine lying position, prone standing position, prone lying position, and standing position.

Supine Standing Position

This position is used for upper back, shoulder, and biceps exercises. For the supine standing position, the handles are adjusted so that they are at shoulder height (figure 7.7). Any grip may be used for exercises performed from this position. If you are a beginner, place your feet close together and under the handles. Grip the handles. Keeping your feet in place, lean backward until your arms are fully extended. If you do this properly, your body should be straight from your ankles all the way to your shoulders.

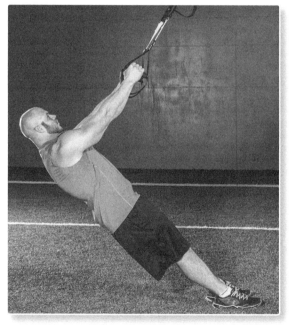

Figure 7.7 Supine standing position.

As you become skilled with these exercises, an easy way to make them more difficult is to change the placement of your feet. You can make supine standing exercises more difficult by moving your feet forward so that part of your body, rather than your feet, is directly under the handles. Moving your feet forward puts you closer to the ground. If you move your feet forward far enough, you will need to adjust the handles so that they hang lower than shoulder height. Even in these positions, you should maintain good posture for the exercises (i.e., maintain a straight line from the ankles to the shoulders).

Supine Lying Position

This position is used in hamstring and core exercises. For the supine lying position, adjust the handles so that they are off the ground. Generally, they will not be higher than knee height (figure 7.8). Next, lie on the ground on your back. Depending on the exercise, you may reach up and grab the handles (so that your shoulders are positioned below the handles) or you may place your feet in the handles.

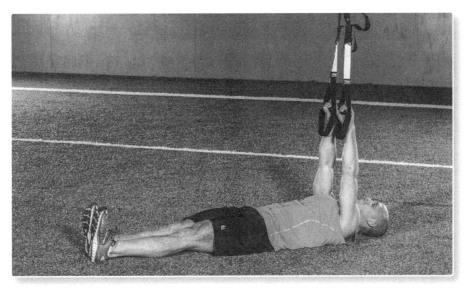

Figure 7.8 Supine lying position.

Prone Standing Position

This position is used in chest and triceps exercises. Adjust the handles so that they are at shoulder height. Depending on the exercise, the prone or neutral grips are most commonly used in conjunction with this position. Grip the handles. Begin with your feet positioned under the handles. Keeping the feet in place, extend your arms and lean forward. Remember that a straight line should run from your ankles to your shoulders (figure 7.9).

To make exercises using this position more difficult, move the feet backward so that they begin farther from the handles. This position forces you to lean forward more, requiring you to support more of your body weight. Even in these advanced positions, you should maintain good posture for the exercises.

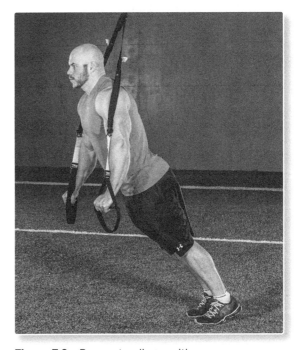

Figure 7.9 Prone standing position.

Prone Lying Position

This variation is used for push-ups, advanced shoulder exercises, and core exercises. For this variation, the handles are adjusted so that they are hanging just above the ground. You assume the push-up position for this exercise, keeping a straight line from your heels to your shoulders (figure 7.10). Depending on the exercise to be performed, either your hands will grip the handles (for a push-up) or you will place your feet in the handles (for a core exercise).

Standing Position

A number of lower-body exercises are performed from a standing position. Adjust the handles so that they are at chest height or shoulder height. Grip the handles and step back until the trainer is tight (figure 7.11). From this position, perform the desired exercise.

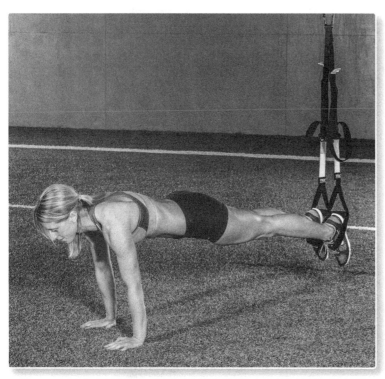

Figure 7.10 Prone lying position.

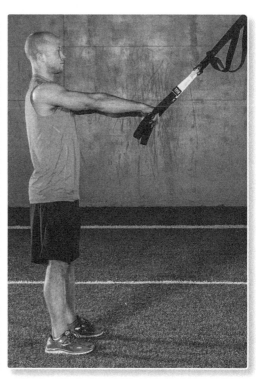

Figure 7.11 Standing position.

FOUNDATIONAL EXERCISES

Every exercise listed in this section should be a mainstay of a maximum interval-training program using the suspension trainer, regardless of your fitness level and experience. Besides their value in enhancing fitness, these exercises have a number of purposes. First, they teach positions, grips, and fundamental movement patterns. Second, they develop your balance and knowledge of your body in space. Finally, they develop many of the stabilizing muscles that support exercise with suspension trainers.

Suspension Chest Press

Intended Uses

The chest press develops the muscles of the chest, shoulders, and triceps. The core helps to stabilize the body during this exercise, so it is trained as well. This exercise is rhythmic in nature and can be used for conditioning.

Prerequisites

- Ability to adjust the straps to the appropriate position.
- Ability to perform exercise from the prone standing position.

Steps

- Grip the handles with a prone grip.
- Assume the prone standing position (*a*).
- From that position, lower yourself toward the handles by flexing your elbows and allowing the handles to move away from each other (*b*).
- From the bottom position, reverse direction until your arms are extended.
- Repeat for the desired number of repetitions.

Key Points

- Maintain a straight line from the heels to the shoulders during this exercise.
- The handles begin the exercise close together, and they move apart as you lower the body toward them.
- During this exercise, you lower the body toward the handles and then push it away from them.

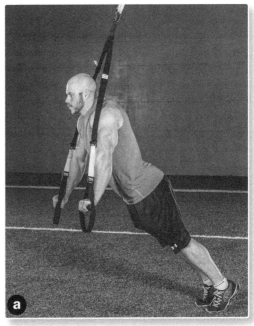

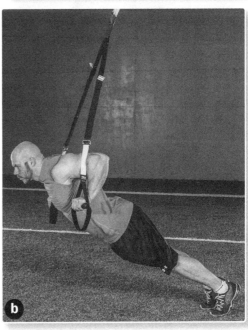

Suspension Row

Intended Uses

This exercise develops the muscles of the upper back, shoulders, and biceps. The core helps to stabilize the body during this exercise, so it is trained as well. This exercise is rhythmic in nature and can be used for conditioning.

Prerequisites

- Ability to adjust the straps to the appropriate position.
- Ability to perform the exercise from the supine standing position.

Steps

- Grasp the handles. Any grip type can be used with the row.
- Assume the supine standing position (*a*).
- From the starting position, pull the body toward the handles (*b*).
- Reverse direction and repeat for the desired number of repetitions.

Key Points

- Maintain a straight line from the heels to the shoulders during this exercise.
- Keep the elbows against the body while pulling the body toward the handles.
- When pulling, focus on bringing the shoulder blades together. When lowering, focus on allowing the shoulder blades to spread apart.

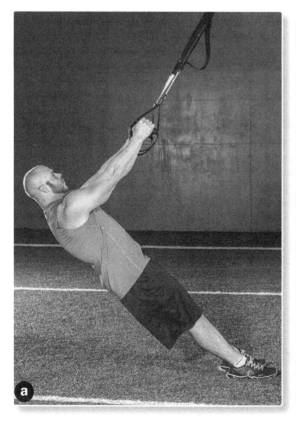
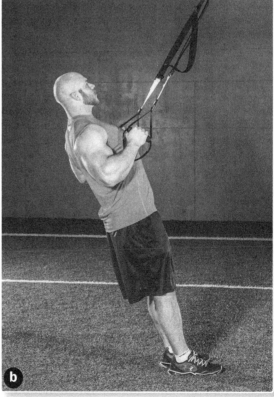

Suspension Biceps Curl

Intended Uses

This exercise develops the biceps muscles. The core must stabilize the body throughout, so the exercise has some benefit to this region as well. It is a rhythmic exercise and lends itself to conditioning.

Prerequisites

- Ability to adjust the straps to the appropriate position.
- Ability to perform the exercise from the supine standing position.

Steps

- Grip the handles with a supine grip.
- Assume the supine standing position.
- Begin the exercise with the feet under the handles and the arms fully extended (*a*).
- Without moving your feet, flex your elbows and pull your body toward the handles (*b*).
- Reverse direction and repeat.

Key Points

- Maintain a straight line from the heels to the shoulders during this exercise.
- Lower the body slowly and under control.

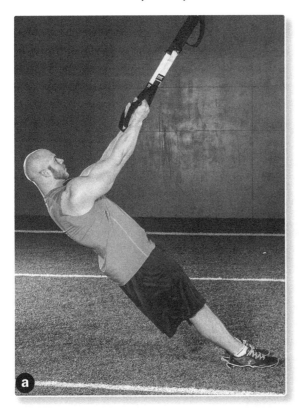

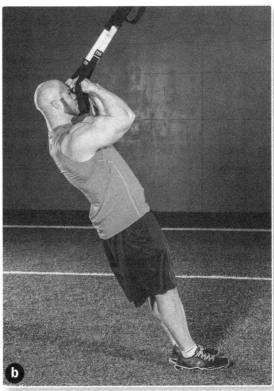

Suspension Triceps Extension

Intended Uses

This exercise develops the triceps muscles. The core must stabilize the body throughout, so the exercise has some benefit to that region as well. It is a rhythmic exercise and lends itself to conditioning.

Prerequisites

- Ability to adjust the straps to the appropriate position.
- Ability to perform the exercise from the prone standing position.

Steps

- Grasp the handles with a prone grip.
- Assume the prone starting position.
- Stand so that your feet are under the handles.
- From that position, extend the arms, pushing the handles out in front of your body (*a*).
- Lean forward until the handles are level with your forehead.
- From that position, flex the elbows and lower your head toward the handles (*b*).
- Keeping the arms locked into position, use the triceps to press the body away from the handles.
- Lower and repeat for the desired number of repetitions.

Key Points

- Maintain a straight line from the heels to the shoulders during this exercise.
- Do not allow the elbows to flare out during this exercise. The elbows should point toward the ground the entire time.

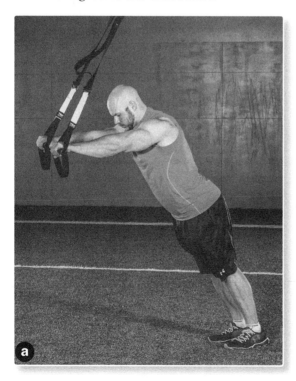 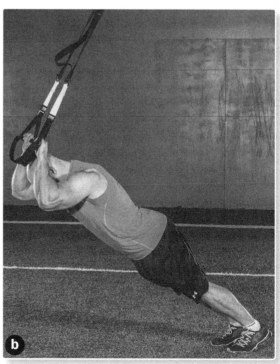

Suspension Squat

Intended Uses

This exercise develops the muscles of the lower body, particularly the quadriceps, hamstrings, and glutes. The exercise requires the core to stability the body. This exercise is also appropriate for a conditioning workout.

Prerequisites

- Ability to assume the standing position.
- Ability to perform a squat exercise while keeping the feet flat on the ground.

Steps

- Grip the handles with a pronated or neutral grip.
- Assume the standing position, with the feet hip-width apart (*a*).
- Set the back.
- Keeping the weight on the heels, push the hips back and flex your knees.
- Squat down until your thighs are parallel to the floor (*b*).
- Reverse direction and repeat for the desired number of repetitions.

Key Points

- Keep your back set throughout the exercise.
- Keep your weight on your heels throughout the exercise.

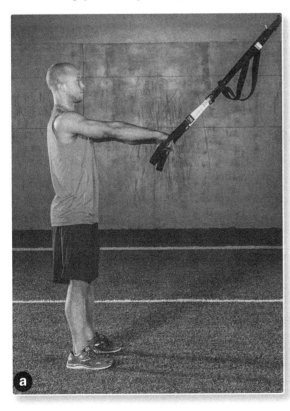 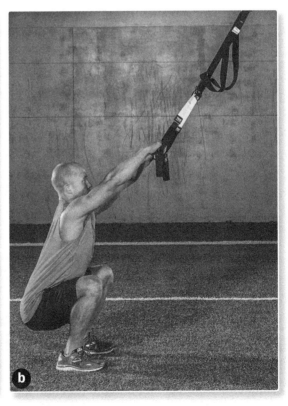

Suspension Reverse Lunge

Intended Uses

This exercise allows you to focus on one leg at a time. It is an excellent exercise for developing the quadriceps, hamstrings, and glutes. In addition, it allows you to work on balance and mobility.

Prerequisites

- Ability to assume the standing position.
- Ability to perform a reverse lunge without a suspension trainer.

Steps

- Grip the handles with a pronated or neutral grip.
- Assume the standing position, with the feet hip-width apart.
- Set the back.
- Take a large step back with your left foot.
- As your left foot steps back, flex your right knee and hip.
- Lower until your right leg is parallel to the floor (a).
- Using your right leg, stand up and step forward with your left foot (b).
- Switch sides.
- Continue alternating legs until you have performed the desired number of repetitions.

Key Points

- During the lunge, the front foot should remain flat on the ground.
- When stepping back, the back knee should not touch the ground.

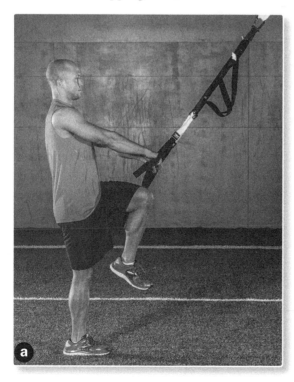 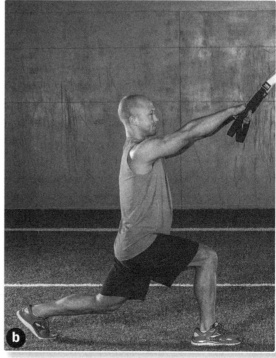

Suspension Hip Up

Intended Uses

The hip up exercise trains the muscles of the core, glutes, and hamstrings.

Prerequisites

- Ability to assume the supine lying position.
- Ability to lift the legs and hold that position.

Steps

- Assume the supine lying position.
- Position yourself so that your feet are under the handles.
- Place the heels in the handles (*a*).
- From this position, lift your hips off the ground (*b*).
- Lower and repeat for the desired number of repetitions.

Key Points

- Keep your legs together while performing this exercise.

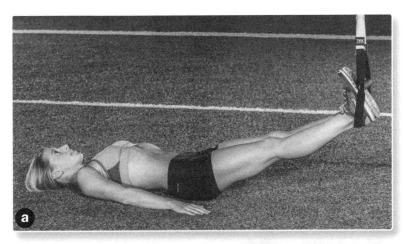

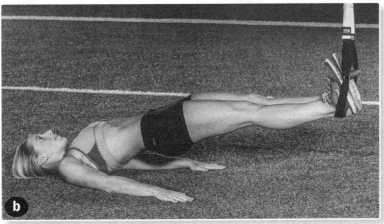

Suspension Leg Curl

Intended Uses

Leg curls with a suspension trainer develop the glutes and hamstrings. Your core muscles will help to get you into position and hold you there, so they will get some benefit as well. Like most suspension-training exercises, this one is great for conditioning workouts.

Prerequisites

■ Ability to assume the supine lying position.

Steps

■ Assume the supine lying position.
■ Place your feet into the handles of the suspension trainer.
■ With your legs straight, lift your hips off the ground (*a*).
■ Keeping your hips off the ground, flex your knees and curl the handles toward your hips (*b*).
■ Reverse direction and repeat for the desired number of repetitions.

Key Points

■ Your hips remain off the ground during the entire exercise.
■ As you curl the handles toward your hips, your hips may lift up higher.

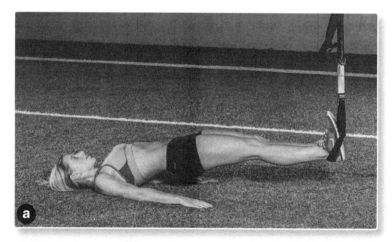

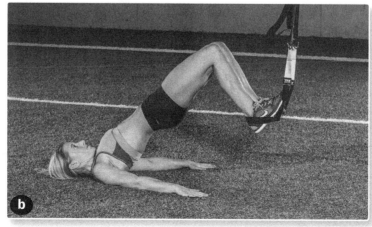

Suspension Knees to Chest

Intended Uses

The knees to chest exercise trains the core muscles and all the abdominal muscles. It primarily uses the upper and lower abdominal muscles to perform the exercise, and the obliques have a stabilizing role. In addition, by forcing you to support yourself using your upper body, those muscles receive some benefit as well.

Prerequisites

- Ability to assume the prone lying position.
- Ability to support yourself using your upper body.

Steps

- Put your feet in the handles.
- Assume the prone lying position (*a*).
- Your arms and legs should be straight.
- While supporting yourself on your arms, bring your knees toward your chest (*b*).
- Reverse direction and repeat for the desired number of repetitions.

Key Points

- As you bring your knees toward your chest, your hips will lift up.

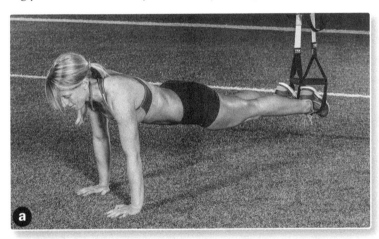

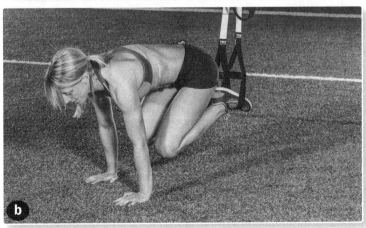

Suspension Lying Leg Raise

Intended Uses

The lying leg raise is another core exercise. This one also uses the upper and lower abdominal muscles to perform the exercise. The obliques have a stabilizing role.

Prerequisites

- Ability to assume the supine lying position.

Steps

- Assume the supine lying position.
- Position yourself so that your eyes are under the handles.
- Reach up and grasp the straps (*a*).
- Keeping your legs straight and together, lift them up a few inches (about 10 cm) off the ground (*b*).
- Lower and repeat for the desired number of repetitions.

Key Points

- Keep the legs straight and together throughout the exercise.

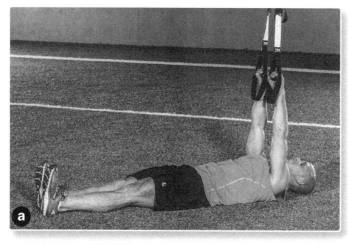

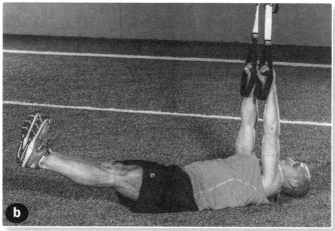

ADVANCED EXERCISES

For the person using the suspension trainer, the advanced exercises are fun and challenging. They require greater levels of fitness, strength, balance, and proprioception. Some of them have the potential to be dangerous. For these reasons, you should perform them only after you have thoroughly mastered the foundational exercises.

Suspension Push-Up

Intended Uses

Push-ups develop the muscles of the chest, shoulders, and triceps. When performing this exercise with a stability trainer, the core and the upper back are involved in a stabilizing role.

Prerequisites

- Ability to perform 20 push-ups with consistent, good form.
- Ability to perform 20 chest presses with consistent, good form.
- Minimum of three months of experience with the stability trainer.

Steps

- Grip the handles with a pronated grip.
- Assume the prone lying position (*a*).
- The upper body should be supporting much of your body weight.
- Flex your elbows and lower yourself toward the floor.
- As you lower yourself, the handles move to the sides.
- Lower until your body is even with the handles (*b*).
- Reverse direction until the arms are fully extended.
- Repeat for the desired number of repetitions.

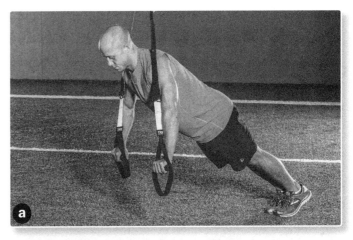

Key Points

- The ankles and shoulders should be in a straight line throughout the exercise.
- The handles may need to move out to the sides some during the exercise.

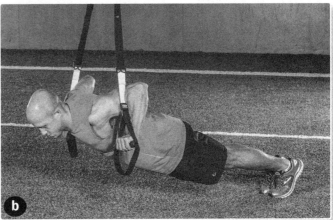

Suspension Fly

Intended Uses

As with dumbbells, the suspension trainer fly isolates the muscles of the chest. It also trains the muscles of the core, which must stabilize the body during performance of the exercise. This is another good exercise for a conditioning workout.

Prerequisites

- Ability to assume the standing prone position.
- Ability to perform 20 repetitions of the chest press with consistent, good technique.
- Minimum of three months of experience with suspension training.

Steps

- Grip the handles with a neutral grip.
- Assume the standing prone position (*a*).
- Maintain a slight bend at the elbows.
- Allow the hands to spread slowly apart, lowering the body toward the floor, until the handles are even with the body (*b*).
- Reverse direction and repeat for the desired number of repetitions.

Key Points

- Maintain a straight line from the heels to the shoulders.
- Maintain a slight bend at the elbows throughout the exercise.
- As the hands are moving to the sides, the body should be lowering.
- This exercise should be performed in a slow and controlled manner.

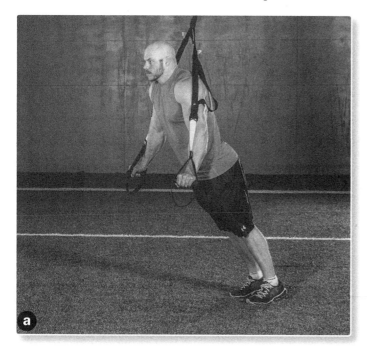

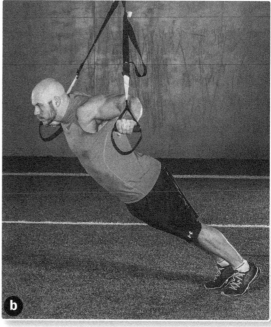

Suspension One-Armed Row

Intended Uses

The one-arm row develops the muscles of the upper back, shoulder, and biceps. It is a more difficult version than the foundational rowing exercise because only one arm is exercising at a time. This variation adds difficulty as well as new balance and stabilization requirements.

Prerequisites

- Ability to adjust the suspension trainer for the one-handed grip.
- Ability to assume the standing supine position.
- Ability to perform 20 repetitions of the row with consistent, good technique.

Steps

- Adjust the suspension trainer for the one-handed grip.
- Grip the handle with a neutral grip.
- Assume the standing supine position (*a*).
- From this position, flex the elbow and pull the body toward the handle (*b*).
- Reverse direction slowly and repeat for the desired number of repetitions. Then switch sides.

Key Points

- Maintain a straight line from the heels to the shoulders throughout the exercise.
- Keep the elbow close to the body while pulling yourself toward the handle.
- Concentrate on retracting your shoulder blade as you pull yourself toward the handle. Then focus on protracting the shoulder blade as you reverse direction.
- Perform this exercise in a slow, controlled manner.

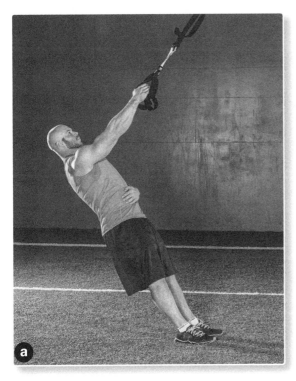 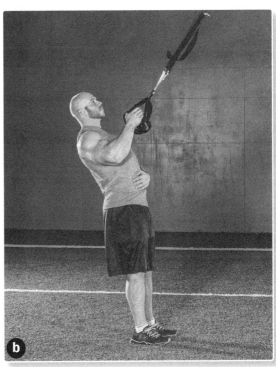

Suspension Reverse Fly

Intended Uses

The reverse fly develops the shoulders and the muscles of the upper back. The muscles of the core work to stabilize the body during this exercise.

Prerequisites

- Ability to assume the standing supine position.
- Ability to perform 20 repetitions on the chest press with good, consistent technique.
- Ability to perform 20 repetitions on the row with good, consistent technique.

Steps

- Grip the handles with a neutral grip. The hands should be close together.
- Assume the standing supine position.
- Flex the elbows slightly and maintain that angle throughout the exercise (*a*).
- Move the handles out to the sides. While this movement is occurring, allow the body to be pulled toward the suspension trainer (*b*).
- Reverse direction and repeat.

Key Points

- Maintain a straight line from the heels to the shoulders throughout the exercise.
- Perform this exercise in a slow, controlled manner.
- Maintain a slight bend at the elbows throughout the exercise.
- As the hands are moving to the sides, the body should be moving closer to the suspension trainer.

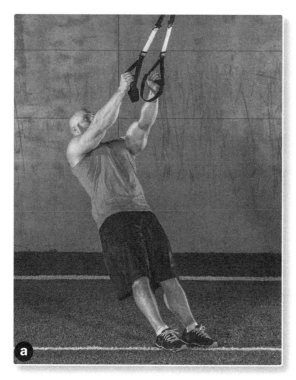 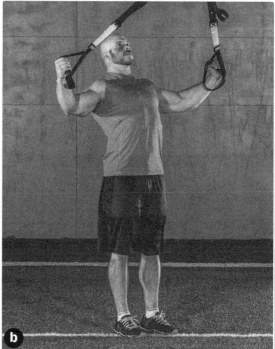

Suspension One-Legged Squat

Intended Uses

Like the squat exercise, this exercise develops the quadriceps, hamstrings, and glutes. Unlike the squat, this variation develops one-legged strength. The one-legged nature of the exercise requires good balance as well as strength in the ankle, foot, and shin to stabilize the body.

Prerequisites

- Ability to perform 20 suspension squats with good, consistent technique.
- Ability to perform 10 reverse lunges on each leg with good, consistent technique.

Steps

- Grip the handles with a neutral grip.
- Assume the standing position.
- Set your back.
- Keeping the left leg straight, lift the left foot off the ground. Lift the foot up so that it is in front of the body (*a*).
- Keeping your weight on your right heel, perform a squat until the thigh is at least parallel to the floor (*b*).
- Reverse direction and repeat for the desired number of repetitions. Then switch legs.

Key Points

- You need to get your balance before attempting the actual squat.
- Keep your back set throughout the exercise.

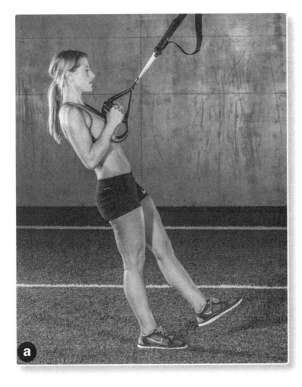 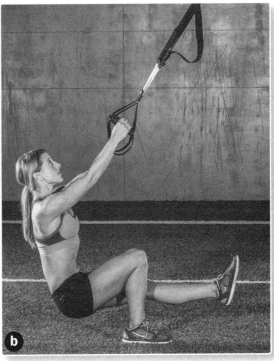

Suspension Foot-in-Trainer One-Legged Squat

Intended Uses

Like the one-legged squat exercise, this exercise develops the quadriceps, hamstrings, and glutes. This variation also develops one-legged strength. This extremely advanced exercise requires a great deal of balance and coordination.

Prerequisites

- Ability to perform 10 one-legged squats on each leg with good, consistent technique.

Steps

- Adjust the suspension trainer for the one-handed grip. The handle should be hanging at knee height from the ground.
- Stand with your back to the suspension trainer.
- Place your right foot into the handle of the trainer and step forward (a).
- Keeping your left foot on the ground and your right foot in the trainer, perform squats using your left leg (b).
- After you have performed the desired number of repetitions, switch legs.

Key Points

- This exercise should be performed in a slow and controlled manner.
- Make sure that you are balanced before performing the squat.

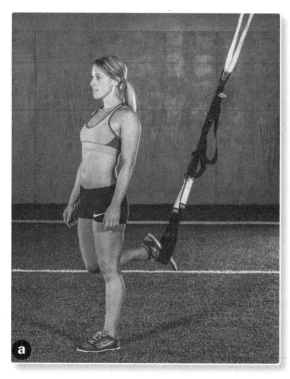
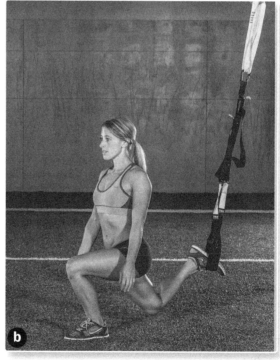

Suspension Foot-in-Trainer One-Legged Hip Bridge

Intended Uses

The one-legged hip bridge primarily trains the glutes and hamstrings. The muscles of the core perform a stabilizing role during this exercise. The one-legged nature makes this a challenging exercise for the lower body.

Prerequisites

- Ability to perform 20 leg curls with good, consistent technique.

Steps

- Adjust the suspension trainer for the one-handed grip.
- Adjust the trainer so that the handles are hanging off the ground at knee height.
- Assume the supine lying position.
- Place the right foot in the handle (*a*).
- The right knee should be slightly bent.
- Extend the right knee and use the right leg to lift both hips off the ground (*b*).
- Lower and repeat for the desired number of repetitions. Switch legs.

Key Points

- When the hips are on the ground, the knee performing the exercise should be flexed to approximately 135 degrees.

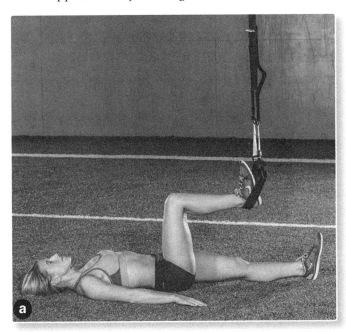

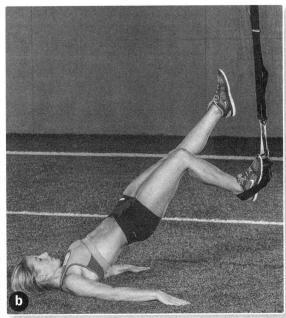

Suspension Foot-in-Trainer One-Legged Leg Curl

Intended Uses

The one-legged leg curl primarily trains the glutes and hamstrings. The muscles of the core perform a stabilizing role during this exercise. The one-legged nature makes this a challenging exercise for the lower body.

Prerequisites

- Ability to perform 20 leg curls with good, consistent technique.

Steps

- Adjust the suspension trainer for the one-handed grip.
- Adjust the trainer so that the handles are hanging off the ground at knee height.
- Assume the supine lying position.
- Place the right foot in the handle (a).
- The right knee should be slightly bent.
- Extend the right knee and use the right leg to lift both hips off the ground.
- Maintaining the elevated position, flex the right knee so that the heel moves toward your hips (b).
- Extend the knee, maintaining the elevated position, and then repeat.
- Perform the desired number of repetitions and then switch legs.

Key Points

- Your hips will remain off the ground during the entire exercise.
- As you curl the handles toward your hips, your hips may lift up higher.

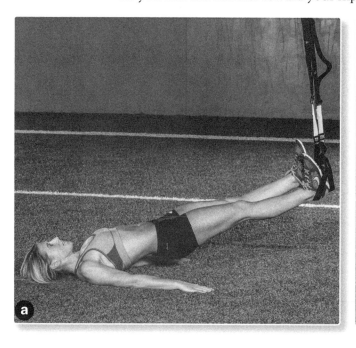
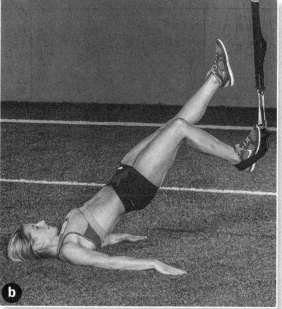

Suspension Pike

Intended Uses

The pike is an advanced exercise for training the muscles of the core. The upper and lower parts of the rectus abdominis perform the exercise, and the obliques stabilize the pelvis. This exercise is challenging from a balance and stability standpoint.

Prerequisites

- Ability to perform 20 repetitions of the knees to chest exercise with good, consistent technique.

Steps

- Place your feet in the handles.
- Assume the prone lying position (*a*).
- Keeping your arms and legs straight, lift your hips high into the air to form an upside-down V with your body (*b*).
- Lower and repeat for the desired number of repetitions.

Key Points

- Keep the arms and legs straight while performing this exercise.
- As you lift the hips, the handles will move toward the arms.

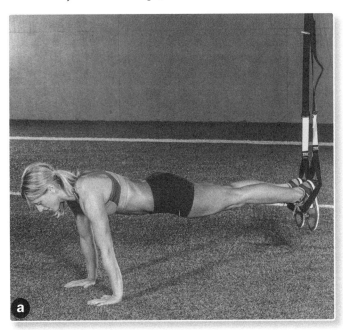
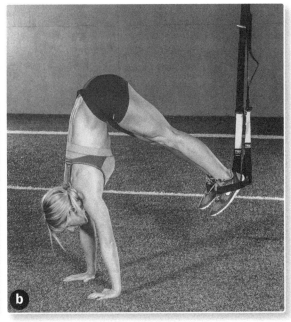

Suspension Clock

Intended Uses

This advanced exercise primarily trains the oblique muscles. People with lower back injuries should not perform this exercise.

Prerequisites

- Ability to perform 20 repetitions of the knees to chest, hips up, and lying leg raise exercises with good, consistent technique.
- At least three months of experience with the chest, hips up, and lying leg raise exercises.

Steps

- Assume the supine lying position.
- Position yourself so that your eyes are located under the handles.
- Reach up and grasp the handles.
- Keeping your legs straight, raise them both up until they are perpendicular to the ground (*a*).
- Keeping your legs straight and together, attempt to lower them to the right side of your body (*b*).
- Reverse direction and attempt to lower them to the left side of your body.
- Repeat for the desired number of repetitions.

Key Points

- Your legs should be as straight as possible throughout this exercise.
- You will need to turn your hips some to lower your legs to the sides.

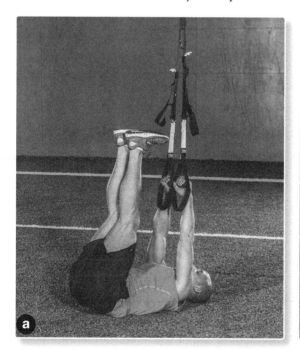 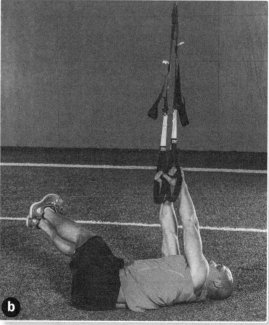

INTRODUCTORY PROGRAM

The introductory program is designed to get you familiar with using the suspension trainer. It will require you to learn how to adjust the trainer, learn the fundamental positions, and learn the grips that are used with it. In addition, it will prepare your body for the more advanced exercises that can be performed with the suspension trainer. This program is meant to be done two times per week. The program should be performed as a circuit. You perform each exercise for a specific time and take as little rest as possible before you perform the next exercise. After you perform the entire list of exercises, start the entire circuit over again. Table 7.2 outlines the introductory program.

Table 7.2 Introductory Suspension-Training Program

Day 1	Day 2
Suspension chest press, p. 111	Suspension squats, p. 115
Suspension rows, p. 112	Suspension reverse lunges, p. 116
Suspension biceps curls, p. 113	Suspension leg curls, p. 118
Suspension triceps extensions, p. 114	Suspension hip ups, p. 117
Suspension squats, p. 115	Suspension chest press, p. 111
Suspension reverse lunges, p. 116	Suspension rows, p. 112
Suspension leg curls, p. 118	Suspension biceps curls, p. 113
Suspension knees to chest, p. 119	Suspension triceps extensions, p. 114

CHAPTER 8

Kettlebells

Over the last several years, kettlebells have moved from being a fringe tool to one that is available in many fitness centers and weight rooms. Today, entry-level strength and conditioning coaches are expected to understand this apparatus and its application to sport. Kettlebells are weighted balls with a handle. Because they come in different weights, they can be used to increase muscle mass, improve strength, and develop power. Their unique shape allows the performance of a wide range of exercises. They are used extensively for interval training because many kettlebell exercises can be performed rhythmically.

Kettlebell exercises have been found to increase heart rate and oxygen consumption in a manner similar to running on a treadmill. These exercises use most of the muscles of the body, so they burn calories. By adjusting the weight, changing the intensity of the workouts is easy, so kettlebells offer flexibility not available with many other types of tools.

Kettlebell exercises require each side of the body to handle the load and develop. Unlike barbell exercises, kettlebell exercises do not permit one side of the body to compensate. These exercises develop the core, shoulder strength and stability, a sense of balance, and spatial awareness. For most kettlebell exercises, you stand on the ground, which means that the exercises are transferable to sport.

Like every tool, kettlebells have drawbacks that you need to be aware of. First, they are much more expensive than free weights. This factor applies not only to your initial investment but also to your acquisition of the heavier kettlebells that will need as you become stronger over time. Second, learning how to perform these exercises takes time. Because of the balance and skill component, you need to invest considerable time in learning the foundational exercises. Several of the advanced exercises can be dangerous if performed improperly. The last drawback is that these exercises are not forgiving of mistakes. Mistakes with kettlebells are painful. They may result in bruising of the forearms or worse if you move incorrectly while attempting to hold a kettlebell overhead.

Kettlebells are used a number of ways. First, any exercise that can be done with a barbell or dumbbell can be done with a kettlebell, so they are an excellent tool for increasing muscle mass, increasing strength, and training for power. Second, their unique design permits you to perform a wide range of unique exercises that you cannot perform well with barbells and dumbbells. Third, they are used for interval training. In general, the exercises are performed for set periods and are usually mixed in with other types of exercise. Table 8.1 shows an example using kettlebells, bodyweight exercises, and heavy ropes. Finally, some people use kettlebells to get an aerobic training effect. This challenging practice requires moving continuously in a rhythmic manner for a long period.

Table 8.1 Sample Program for Integrating Kettlebell Training With Other Forms of Training

Bodyweight jumping jacks, p. 13	Suspension squat, p. 115
Kettlebell two-handed swing, p. 135	Kettlebell clean, p. 138
Heavy ropes one-handed slam, p. 88	Heavy ropes one-handed slam, p. 88
Bodyweight mountain climber for 10 yards, p. 17	Bodyweight inchworm for 10 yards, p. 15
Kettlebell snatch, p. 136	Kettlebell goblet squat, p. 140
Heavy ropes one-handed slam, p. 88	Heavy ropes one-handed slam, p. 88

Unless otherwise noted, perform each exercise for 30 seconds. Repeat the circuit as many times as needed. Rest 1 to 2 minutes after each repetition of the circuit.

GETTING STARTED

Learning how to grip and hold the kettlebell properly will save a lot of time, frustrations, and bruises. Before jumping into the exercises, take some time to learn the basic grips and holds. This book explains three grips and one hold.

The grip used most often for the exercises in this book is the inside handle grip. Users will be strong with this grip. Begin with the kettlebell on the ground with the handle facing up. Looking down at the kettlebell, use the right hand to grip it. The right hand grips the left top corner of the handle. Make sure to use the fingers and thumb to grip the kettlebell (figure 8.1). To grip with the left hand, grip the right top corner of the handle.

On the snatch and overhead squat, you use a different type of grip, the middle handle grip, to prevent those exercises from bruising the forearm. For this grip, begin with the kettlebell on the ground with the handle facing up. Use the fingers and thumb of the right hand to grip the handle at its middle (figure 8.2).

With some exercises, you use a two-handed grip. For this grip, grasp the middle of the kettlebell's handle with both hands. Position the hands next to each other, touching, and use the thumbs and fingers to grip the handle (figure 8.3).

The hold relates to how to stand with the kettlebell on the shoulder. The hold is important because it is how you receive the kettlebell during the clean and it sets up presses and

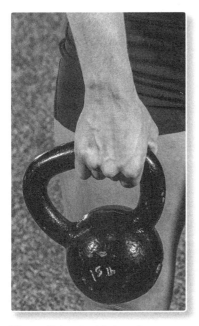

Figure 8.1 Inside handle kettlebell grip.

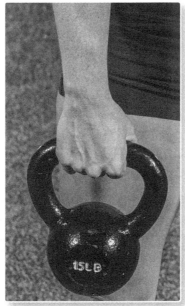

Figure 8.2 Middle handle kettlebell grip.

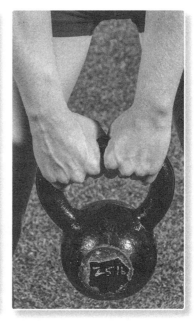

Figure 8.3 Two-handed kettlebell grip.

jerks. Performing the hold properly will keep the shoulders healthy. Performing it improperly will needlessly increase the difficulty of the exercises and could lead to injury! First, realize that the kettlebell won't actually fit on the shoulder. As a result, it sits outside the shoulder and forearm in the crook between the two. Second, when holding the kettlebell on the shoulder, use an inside handle grip but have the palm facing up toward the sky. Third, when the kettlebell is in this position, the elbow needs to be pointed toward the front of the body, not flared out to the side (figure 8.4). This position keeps the shoulder ready for any impending overhead work.

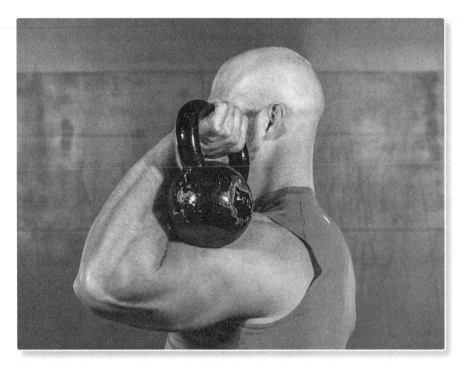

Figure 8.4 Proper positioning of kettlebell on the shoulder when standing.

FOUNDATIONAL EXERCISES

These exercises make up the bulk of strength and conditioning programs that use kettlebells. They teach critical techniques that have application to other, more advanced kettlebell exercises. They are also important for preparing the body to perform more advanced exercises.

Kettlebell Two-Handed Swing

Intended Uses

The two-handed swing uses most of the muscles of the body. It can be performed to develop strength, power, and the horizontal application of force. It is also a rhythmic exercise, so it can be performed for time to develop conditioning.

Prerequisites

- Ability to use the hips in a squatting motion.
- Ability to squat while keeping the weight on the heels.
- Ability to maintain correct back posture.

Steps

- The kettlebell is on the floor.
- Stand over the kettlebell so that the feet are shoulder-width apart and the kettlebell is between the feet.
- Set the back.
- Keeping the weight on the heels, push the hips back and squat down until you can grip the kettlebell using a two-handed grip.
- Stand up, holding the kettlebell on straight arms.
- Keeping the arms straight, push the hips back, allowing the kettlebell and arms to swing back between the knees (*a*).
- Without pausing, extend the knees and hips, allowing the kettlebell to swing forward until the arms are a little more than parallel to the floor (*b*).
- Reverse direction and repeat.

Key Points

- Keep the weight on the heels.
- Maintain a tight back during this exercise.
- Use the hips as a hinge to help perform this exercise.
- Keep the arms straight throughout.
- Swing the arms only until they are parallel to the floor.

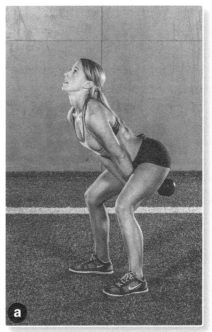

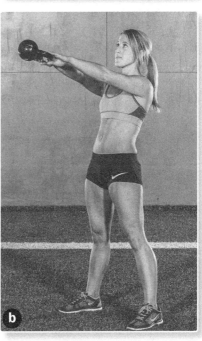

Kettlebell Snatch

Intended Uses

The snatch uses most of the muscles of the body. It is a ground-based exercise that develops balance and proprioception. It is also a rhythmic exercise that can be performed for time to develop conditioning

Prerequisites

- Ability to use the hips in a squatting motion.
- Ability to squat while keeping the weight on the heels.
- Ability to maintain correct back posture.
- Sufficient strength to hold the kettlebell overhead on a straight arm.
- Ability to position the kettlebell in line with the hips for balance when overhead.

Steps

- The kettlebell is on the floor.
- Stand over the kettlebell so that the feet are shoulder-width apart and the kettlebell is between the feet.
- Set the back.
- Keeping the weight on the heels, push the hips back and squat down until you can grip the kettlebell with the right hand using a middle handle grip.
- Stand up, holding the kettlebell with a straight arm.
- Hold the left arm out to the side for balance.
- Keeping the right arm straight, push the hips back, allowing the kettlebell and arm to swing back between the knees.
- Without pausing, extend the knees and hips, allowing the kettlebell to swing forward.
- As the kettlebell swings forward, flex the right elbow, allowing the kettlebell to travel up the body. When the right elbow is positioned beneath the kettlebell, punch the right hand up through the kettlebell (a).
- While punching up, move into a squat (b).
- The kettlebell should end up slightly behind the head and in line with the hips.
- Reverse direction and repeat.
- Switch arms after you perform the desired number of reps.

Key Points

- Keep the weight on the heels.
- Maintain a tight back during this exercise.
- Use the hips as a hinge to help perform the exercise.
- Use the middle grip throughout.
- Punch upward when the elbow is beneath the kettlebell.
- The kettlebell must be in line with the hips for balance.

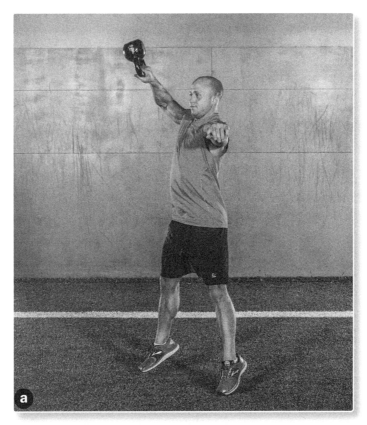

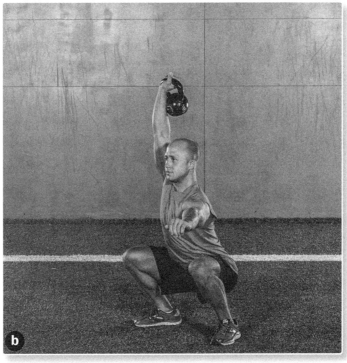

Kettlebell Clean

Intended Uses

Like many of the exercises in this chapter, the clean uses most of the muscles of the body and is a ground-based exercise. It is rhythmic in nature, so it can be performed for time to develop conditioning. In addition, by teaching you how to bring the kettlebell to the shoulders, the clean serves as preparation for other exercises.

Prerequisites

- Ability to use the hips in a squatting motion.
- Ability to squat while keeping the weight on the heels.
- Ability to maintain correct back posture.
- Ability to hold the kettlebell on the shoulder.

Steps

- The kettlebell is on the floor.
- Stand over the kettlebell so that the feet are shoulder-width apart and the kettlebell is between the feet.
- Set the back.
- Keeping the weight on the heels, push the hips back and squat down until you can grip the kettlebell with the right hand using an inside handle grip.
- Stand up, holding the kettlebell with a straight arm (*a*).
- Keeping the right arm straight, push the hips back, allowing the kettlebell and arm to swing back between the knees.
- Without pausing, extend the knees and hips, allowing the kettlebell to swing forward.
- As the kettlebell swings forward, flex the right elbow.
- Move into a squat, receiving the kettlebell on the right shoulder (*b*).
- Lower and repeat for the desired number of reps and then switch arms.

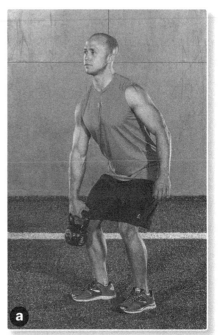

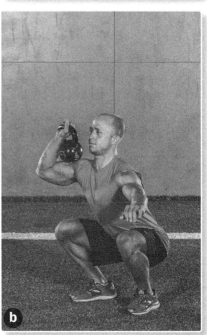

Key Points

- Keep the weight on the heels.
- Maintain a tight back during this exercise.
- Use the hips as a hinge to help perform the exercise.
- Use the inside handle grip throughout.
- After you receive the kettlebell, it should rest on the outside of the forearm and shoulder.
- The elbow should face toward the front.

Kettlebell Jerk

Intended Uses

The jerk is another ground-based, rhythmic exercise that uses most of the muscles of the body. It can be used to develop power and upper-body strength. In addition, it develops balance and proprioception.

Prerequisites

- Ability to use the hips in a squatting motion.
- Ability to squat while keeping the weight on the heels.
- Ability to maintain correct back posture.
- Ability to hold the kettlebell on the shoulder properly.
- Sufficient strength to hold the kettlebell overhead on a straight arm.
- Ability to position the kettlebell in line with the hips for balance when overhead.

Steps

- Clean the kettlebell to the right shoulder.
- The right elbow should face forward.
- Keeping the weight on the heels, move quickly into a quarter squat (*a*).
- Without pausing, use the legs to drive the kettlebell off the shoulder (*b*).
- Press the kettlebell up and slightly behind the head.
- The kettlebell should end up in line with the hips.
- Lower and repeat for the desired number of reps and then switch sides.

Key Points

- The dip and drive need to be performed quickly, with no pauses.
- Keep the kettlebell on the shoulder during the dip.
- Ensure that the elbow faces forward during the dip and drive.
- The kettlebell should end up slightly behind the head, in line with the hips.

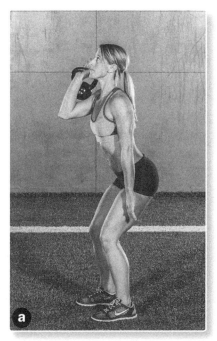

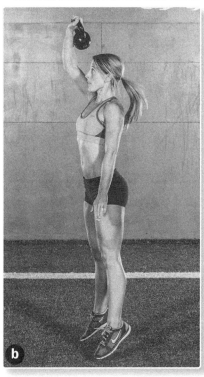

Kettlebell Goblet Squat

Intended Uses

The goblet squat develops the muscles of the lower body and core. This exercise can be performed rhythmically and used in a conditioning workout. The goblet squat can also be used with heavier weights to develop lower-body strength.

Prerequisites

- Ability to use the hips in a squatting motion.
- Ability to squat while keeping the weight on the heels.
- Ability to maintain correct back posture.

Steps

- Feet should be between hip-width and shoulder-width apart.
- Grip the kettlebell with both hands, with one hand on each side of the handle.
- Hold the kettlebell against the body at chest level, keeping the elbows down (*a*).
- Set the back.
- Keeping the weight on the heels, squat down by pushing the hips back (*b*).
- Squat down as far as is comfortable.
- Reverse direction and repeat for the desired number of repetitions.

Key Points

- The hips should initiate the squat.
- Keep the weight on the heels while squatting.
- Maintain proper back positioning.

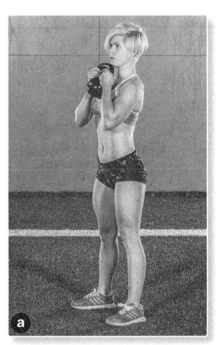

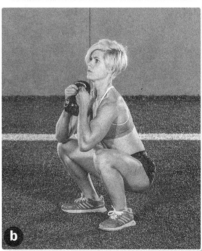

Kettlebell Deadlift

Intended Uses

Like the barbell variation, the kettlebell deadlift is used for the lower body and core. It can be performed rhythmically and used in a conditioning routine. It can also be used to develop strength.

Prerequisites

- Ability to use the hips in a squatting motion.
- Ability to squat while keeping the weight on the heels.
- Ability to maintain correct back posture.

Steps

- The kettlebell is on the floor.
- Stand over the kettlebell so that the feet are shoulder-width apart and the kettlebell is between the feet.
- Set the back.
- Keeping the weight on the heels, push the hips back and squat down until you can grip the kettlebell with a two-handed grip (*a*).
- Keeping the arms straight and back set, stand up while holding the kettlebell (*b*).
- Reverse direction and repeat.

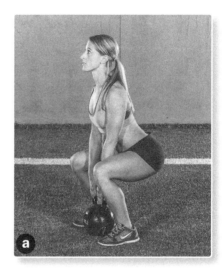

Key Points

- Keep the weight on the heels throughout.
- Keep the back tight during this exercise.
- While standing up, the hips and shoulders should rise at the same speed.
- The arms should remain straight throughout.

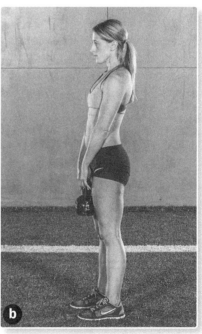

Kettlebell Romanian Deadlift

Intended Uses

Like the barbell variation of this exercise, the kettlebell Romanian deadlift develops the hamstrings, glutes, and lower back. It strengthens the hamstrings in the lengthened position, which is important for sprinting and jumping. It can be performed rhythmically for conditioning, or it can be performed as a strengthening exercise.

Prerequisites

- Ability to maintain correct back posture.

Steps

- Stand up holding a kettlebell with both hands.
- Hold the kettlebell in front of the body so that it rests on the thighs (*a*).
- Use a middle handle grip on the kettlebell.
- Feet should be hip-width apart.
- Set the back.
- Unlock the knees.
- Maintaining the knee angle, push the hips back.
- As you push the hips back, bend forward, allowing the kettlebell to slide down the thighs (*b*).
- Lower the kettlebell as far as is comfortable, reverse direction, and repeat.

Key Points

- This exercise is performed from the hips, not the knees or the back.
- The arms should remain straight throughout.
- Keep the back tight during this exercise.

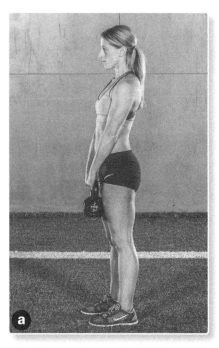

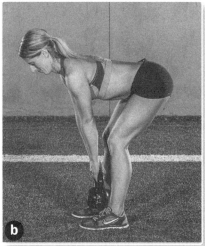

Kettlebell Push-Up

Intended Uses

This variation of the push-up develops the muscles of the chest, shoulders, and triceps. This is a great exercise for conditioning workouts.

Prerequisites

- Ability to perform 20 regular push-ups with good form.

Steps

- Begin with a kettlebell on the ground. The handle should face up.
- Assume the push-up position and have the left hand gripping the kettlebell (a).
- Hands should be wider than shoulder-width apart.
- Hands should be positioned at a level even with the middle or lower chest.
- From the starting position, lower the body until the chest is even with the kettlebell (b).
- Reverse direction until the arms are extended.
- After you have performed the desired number of repetitions, switch the hand that is grasping the kettlebell. Repeat with the other hand grasping the kettlebell.

Key Points

- A straight line should run from the heels to the shoulders throughout the exercise.
- Lower the body only until it is even with the kettlebell.
- Perform this exercise with both sides grasping the kettlebell.

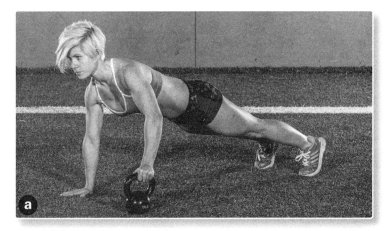

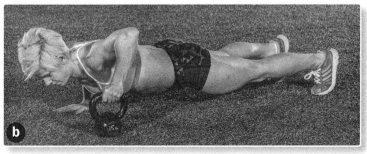

Kettlebell Bent-Over Row

Intended Uses

The kettlebell variation of this exercise develops the muscles of the upper back, shoulders, and biceps. It can be used to develop upper-body strength. It can also be performed rhythmically as part of a conditioning routine.

Prerequisites

- Ability to maintain proper back posture.

Steps

- Stand up with a kettlebell in each hand.
- Grip the kettlebells with a middle handle grip.
- Feet should be hip-width apart.
- Set the back.
- Unlock the knees. Maintain this knee angle throughout the exercise.
- Keeping the weight on the heels, push the hips back and lean forward, allowing the kettlebells to slide down the thighs (*a*).
- When the upper body is just above parallel to the floor, stop leaning forward.
- Maintaining the position of the upper body, pull the kettlebells toward the sides of the body at a level even with the belly (*b*).
- Lower and repeat for the desired number of repetitions.

Key Points

- Maintain a tight back throughout.
- Avoid swinging the upper body.
- As you pull the kettlebells toward the body, the upper arms should remain tight to the body and should brush the body.
- As you pull the kettlebells toward the body, concentrate on drawing the shoulder blades together.
- As you lower the kettlebells, concentrate on allowing the shoulder blades to spread apart.

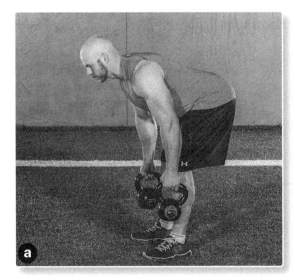
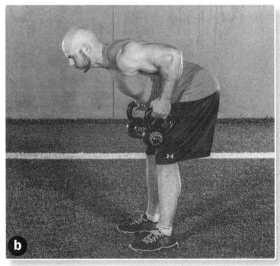

Kettlebell Press

Intended Uses

The kettlebell press develops the shoulders and triceps. In addition, it requires the muscles of the core to stabilize the trunk. This is an upper-body strengthening exercise.

Prerequisites

- Ability to maintain proper back posture.
- Ability to hold the kettlebell on the shoulder properly.
- Sufficient strength to hold the kettlebell overhead on a straight arm.
- Ability to position the kettlebell in line with the hips for balance when it is overhead.

Steps

- Clean the kettlebell to the right shoulder (*a*).
- Feet should be hip-width apart.
- Set the back.
- Hold the left arm out for balance.
- Keeping the right elbow pointing forward, press the kettlebell up (*b*).
- The kettlebell should travel up and slightly behind the head so that it ends up in line with the hips.
- Lower and repeat. Switch sides after you perform the desired number of repetitions.

Key Points

- Maintain a tight back throughout.
- Avoid using the legs to perform the exercise.
- The elbow must remain in position and not flare out to the side during the exercise.
- The kettlebell should end up in line with the hips for balance.

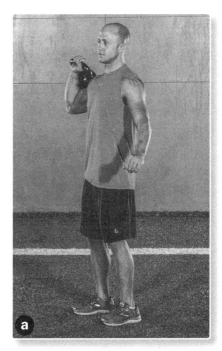

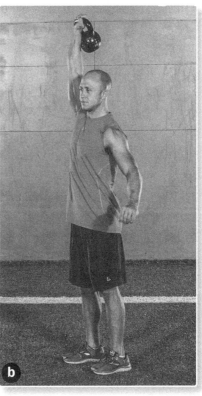

ADVANCED EXERCISES

The advanced exercises described in this chapter build on the foundational exercises that have already been covered. To perform these advanced exercises safely and effectively, you need solid technique and a base level of strength and fitness. In other words, you cannot skip straight to the advanced exercises without paying your dues with the foundational ones. Use the advanced exercises described here only after you have met their prerequisites.

Kettlebell One-Handed Swing

Intended Uses

The one-handed swing requires one arm to work at a time, which creates unique demands. Like the two-handed variation, it develops the ability to apply force horizontally. This exercise can be used to develop strength, or it can be performed rhythmically for conditioning.

Prerequisites

- Ability to execute the two-handed swing with consistent, good technique.
- Ability to perform 10 two-handed swings with 20 percent of body weight.

Steps

- Place the kettlebell on the floor with the handle facing up.
- Stand over the kettlebell and straddle it. Feet should be shoulder-width apart.
- Set the back.
- Keeping the weight on the heels, squat down until you can grasp the kettlebell with the right hand. Use an inside handle grip.
- Keeping the arm straight, stand up with the kettlebell.
- Push the hips back, allowing the kettlebell and arm to swing backward between the knees (a).
- Without pausing, reverse direction and swing the kettlebell forward until the right arm is parallel to the floor (b).
- Repeat for the desired number of repetitions.
- Switch arms and repeat.

Key Points

- Keep the weight on the heels throughout.
- Maintain a tight back.
- Use the hips as a hinge to lower and raise the kettlebell.
- Keep the arm that is attached to the kettlebell straight.
- Avoid allowing the arm to rise to a level above parallel to the floor.

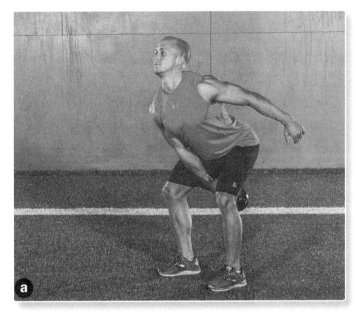

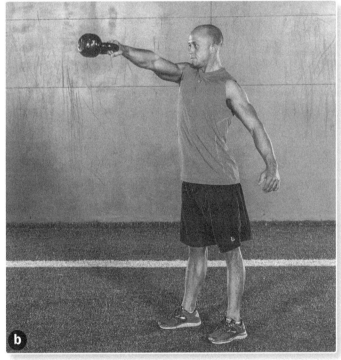

Kettlebell Two-Handed Snatch

Intended Uses

This variation also uses most of the muscles of the body. It develops both sides of the body at the same time, along with balance and proprioception. This variation requires a lot more coordination and flexibility than the one-handed snatch does.

Prerequisites

■ Ability to execute the one-handed snatch with good, consistent technique.

■ Minimum of six months of experience performing one-handed snatches.

■ Ability to perform 10 one-handed snatches with 20 percent of body weight.

Steps

■ Place the kettlebells on the floor.

■ Stand over the kettlebells so that the feet are shoulder-width apart and the kettlebells are between the feet.

■ Set the back.

■ Keeping the weight on the heels, push the hips back and squat down until you can grip each kettlebell using a middle handle grip.

■ Stand up, holding the kettlebells with straight arms.

■ Keeping the arms straight, push the hips back, allowing the kettlebells and arms to swing back between the knees.

■ Without pausing, extend the knees and hips, allowing the kettlebells to swing forward (*a*).

■ As the kettlebells swing forward, flex the elbows, allowing the kettlebells to travel up the body. When the elbows are positioned beneath the kettlebells, punch each hand up through the kettlebell.

■ While punching up, move into a squat (*b*).

■ The kettlebells should end up slightly behind the head and in line with the hips.

■ Reverse direction and repeat.

Key Points

■ Keep the weight on the heels.

■ Maintain a tight back during the exercise.

■ Use the hips as a hinge to help perform this exercise.

■ Use the middle grip throughout.

■ Punch upward when the elbows are beneath the kettlebell.

■ The kettlebells must be in line with the hips for balance.

■ Controlling the kettlebells overhead is easier if they are moved toward each other while above the head.

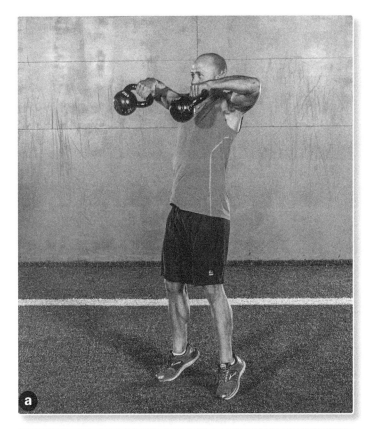

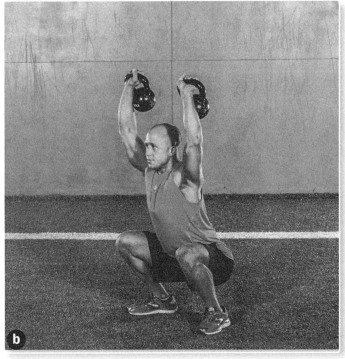

Kettlebell Two-Handed Clean

Intended Uses

The two-handed clean has many of the same uses as the two-handed snatch. One important difference is that (like the one-handed variation of the clean) this one brings the kettlebells to both shoulders, an action that serves as preparation for future exercises.

Prerequisites

- Ability to execute the one-handed clean with good, consistent technique.
- Minimum of six months of experience performing one-handed cleans.
- Ability to perform 10 one-handed cleans with 20 percent of body weight.

Steps

- Place the kettlebells on the floor.
- Stand over the kettlebells so that the feet are shoulder-width apart and the kettlebells are between the feet.
- Set the back.
- Keeping the weight on the heels, push the hips back and squat down until you can grip each kettlebell using an inside handle grip.
- Stand up, holding the kettlebells with straight arms.
- Keeping arms straight, push the hips back, allowing the kettlebells and arms to swing back between the knees.
- Without pausing, extend the knees and hips, allowing the kettlebells to swing forward, traveling up the body (*a*).
- As the kettlebells swing forward, flex the elbows.
- Move into a squat, receiving the kettlebells on the shoulders (*b*).
- Lower and repeat for the desired number of reps.

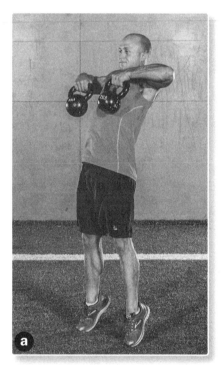

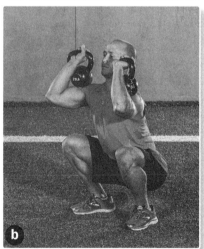

Key Points

- Keep the weight on the heels.
- Maintain a tight back during this exercise.
- Use the hips as a hinge to help perform the exercise.
- Use the inside handle grip throughout.
- After receiving the kettlebells, they should rest on the outside of the forearms and shoulders.
- The elbows should face toward the front.

Kettlebell Two-Handed Jerk

Intended Uses

In terms of power, strength, and developing most of the muscles of the body, this exercise has many of the same uses as the one-handed jerk. Using two kettlebells requires more skill than performing the one-handed variation.

Prerequisites

- Ability to execute the one-handed jerk with good, consistent technique.
- Minimum of six months of experience performing one-handed jerks.
- Ability to perform 10 one-handed jerks with 20 percent of body weight.

Steps

- Clean the kettlebells to the shoulders.
- The elbows should face forward.
- Keeping the weight on the heels, move quickly into a quarter squat (*a*).
- Without pausing, use the legs to drive the kettlebells off the shoulders.
- Press the kettlebells up, toward each other and slightly behind the head (*b*).
- The kettlebells should end up in line with the hips.
- Lower and repeat for the desired number of reps.

Key Points

- The dip and drive must be performed quickly, with no pauses.
- Keep the kettlebells on the shoulders during the dip.
- Ensure that the elbows face forward during the dip and drive.
- The kettlebells should end up slightly behind the head, in line with the hips.
- Moving the kettlebells toward each other while they are overhead makes balance and control easier.

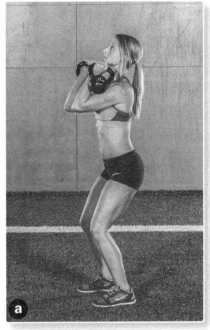

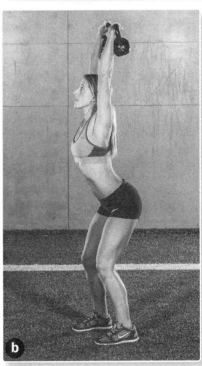

Kettlebell Overhead Squat

Intended Uses

The overhead squat requires a great deal of balance and proprioception. It develops mobility at the shoulders, knees, hips, and ankles. It also develops the muscles of the upper body. This exercise can be used as a strength exercise, or it can be performed rhythmically for a conditioning exercise.

Prerequisites

- Ability to perform squats while keeping the weight on the heels.
- Ability to maintain proper back posture.
- Ability to perform one-handed snatches and one-handed jerks with good, consistent technique.
- Minimum of six months of experience with one-handed snatches and one-handed jerks.

Steps

- Using the right hand, snatch the kettlebell overhead (*a*).
- Ensure that the kettlebell is positioned slightly behind the head.
- Move the feet until they are at least shoulder-width apart.
- Keeping the kettlebell overhead, squat down as far as is comfortable (*b*).
- Reverse direction and repeat for the desired number of repetitions.
- Switch arms.

Key Points

- Hold the opposite arm out to the sides to assist with balance.
- The kettlebell has to be in line with the hips.
- Push against the kettlebell during the squat to keep the arm straight.
- Keep the weight on the heels during the squat.

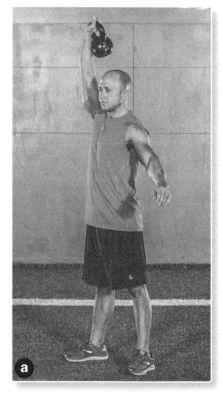

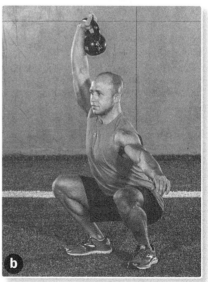

Kettlebell Overhead Lunge

Intended Uses

Like any lunge, the overhead lunge develops the lower body, and it does so by focusing on one leg at a time. Unlike other lunges, it develops shoulder mobility. It also requires balance and proprioception.

Prerequisites

- Ability to perform lunges without extra weight.
- Ability to perform one-handed snatches and one-handed jerks with good, consistent technique.
- Minimum of six months of experience performing one-handed snatches and one-handed jerks.

Steps

- Using the left hand, snatch the kettlebell overhead (*a*).
- Ensure that the kettlebell is positioned slightly behind the head.
- Hold the right arm out to the side for balance.
- Keeping the kettlebell overhead, take a large step forward with the right foot.
- Step forward in a heel-to-toe manner.
- As the foot strikes the ground, flex the right hip and knee until the thigh is parallel to the floor (*b*).
- Reverse direction.
- Repeat with the right leg for the desired number of repetitions.
- Switch the arm that is holding the kettlebell, switch legs, and perform lunges with the other side.

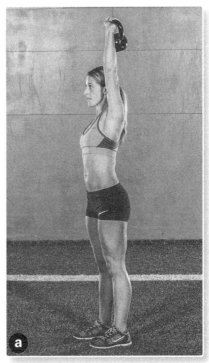

Key Points

- Keep the back tight.
- The kettlebell must be in line with the hips.
- Push against the kettlebell during the lunges.
- Step forward in a heel-to-toe manner.
- The step should be long enough so that the front thigh is parallel to the floor and the front shin is perpendicular to the ground.

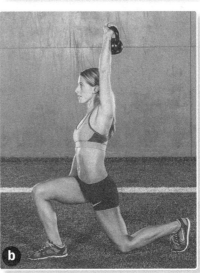

Kettlebell One-Legged Romanian Deadlift

Intended Uses

Like the regular variation, the one-legged Romanian deadlift develops the hamstrings, glutes, and lower back. It also strengthens the hamstrings in the lengthened position. The fact that this is a unilateral exercise means that it may provide a little more transfer to some real-life activities like sprinting, and it is helpful in developing balance and proprioception.

Prerequisites

- Ability to perform kettlebell Romanian deadlifts with good, consistent technique.
- Minimum of six months of experience performing Romanian deadlifts.

Steps

- Stand up with the kettlebell in the right hand.
- Grip the kettlebell with a middle handle hold.
- Feet should be hip-width apart.
- Set the back.
- From the starting position, lift one leg (*a*) and being to hinge forward using the hips.
- Lean the upper body forward while picking the left leg off the ground and lifting it behind the body.
- As you lean your body forward, allow the kettlebell to slide down the right thigh as far as is comfortable (*b*).
- Reverse direction and repeat for the desired number of repetitions. Then switch sides.

Key Points

- Keep the arm holding the kettlebell straight.
- Keep the weight on the heel.
- The lifting of the leg should parallel the lowering of the upper body.

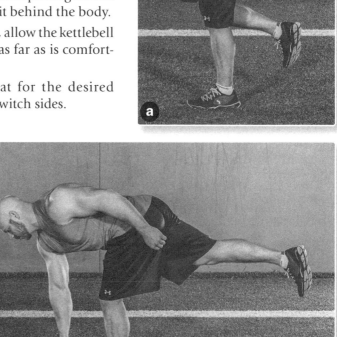

Kettlebell Prone Row

Intended Uses

The prone row is another exercise that develops the muscles of the upper back, shoulder, and biceps. In addition, it requires the shoulders and core to act in a stabilizing role.

Prerequisites

- Ability to perform 20 kettlebell push-ups with good, consistent technique.
- Ability to perform five pull-ups without swinging or kipping.

Steps

- Assume the push-up position.
- The kettlebell should be next to the left hand.
- Shifting the weight to the right arm, grip the kettlebell with the left hand (*a*).
- While maintaining the push-up position, pull the kettlebell toward the left side of the body (*b*).
- Lower and repeat for the desired number of repetitions and then switch sides.

Key Points

- Keep the support arm straight during the performance of this exercise.
- A straight line should run from the heels to the shoulders during the exercise.

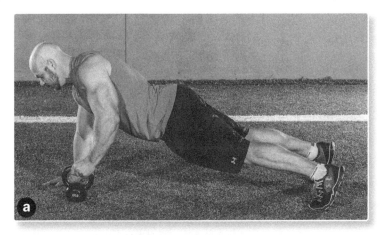

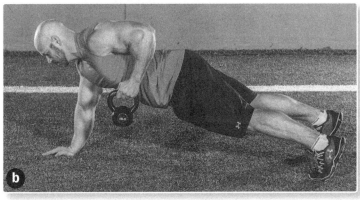

Kettlebell Get-Up

Intended Uses

The get-up develops several abilities and areas of the body. It develops balance and proprioception. It strengthens the shoulder and requires it to act in a stabilizing function. It enhances the strength and stability of the core muscles and trains the muscles of the lower body.

Prerequisites

- Ability to perform 10 overhead squats with 20 percent of body weight.
- Ability to perform overhead lunges with good, consistent technique.
- Minimum of six months of experience with overhead squats and lunges.

Steps

- Lie on the ground, face up.
- The kettlebell should lie on the ground next to your right shoulder.
- Flex your right knee and hip, drawing your right foot toward your hips.
- Your right foot should be flat on the ground.
- Gripping the kettlebell with a pronated, inside handle grip, press it so that it is above the right shoulder (a).
- The right arm should be straight.
- Keeping the right arm fully extended, place the left arm on the ground at a 90-degree angle to the body
- Pushing against the ground with the right foot, roll the body toward the left (b).
- As you roll the body to the left, the kettlebell should remain in a position perpendicular to the ground.
- Using the left arm, push the upper body into a sitting position.
- The kettlebell should now be overhead, still perpendicular to the ground.
- Slide the right leg forward into a lunge position (c).
- Stand up, keeping the kettlebell overhead (d).
- Lower and repeat. Then switch sides.

Key Points

- This exercise has several complicated phases, so you should perform it slowly and carefully.
- This exercise is not forgiving of mistakes.
- After you press the kettlebell up initially, the arm must remain straight throughout the exercise.
- Allowing the kettlebell to drift out of position during the exercise will result in a loss of control and possible injury.

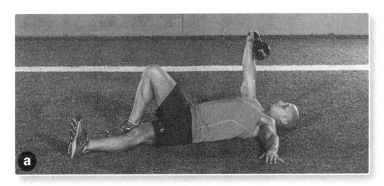

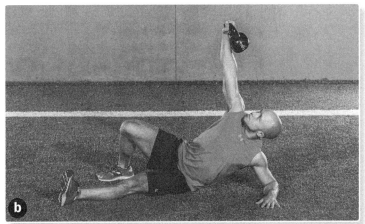

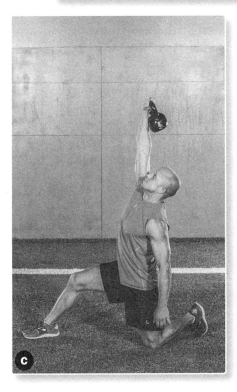

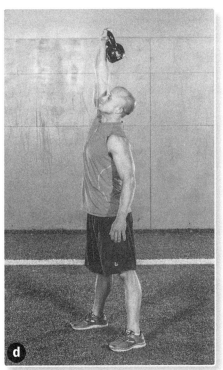

Kettlebell Windmill

Intended Uses

The windmill develops the strength of the shoulder while also requiring it to act in a stabilizing role. It enhances core strength and endurance. The windmill also develops balance and proprioception.

Prerequisites

- Ability to perform 10 overhead squats with 20 percent of body weight.
- Minimum of six months of experience with overhead squats.

Steps

- Clean the kettlebell to the left shoulder.
- Press or jerk the kettlebell overhead.
- Turn the feet toward the left so that they are at a 45-degree angle.
- The hips should point straight ahead.
- Keeping the kettlebell overhead, push the hips toward the left and lean the body toward the right.
- As you are leaning toward the right, slide the right hand down the right leg.
- Bend forward as far as is comfortable.
- Reverse direction and repeat.
- Switch sides.

Key Points

- The feet should be pointed in the direction in which the body will lean.
- The hips should face forward during the exercise.
- The arm holding the kettlebell should remain straight throughout.
- Allowing the kettlebell to move out of position will result in loss of control and possible injury.

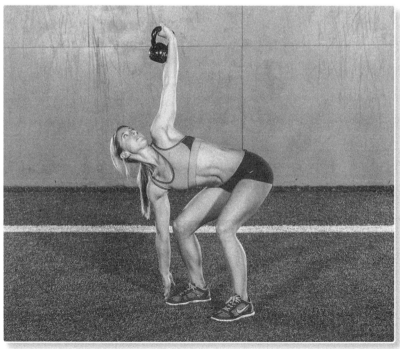

INTRODUCTORY PROGRAM

If you are going to use kettlebells as part of a conditioning program, you need to take the time to learn the exercises. Learning good, consistent technique on these exercises will ensure that they are safe and effective. Table 8.2 provides a sample introductory program to help you become familiar with many of these exercises. You can do this program as part of a warm-up for strength training or for a conditioning workout.

Table 8.2 Introductory Kettlebell Program

Day 1	Day 2
Kettlebell two-handed swing, 10×, p. 135	Kettlebell jerk, 5× (right hand), p. 139
Kettlebell snatch, 5× (right hand), p. 136	Kettlebell push-up, 10× (right hand grips kettlebell), p. 143
Kettlebell two-handed swing, 10×, p. 135	Kettlebell jerk, 5× (left hand), p. 139
Kettlebell snatch, 5× (left hand), p. 136	Kettlebell push-up, 10× (left hand grips kettlebell), p. 143
Kettlebell goblet squat, 10×, p. 140	Kettlebell bent-over row, 5×, p. 144
Kettlebell clean, 5× (right hand), p. 138	Kettlebell press, 5× (right hand), p. 145
Kettlebell deadlift, 5×, p. 141	Kettlebell bent-over row, 5×, p. 144
Kettlebell clean, 5× (left hand), p. 138	Kettlebell press, 5× (left hand), p. 145
Kettlebell Romanian deadlift, 10×, p. 142	

Repeat as many times as needed.

CHAPTER 9

Sandbags

The use of sandbags as a strength-training implement has increased dramatically in popularity in the last several years. They are versatile, can be dropped without causing significant damage or injuries, and, depending on the type of bag used, are relatively affordable. Many sandbags designed for fitness training are made of vinyl, canvas, or other rugged material and have handles sown into them that allow a variety of grips.

Sand provides a unique training stimulus when compared with traditional forms of resistance training. As sandbags are moved or lifted, the sand inside shifts. The shifting creates a dynamic, or active, form of resistance similar to what is experienced in many sports, especially those that are combative in nature or require redirecting an opponent's body mass (e.g., American football, rugby). In contrast to barbell and dumbbells, sandbags create an uneven disbursement of weight when moved. This off-center loading makes sandbags excellent tools for improving balance, coordination, body awareness, and muscular fitness.

The amount of active resistance presented by sand-filled implements varies not only by size and weight but also by construction. Many sandbags are relatively pliable, which allows the sand within the implement to shift position. But after the bags are in position, they may act as a sort of dead weight. Sand-filled tubes are a bit more dynamic than sand-filled bags for two reasons. First, the relatively greater amount of dead space within a tube encourages more movement. Second, the particles of sand bounce off the sides of the more solidly constructed tube, increasing the amount of kinetic energy, whereas the particles of sand within a bag are deadened as they work to reshape the sides of the bag. This difference in resistance must be accounted for when determining training load. Most people can lift more weight when using bags than tubes because after the bags are in position they tend to be more stable.

GETTING STARTED

Sandbags lend themselves well to performing a wide variety of basic and more complex exercises. After perfecting the basic exercises, you can add more elements to your routine by combining exercises to make combination movements. For example, the clean exercise can be combined with the front squat followed by the overhead press to create a total-body exercise. Another combination could involve performing a Romanian deadlift and immediately transitioning into a high pull or upright row. In table 9.1 you will find some combinations movements that work well together. Including complexes is another way to create a fun and challenging workout. Complexes consist of several (generally four to six) exercises performed in sequential order for a set number of repetitions before you move to the next exercise. Table 9.1 provides sample complex workouts that you can use after you have mastered basic exercise techniques and improved your fitness.

Table 9.1 Sample Combination Movements

Clean + front squat
Front squat + Y press
Front squat + forward lunge
Romanian deadlift + high pull
Overhead press + overhead squat

When creating various movement combinations, or complexes, a few key points should be considered.

- **Make certain that you are able to transition smoothly from one exercise to the next.** Use similar hand grips so that you do not waste time transitioning from one grip to another.

- **Adjust the training load based on the weakest exercise movement in the combination or series.** For instance, in most cases people are able to squat more than they can overhead press. Therefore, if you create a combination movement using these two exercises, you would be limited to the weight you could use to perform the overhead press safely for the desired number of repetitions.

- **Do not put the sandbag down until you have completed the entire set or complex.** Holding the sandbag throughout the set or complex increases the metabolic demands and builds endurance in the muscles used for gripping.

FOUNDATIONAL EXERCISES

The first group of exercises featured in this section focus on basic foundational movement patterns that will set the stage for more complex variations later. You need to master these exercises before moving on to the advanced sandbag exercises featured in this chapter or performing combination movements and complexes.

Sandbag Romanian Deadlift

Intended Uses

Romanian deadlifts improve lower-body muscular endurance and dynamic flexibility in the hamstrings, as well as develop trunk stability. Additionally, this exercise helps develop a basic hip hinge movement pattern that is essential for performing many basic and advanced level progressions.

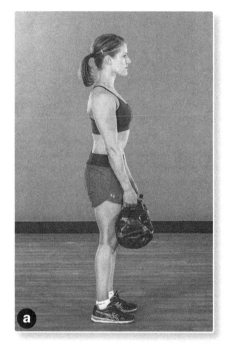

Prerequisites

- Ability to perform a hip hinge correctly.
- No previous history of lower back injury or pain.

Steps

- Begin by standing in the universal athletic position (chest up, shoulders back, and a slight bend in the ankles, knees, and hips).
- Using a neutral grip, hold the sandbag across the midthighs (*a*).
- While keeping the trunk braced and knees slightly bent, push the hips back and flex forward at the waist.
- While keeping the sandbag in contact with the legs, allow the sandbag to travel downward until you feel mild discomfort in the hamstrings or the sandbag touches the base of the ankles (*b*).
- Extend the hips and return to the starting position.

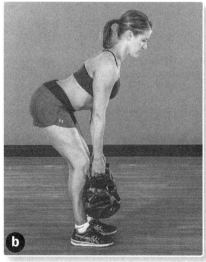

Key Points

- Maintain a slight arch in the lower back throughout the duration of this exercise.
- Do not allow the sandbag to lose contact with the legs because doing so increases the stress placed on the lower back.

Sandbag Front Squat

Intended Uses

This exercise improves lower-body and trunk muscular endurance and helps improve range of motion in the ankle, knees, and hips.

Prerequisites

- Good range of motion in the ankles, knees, hips, and shoulders.
- Ability to maintain an upright torso throughout the entire exercise movement.

Steps

- Begin by standing with the feet approximately shoulder-width to hip-width apart while holding the sandbag with either an overhand or neutral grip.
- Lift the sandbag to shoulder level.
- Rotate the elbows forward, pushing them up toward the ceiling, until the upper am is parallel to the ground and the sandbag is resting on your collarbone (a). This position may be referred to as the rack position.
- While maintaining this position, squat downward until the top of the thighs is parallel to the ground (b).
- Extend the ankles, knees, and hip and return the starting position.

Key Points

- Maintain an upright torso and a slight arch in the lower back throughout the duration of this movement.
- To ensure equal weight distribution throughout the forefoot and heel, the knees should remain in alignment with the toes and the whole foot should remain flat on the floor during the entire movement.

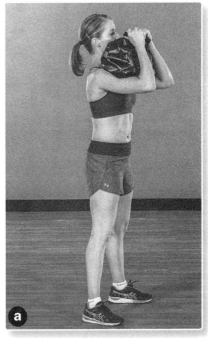

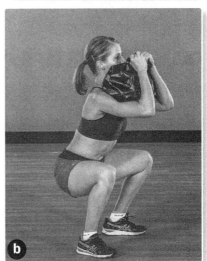

Sandbag Deadlift

Intended Uses

This multijoint exercise provides a sport-specific option for developing muscular endurance in the lower body.

Prerequisites

- Ability to perform a bodyweight squat with proper form and technique.

Steps

- Begin by squatting downward and grabbing the sandbag with an overhand or neutral grip (*a*).
- Keep the arms fully extended and, while maintaining a slight arch in the lower back, stand up until the knees, hips, and torso are fully extended (*b*).

Key Points

- To ensure equal weight distribution throughout the forefoot and heel, the knees should remain in alignment with the toes and the whole foot should remain flat on the floor during the entire movement.
- Do not allow the back to flex or shoulders to round during this movement.

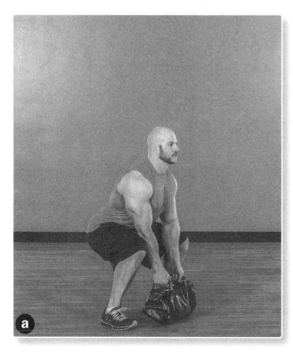
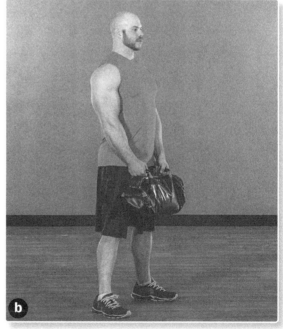

Sandbag Split Squat

Intended Uses

This exercise improves lower-body muscular endurance, reduces strength and endurance discrepancies between the right and left legs, and enhances balance.

Prerequisites

- Ability to perform the front squat.
- Good shoulder range of motion.
- Good trunk stability.
- No current lower-body injuries.

Steps

- Begin by standing with the feet approximately shoulder-width to hip-width apart while holding the sandbag in the rack position with either an overhand or neutral grip.
- Without rotating the hips, step back with one foot and assume a staggered stance (*a*). Both the back and front foot should be in full contact with the ground at this point.
- While keeping the trunk braced, the chest up, and the shoulder blades together, allow the hips, knees, and ankles to flex until the back-leg knee almost touches the ground (*b*).
- When the top of the front-leg (working) thigh is parallel to the ground, extend the hips, knees, and ankles and return to the starting position.
- Perform the desired number of repetitions and then switch legs.

Key Points

- Keep the lead knee in alignment with the second toe of the led foot.
- Do not allow the trunk to flex during the movement.

Variations

- To increase the stability demands of the trunk and shoulders, lift the sandbag overhead during this movement.

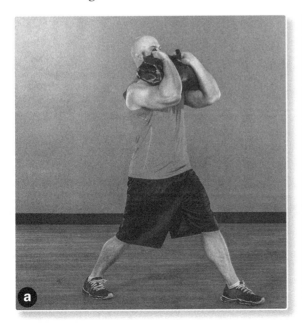
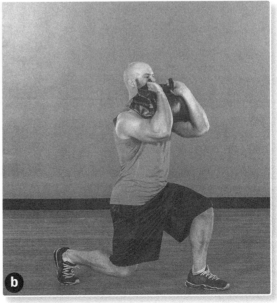

Sandbag In-Place Lunge

Intended Uses

The in-place lunge is a progression to the split squat exercise previously described. This exercise improves lower-body muscular endurance, reduces strength and endurance discrepancies between the right and left legs, and improves balance. Additionally, it would be considered a sport-specific movement for those who participate in sports that require running or that require the legs to act in a reciprocating fashion.

Prerequisites

- Ability to perform the front squat.
- Good shoulder range of motion.
- Good trunk stability.
- No current lower-body injuries.

Steps

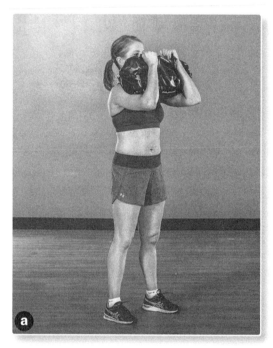

- Begin by standing with the feet approximately shoulder-width to hip-width apart while holding the sandbag in the rack position with either an overhand or neutral grip (*a*).
- Take an exaggerated step forward with one leg.
- When the entire foot of the lead leg makes contact with the ground, flex at the knee, hips, and ankle until the front-leg thigh is parallel to the floor (*b*).
- Keep the front foot flat and the knee in line with the second toe of the front foot.
- Forcefully push back off the front leg to return to the starting position.
- Alternate leading first with the right leg and then with the left leg.

Key Points

- Make certain each leg gets an equal amount of work.

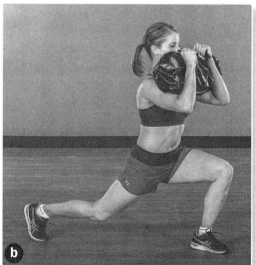

Sandbag Overhead Press

Intended Uses

The overhead press is a good exercise for developing upper-body muscular endurance, specifically within the shoulders and triceps.

Prerequisites

- Good shoulder stability.
- No previous shoulder injuries.

Steps

- Begin by standing in the universal athletic position (chest up, shoulders back, and a slight bend in the ankles, knees, and hips) while holding the sandbag in the rack position using a neutral or overhand grip (a).
- Set the back.
- Extend the arms and press the sandbag directly overhead (b).
- Allow the arms to flex and return the sandbag back to the starting position.

Key Points

- Keep the back set throughout the duration of the exercise.
- If at any time you lose control of the weight while it is overhead, simply let go and let the bag fall to the floor either behind or in front of you. Do not attempt to save the lift.

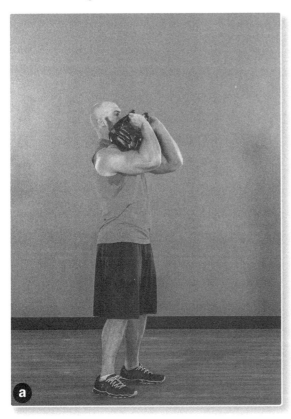
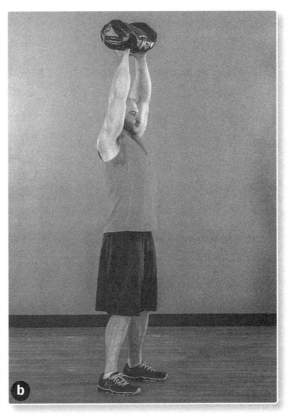

Sandbag Bent-Over Row

Intended Uses

The bent-over row is used primarily to strengthen the muscles of the upper back and increase trunk stability.

Prerequisites

- Ability to perform the Romanian deadlift with good form and technique.
- No lower back injuries.
- Good trunk stability.

Steps

- Begin by standing in the universal athletic position (chest up, shoulders back, and a slight bend in the ankles, knees, and hips).
- Using a neutral grip, hold the sandbag across the midthighs.
- While keeping the trunk braced and knees slightly bent, push the hips back and flex forward at the waist.
- While keeping the sandbag in contact with the legs, allow the sandbag to travel downward until you feel a mild discomfort in the hamstrings or the sandbag touches the ankles (a).
- Set the back and maintain this position.
- Bend the arms and pull the sandbag toward the navel (b). Then allow the shoulders and arms to extend and return the bag back to the starting position.
- Repeat for the desired number of repetitions.

Key Points

- Maintain a slight arch in the lower back throughout the duration of this exercise.
- Keep the sandbag over the feet throughout the duration of this exercise.
- Maintain a slight bend in the knees.
- Keep the shoulder blades squeezed together and pushed slightly downward throughout this exercise.

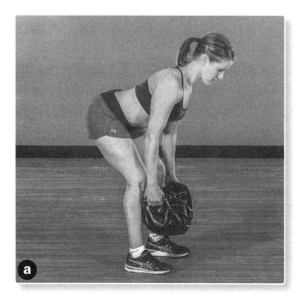 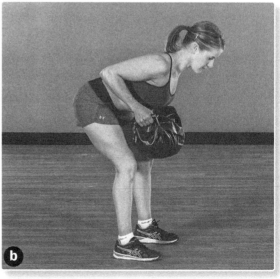

Sandbag Upright Row

Intended Uses

The upright row can be used to improve muscular endurance in the shoulders and trapezius muscles.

Prerequisites

- No preexisting shoulder injuries.

Steps

- Begin by standing in the universal athletic position (chest up, shoulders back, and a slight bend in the ankles, knees, and hips) while holding the sandbags across the thighs using a neutral or overhand grip (a).
- Set the back.
- Bend the arms and flex the shoulders to lift the sandbags up to chest level (b).
- Allow the shoulders and arms to extend and return the sandbags back to the starting position.

Key Points

- Keep the back set throughout the exercise.
- Raise the sandbags only to the chest, rather than the chin, to reduce the risk of shoulder impingement.

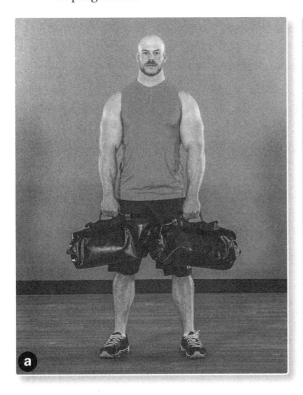
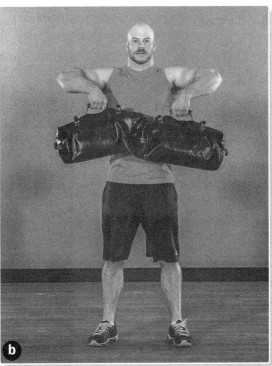

ADVANCED EXERCISES

The following exercises are considered advanced because they require more skill, strength, or both skill and strength. Perform these exercises only after you have perfected the basic exercises in this chapter.

Sandbag Overhead Squat

Intended Uses

This exercise is excellent for improving shoulder stability and trunk stability while also enhancing lower-body muscular endurance.

Prerequisites

- Good shoulder and trunk stability.
- No previous shoulder injury.
- Good shoulder range of motion.

Steps

- Begin by holding the sandbag overhead using a neutral or overhand grip (*a*).
- Maintain a rigid torso and squat downward until the upper thighs are approximately parallel to the floor (*b*).
- At the bottom of the movement, the arms should remain fully extended.
- While keeping the bag overhead, extend the ankles, knees, and hip to return to the starting position. Picture yourself pushing your feet through the floor while you keep the arms and shoulders locked, keep the chest up, and extend the hips.

Key Points

- To ensure equal weight distribution throughout the forefoot and heel, the knees should remain in alignment with the toes and the whole foot should remain flat on the floor during the entire movement.

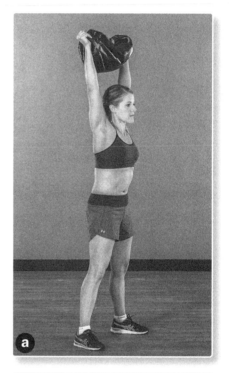

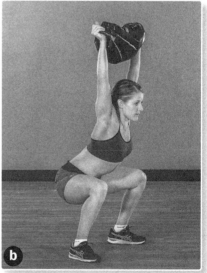

Sandbag Farmer's Walk

Intended Uses

Farmer's walks are used primarily for developing trunk stability and grip strength. The dynamic shifting of the sand within the tubes creates active resistance similar to what many athletes experience during competition.

Prerequisites

- Good trunk stability and grip strength.
- Ability to perform a deadlift.
- Sufficient strength to lift two sandbags simultaneously.

Steps

- Begin by standing with one sandbag just outside each foot.
- Squat down, set the back, and using an overhand grip simultaneously pick up both sandbags.
- Walk 30 feet (10 m) to a predetermined marker while carrying a sandbag in each hand (a-b).
- Round the marker and return to the starting line before dropping the bags.

Variations

- Increase the weight of each bag.
- Travel a greater distance.
- Lift the bags by the ends and lift them overhead to increase the stability demands placed on the trunk and shoulders as the bags swing back and forth.
- Perform a suitcase carry in which you use only one bag. This variation increases the demands on the trunk to stabilize on the side opposite the weight (if you are carrying the weight in the right hand, the left side of the trunk must work harder to stabilize).

Key Points

- Keep the back set throughout the duration of this movement.

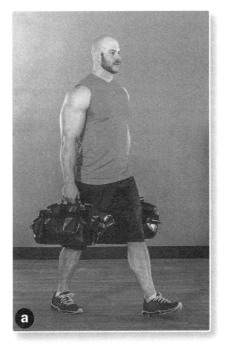

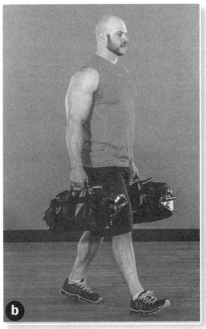

Sandbag Push-Up to Overhead Press

Intended Uses

This exercise is a total-body agility and coordination drill that can be used to improve trunk stability and overall upper-body muscular endurance.

Prerequisites

- No preexisting shoulder injuries.
- Ability to perform a push-up with good form and technique.

Steps

- Begin by assuming a push-up position while using a neutral grip to hold the sandbag (*a*).
- Perform a push-up (*b*) and then rapidly drive the knees toward the chest (*c*). Stand up while simultaneously lifting the sandbag to the rack position (*d*).

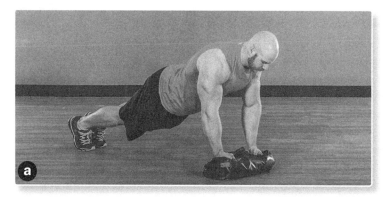

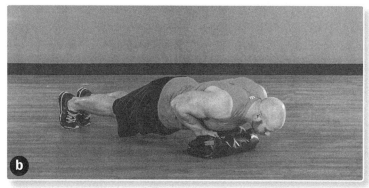

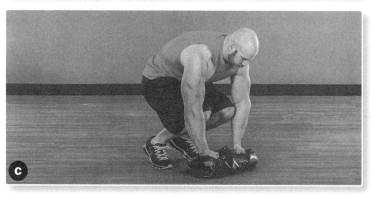

- When standing, perform an overhead press (*e*).
- Keep the sandbag close to the body and lower it to the knees. Then lower it back to the ground and return to the starting position.

Key Points

- Keep the sandbag close to the body while lifting it from the ground to reduce the stress placed on the lower back.

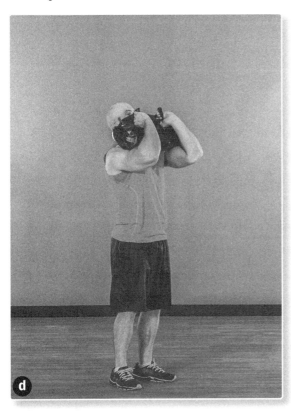

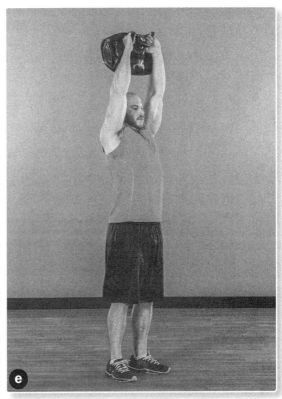

Sandbag Y Press

Intended Uses

The Y press adds a rotational element to the overhead press and can be used to enhance trunk stability and mobility.

Prerequisites

- No preexisting shoulder injuries.
- Ability to perform an overhead press correctly.
- Good trunk range of motion.

Steps

- Grab the sandbag using a neutral grip (*a*). Then assume a three-quarter squat position and rest the bag on the midthighs.
- In one smooth and controlled movement, lift the bag to shoulder level and then press it overhead while pivoting on the right foot, allowing the trunk to turn so that the torso is facing the left (*b*).
- When the bag is overhead, allow the arms to bend while simultaneously pivoting the right foot and lowering the bag back to the starting position.
- Repeat pivoting on the left foot and turning the trunk to the right while pressing the bag overhead.

Key Points

- When pivoting the back foot, think about what it is like to squash a bug when executing this movement.
- Keep the trunk braced and the back set throughout the exercise.
- Allow the back hip to pivot while keeping the front-leg foot positioned straight ahead.

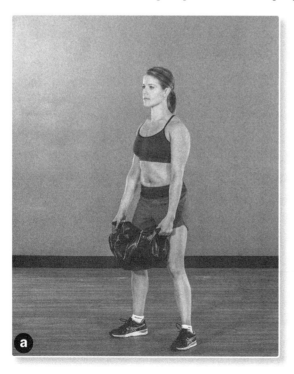

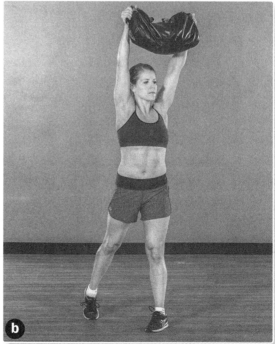

Sandbag Walkover Lunge

Intended Uses

This exercise is great for improving balance and trunk and hip stability while using an off-center load.

Prerequisites

- Ability to perform a lunge with proper technique.
- Ability to balance on one leg.

Steps

- Either position the sandbag on one shoulder or in the rack position.
- Set the back and keep the trunk braced.
- Take an exaggerated step backward with the right leg and perform a reverse lunge (*a*).
- Immediately push off with the left leg and lift the right leg up, driving the right knee toward the chest while maintaining good posture and alignment (*b*).
- Quickly step forward with the right leg into a forward lunge position.
- Push off the right leg, drive the left knee back toward the chest, and immediately repeat this sequence.
- Perform for the desired number of repetitions. If using rack position, then place the bag on the left shoulder and repeat on the opposite leg.

Key Points

- Always make certain that both legs receive equal amounts of work.
- Keep the hips squared the entire time and do not let the trunk or pelvis rotate.

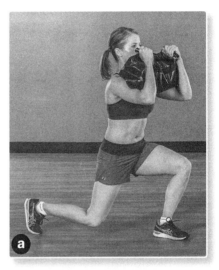

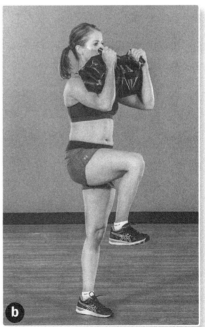

Sandbag Swing and Lift

Intended Uses

This exercise helps improve trunk mobility and rotational power. This drill is a prerequisite to the squat and lift exercise.

Prerequisites

- No preexisting back injuries.
- Good range of motion through the trunk.

Steps

- While holding the bag with a neutral grip, assume a three-quarter squat position and rest the bag on the right hip (*a*).
- While keeping the sandbag close to the torso, rotate the trunk and lift the bag across the body, allowing it to land on the left shoulder (*b*).
- Swing the bag back to the starting position and repeat for the desired number of repetitions. Then reposition the bag on the opposite hip and lift it to the right shoulder for the same number of reps.

Key Points

- Keep the trunk braced.
- Do not allow the shoulders to round while performing this movement.

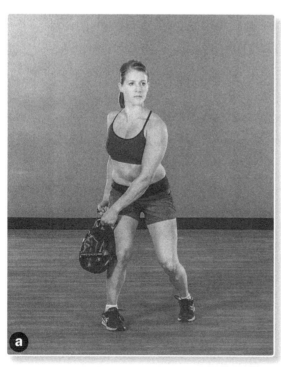
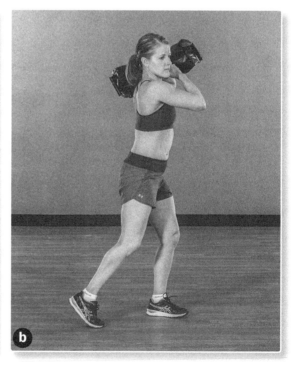

Sandbag High Pull

Intended Uses

This exercise looks similar to the upright row, but the sandbag high pull emphasizes greater speed of movement.

Prerequisites

- No preexisting shoulder injuries.

Steps

- Begin by standing in the universal athletic position (chest up, shoulders back, and a slight bend in the ankles, knees, and hips) while holding the sandbags just below the knees using an overhand grip (*a*).
- Keep the arms straight and set the back.
- Simultaneously extend the ankles, knees, and hips while explosively shrugging the shoulders.
- Allow the arms to bend and drive the elbows straight up until the sandbags are at chest level (*b*).
- While maintaining good body alignment and control, lower the sandbags back to the starting position.

Key Points

- Keep the arms straight and allow the force generated by the ankles, knees, and hips to propel the sandbags upward.
- Generate enough force so that the arms can passively bend to get the sandbags to chest level (unlike the upright row, in which the muscles of the arms and shoulders predominately lift the weight).

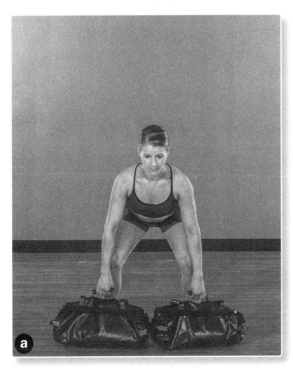
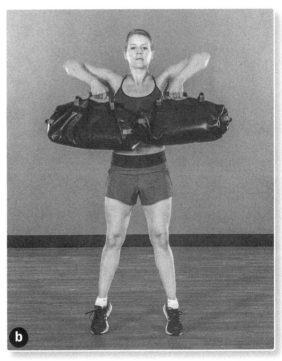

Sandbag Push Press

Intended Uses

The sandbag push press is an effective exercise for training the shoulders and building total-body coordination and power.

Prerequisites

- Good shoulder and trunk stability.
- Good shoulder range of motion.
- No current shoulder injuries.

Steps

- Grab the sandbag using an overhand or neutral grip.
- Set the back and lift the sandbag to shoulder level.
- Move the sandbag into the rack position.
- Quickly dip about 6 inches (15 cm) by simultaneously bending the ankle, knees, and hips (*a*).
- Without pausing, quickly drive, or push, the sandbag overhead by extending the hips, knees, and arms (*b*).
- Allow the arms to bend, returning the sandbag to its starting position.

Key Points

- Remember this technique by using the mnemonic "Dip and drive."

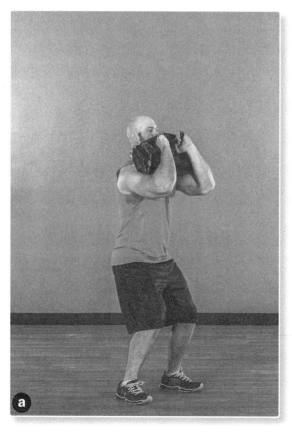 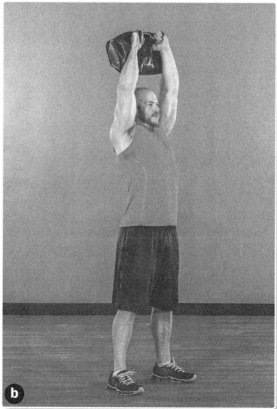

Sandbag Jerk

Intended Uses

Like the sandbag push press, this exercise is excellent for developing total-body coordination and power.

Prerequisites

- Good trunk and shoulder stability.
- Good shoulder range of motion.
- No preexisting shoulder injuries.
- Ability to perform the sandbag push press.

Steps

- Grab the sandbag using an overhand or neutral grip.
- Set the back and lift the sandbag to shoulder level.
- Move the sandbag into the rack position.
- Quickly dip about 6 inches (15 cm) by simultaneously bending the ankle, knees, and hips (*a*).
- Without pausing, quickly drive, or push, the sandbag overhead by extending the hips, knees, and arms.
- As the sandbag is traveling upward, rapidly drop the body 6 to 8 inches (15 to 20 cm) underneath the sandbag while allowing the arms to reach full extension (*b*).
- Stand up straight while keeping the sandbag overhead with the arms fully extended.
- Allow the arms to bend, returning the sandbag to its starting position.

Key Points

- Remember this technique by using the mnemonic "Dip, drive, and then drop."
- When dropping beneath the sandbag, concentrate on pushing yourself *under* the sandbag, rather than pushing the sandbag overhead.

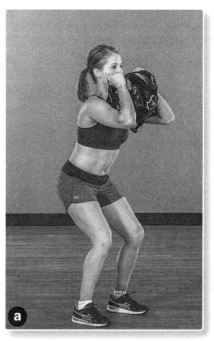

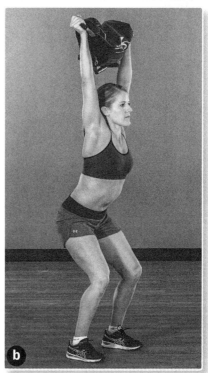

Sandbag Clean

Intended Uses

The sandbag clean is an advanced exercise that helps to improve total-body coordination and power.

Prerequisites

- Ability to perform the high pull and front squat exercises.

Steps

- Begin by squatting down to hold the sandbag just below the knees using an overhand grip (*a*).
- Keep the arms straight and set the back.
- Simultaneously extend the ankles, knees, and hips while explosively shrugging the shoulders.
- Allow the arms to bend and drive the elbows straight up until the sandbag is at chest level (*b*).
- As the bag is traveling upward, quickly drop the body 6 to 8 inches (15 to 20 cm) downward.
- When the bag is at its maximal height, rotate the elbows forward and up toward the sky to catch the sandbag in a rack position (*c*).
- While maintaining good body alignment and control, lower the sandbag back to the starting position.

Variations

- To add variety and increase the difficulty of this exercise, combine the sandbag clean with a push press or jerk.

Key Points

- Maintain proper posture and good body control throughout the duration of this exercise.
- Keep the knees aligned with the second toes and keep the hips aligned with the knees.
- Never sacrifice technique for greater speed or volume when using this exercise.

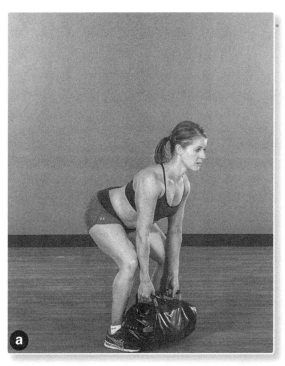

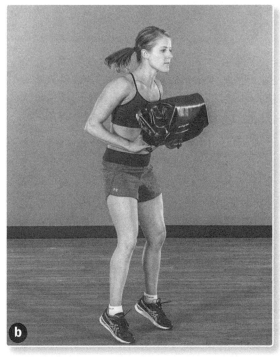

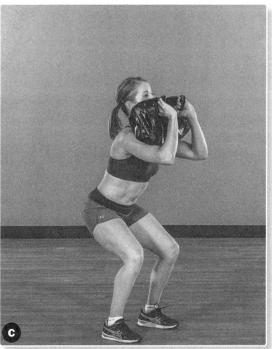

Sandbag Squat to Carry

Intended Uses

This exercise provides asymmetrical loading, which helps to improve balance and trunk stability.

Prerequisites

- Good trunk stability and range of motion.
- No preexisting back injuries.

Steps

- Begin by placing the sandbag on the ground between the feet.
- Squat down and grab the bag using a neutral grip (*a*).
- Lift the bag as quickly as possible to shoulder height.
- Allow the sandbag to land on the shoulder (*b*).
- Return the bag to the beginning position and then repeat this procedure, lifting it to the opposite shoulder.

Key Points

- Do not allow the trunk to flex when lifting the bag from the floor.
- Use a rapid extension of the hips and glutes to generate the force needed to lift the bag to shoulder level.

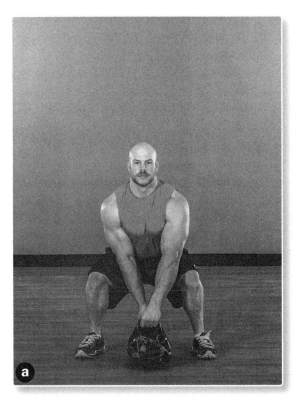
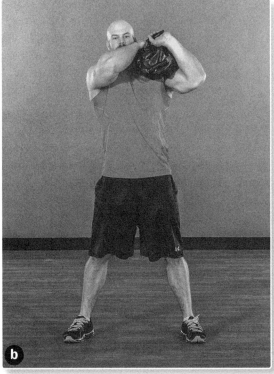

INTRODUCTORY PROGRAM

The introductory program is designed to familiarize you with using sandbags. This program requires you to learn how to adjust and shift your weight to control the active resistance created by the sandbags. You should perform this program twice a week. Because it is a circuit program, you perform each exercise for a specific time. Then, with as little rest as possible, you perform the next exercise. After you have performed each of the exercises, rest for one to two minutes and then do another round of the circuit. The introductory program is shown in table 9.2.

Table 9.2 Sample Introductory Program

Exercise	Repetitions
Sandbag Romanian deadlift, p. 162	10
Sandbag upright row, p. 169	10
Sandbag front squat, p. 163	10
Sandbag bent-over row, p. 168	10
Sandbag overhead press, p. 167	10

CHAPTER 10

Alternative Training Formats

Chapters 4 through 9 cover a wide variety of training formats. Although the exercises in these chapters are some of our favorites, we have only scratched the surface of training possibilities. Several other implements can be used for maximal interval training. As with the exercises already covered, the drills in this chapter can be used as a stand-alone method of training or combined with other types to add variety to a training session.

RESISTANCE BANDS

Resistance bands are extremely versatile and portable pieces of equipment. They take up little space, easily fit in a backpack or suitcase, and allow you to take your workout on the go. For these reasons, they are an ideal piece of equipment for frequent travelers.

Another benefit of resistance bands is that users can adjust the intensity, or training load, to their strength and fitness levels. Thicker bands typically provide more resistance, whereas thinner bands provide less resistance (figure 10.1). But by simply shortening the length of the band or increasing the distance between the attachment point and distal end of the band, resistance can be increased. Thus, these bands can be adjusted to suit a wide range of people with varying abilities. The following are just a few examples of the many options available when using resistance bands.

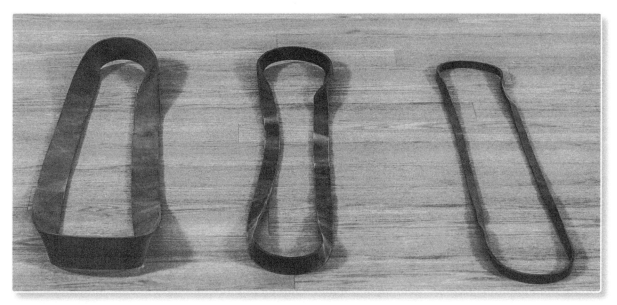

Figure 10.1 Resistance bands with varying degrees of resistance.

Heavy Resistance Band Standing Row

Intended Uses

The purpose of the heavy band row is to increase local muscular endurance in the muscles of the rhomboids and middle trapezius.

Prerequisites

- Good shoulder strength and stability.
- Good trunk stability.

Steps

- Wrap the heavy band around a stationary object, such as a squat rack or pole.
- While holding each end of the band, assume an athletic position by bending the ankles, knees, and hips slightly and setting the back.
- Back away from the attachment point until the arms are fully extended (*a*).
- Pull the band toward the middle of the torso (*b*) and then extend the arms in a controlled manner until the bands return to the staring position.
- Repeat for the desired number of repetitions.

Key Points

- Perform this exercise as quickly as possible while maintaining control of the resistance band. Do not allow the band to snap back; instead, control the eccentric (lowering) portion of the movement.
- Select a band that creates enough tension so that you are able to perform only 20 to 25 repetitions with proper form and technique before fatiguing.

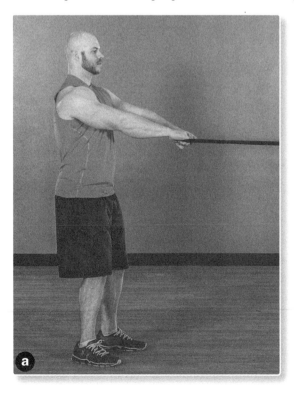

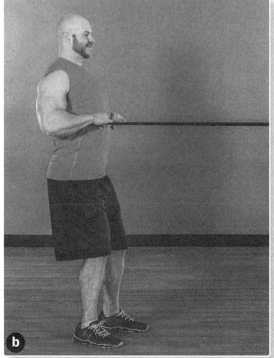

Heavy Resistance Band Standing Chest Press

Intended Uses

The purpose of the band press is to improve local muscular endurance in the muscles of the chest, shoulders, and triceps.

Prerequisites

- Good shoulder strength and stability.
- Good trunk stability.

Steps

- Place the heavy band across the upper portion of your back.
- While holding each end, position the band so that the hands are just under the armpits (*a*).
- Assume an athletic position by bending the ankles, knees, and hips slightly and setting the back.
- Extend both arms and press the ends of the band away from the body, while using your torso as an anchor (*b*).
- Return to the starting position in a controlled manner and repeat for the desired number of repetitions.

Key Points

- Perform this exercise as quickly as possible while maintaining control of the resistance band. Do not allow the band to snap back; instead, control the downward phase of the movement.
- Select a band that creates enough tension so that you are able to perform only 20 to 25 repetitions with proper form and technique before fatiguing.

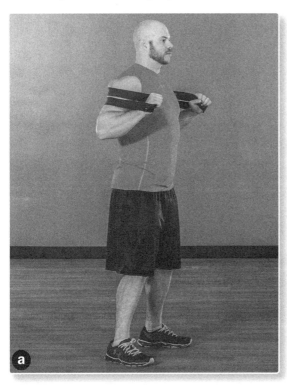
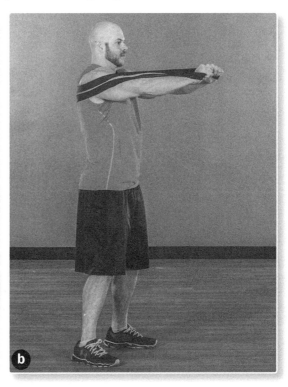

Resistance Band Push-Up

Intended Uses

The purpose of the band push-up is to increase the intensity and resistance used when performing a traditional push-up.

Prerequisites

- Good upper-body strength.

Steps

- Assume a push-up position and, while stabilizing the ends of a band under each hand, stretch the middle portion of the band around your back, across the shoulder blades (*a*).
- In a controlled manner, lower yourself to the ground and begin performing push-ups as described in chapter 3 (*b*).

Key Points

- Maintain a rigid torso throughout the exercise movement (i.e., do not allow the hips to sag or the back to arch).
- Lower yourself in a slow, controlled manner and then explode when extending the arms and pressing yourself away from the floor.

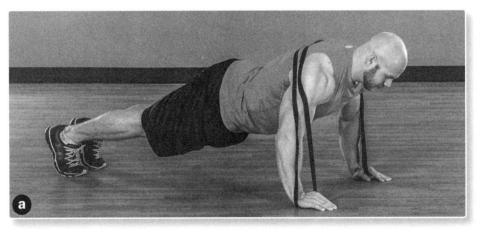

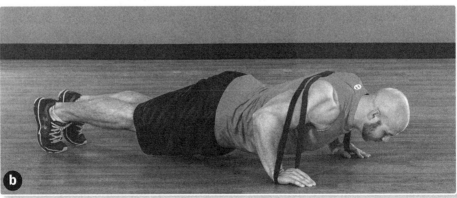

Resistance Band Assisted Pull-Up

Intended Uses

This exercise can be used to strengthen the muscles of the upper back.

Prerequisites

- No preexisting shoulder injuries.

Steps

- Lay the middle of a resistance band over the top of a pull-up bar. Then take one end of the band and pull it through the center of the other end so that it secures the band to the bar.
- Place one foot through the loop and allow the end of the band to hook under the foot.
- Reach overhead and grab the pull-up bar using an overhand grip (*a*).
- Allow the tension created on the band to assist you in performing the pull-up (*b*).

Key Points

- Be careful getting in and out of the band attachment. If you perform the exercise incorrectly, the band may inadvertently slip and cause injury.
- Keep the ankle of the band leg flexed at all times (i.e., pull the toes toward the shins).

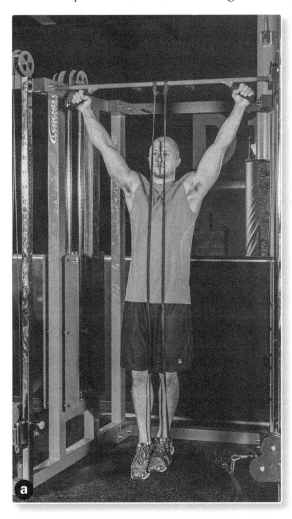 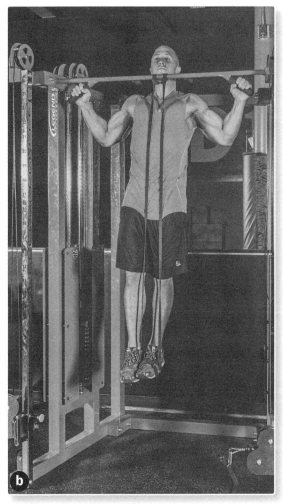

Heavy Resistance Band Squat

Intended Uses

This exercise is primarily used to increase lower-body muscular endurance.

Prerequisites

■ Good form and technique when performing the squat exercise with body weight.

Steps

■ Take a heavy band and drape it over your neck so that the center portion is resting on the back of the neck.

■ Squat down and bring the band around the outside portion of the feet, anchoring the band under the middle portion of each foot (*a*).

■ Set the back and extend the knees and hips until you are back in a standing position (*b*).

■ Repeat for the desired number of repetitions.

Key Points

■ At the lowest portion of the squat exercise, minimal to no tension should be on the band. As you begin to stand, the tension of the band should progressively increase.

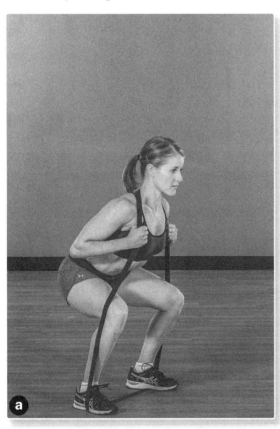
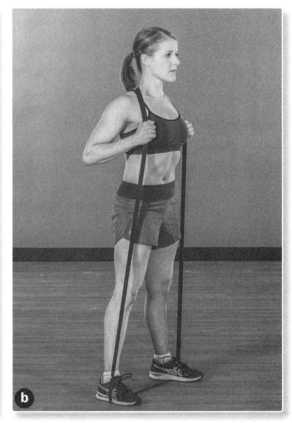

WATER-FILLED STABILITY BALLS

Similar to sandbag training, training with water-filled items provides a dynamic resistance that is inherently unstable when moved. Kegs, log bars, and slosh pipes are commonly incorporated into traditional resistance-training programs as a way to unload the joints after heavy training, improve joint and trunk stability, and add novel training stimuli to reduce boredom and staleness that may lead to overtraining. In many cases, however, water-filled implements may be expensive or difficult to come by. The following exercises were designed for use with water-filled stability balls. When filled with water, stability balls afford the user many of the benefits seen with the use of the implements previously mentioned, but they typically cost much less and if dropped they are less likely to cause damage to property or injuries to people.

The following exercises using a water-filled stability ball incorporate many large-muscle groups and diverse movement patterns.

Creating a Water-Filled Stability Ball

Step 1: Air up the ball to three-quarters of its capacity.

Step 2: Hold the nozzle of a garden hose firmly against the inflation site and then slowly turn the water on until the ball is at the desired weight. The water be must turned on slowly and the nozzle held firmly against the ball to minimize the amount of water spilled. Do this outdoors so that spillage is not a problem.

Step 3: Use a bathroom scale to ensure that the ball is filled to the desired weight.

Step 4: After the ball is filled to the desired level, pressurize it using an air pump.

Step 5: Insert the plug into the inflation site.

Water-Filled Stability Ball Lift

Intended Uses

This exercise improves lower-body and trunk endurance, strength, and stability.

Prerequisites

- Ability to perform a squat correctly.

Steps

- Fill a Swiss ball with water to the desired weight.
- Squat down (a), set the back, and pick up the ball (b).
- When you are in a full upright and standing position, drop the ball and repeat the process.

Key Points

- Keep the back set throughout the duration of the exercise.
- Maintain proper squatting technique throughout the movement.

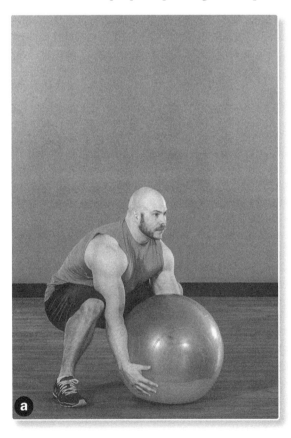
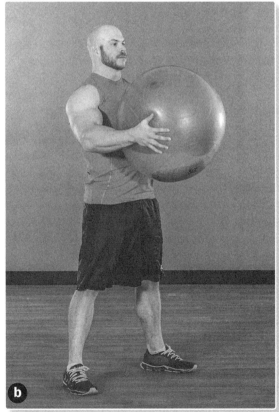

Water-Filled Stability Ball Squat

Intended Uses

This exercise improves lower-body and trunk endurance, strength, and stability.

Prerequisites

- Ability to perform a squat correctly.

Steps

- Fill a Swiss ball with water to the desired resistance.
- Squat down, set the back, and pick up the ball (*a-b*).
- While keeping the back set, repeat this action for a set time or the desired number of repetitions.

Key Points

- Keep the back set throughout the duration of the exercise.
- Maintain proper squatting technique throughout the movement.

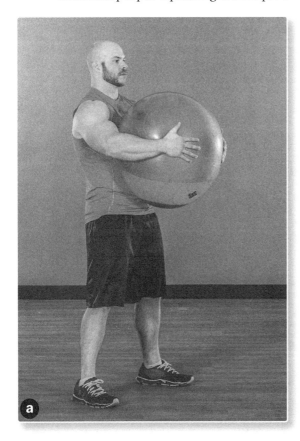
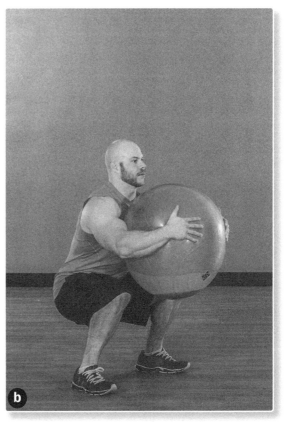

Water-Filled Stability Ball Carry

Intended Uses

The water-filled stability ball carry is an alternative to the classic Atlas stone carry seen in strong-man competitions.

Prerequisites

- Good trunk strength and stability.

Steps

- Fill a Swiss ball with water to the desired resistance.
- Squat down, set the back, and pick up the ball.
- Place two markers approximately 10 meters apart.
- While carrying the ball, walk back and forth between the two markers as many times as possible during a set time (*a-b*).

Key Points

- Maintain a rigid torso throughout the duration of the exercise.
- Do not run during this exercise because doing so may cause an injury. The sloshing water creates an active resistance that you must control and stabilize to perform the exercise safely. Make certain that one foot is in contact with the ground at all times.

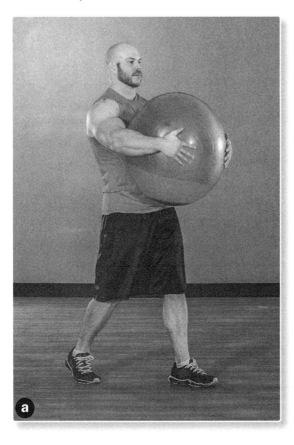

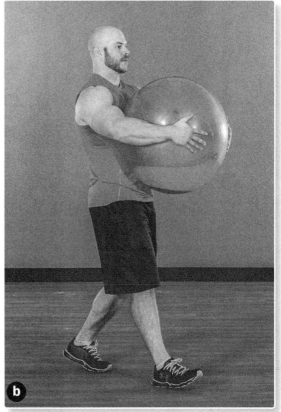

WEIGHTED TRAINING SLEDS

Training sleds are generally used for speed development, but when they are loaded above 10 percent of total body weight, the emphasis shifts from speed of movement to training the glycolytic energy system. The following sled drills combine traditional weight plates, ropes, and suspension-training systems that can challenge even the strongest people.

Sled Push

Intended Uses

This exercise improves force production capabilities and mimics certain combative and sport situations in which people attempt to move or redirect an opponent.

Prerequisites

- No preexisting lower back, ankle, knee, or hip injuries.

Steps

- Load a training sled with approximately 20 to 30 percent of your body weight.
- Grab the handlebars, set the back, and drive the knee of one leg toward the chest while forcefully extending the ankle, knee, and hip of the other leg to drive the sled forward (*a-b*).
- Push the sled for a set distance or a predetermined time.

Key Points

- Maintain a rigid trunk throughout the duration of the exercise.
- Do not round the shoulders while driving the sled forward.
- Focus on pushing the ground away with every stride.

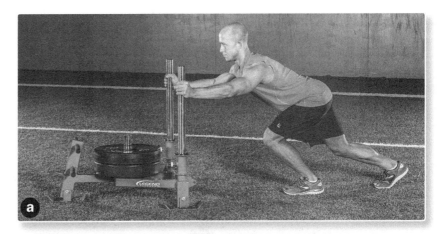

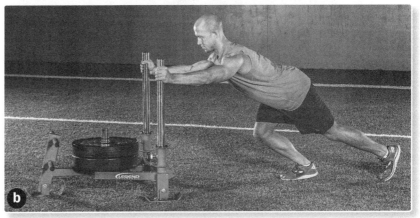

Sled Pull

Intended Uses

Sled pulls increase muscular endurance in the muscles of the upper back and biceps.

Prerequisites

- Ability to perform three to five pull-ups.

Steps

- Attach a 25- to 30-foot (8 to 9 m) rope to a training sled.
- Pull the rope until it is taut. Then, facing the sled, set the back and assume an athletic stance (chest up, shoulders back, and a slight bend in the ankles, knees, and hips).
- Using an overhand grip, pull the sled toward you using a hand-over-hand grip (*a-b*).

Key Points

- Maintain a rigid torso and do not allow the back to round.

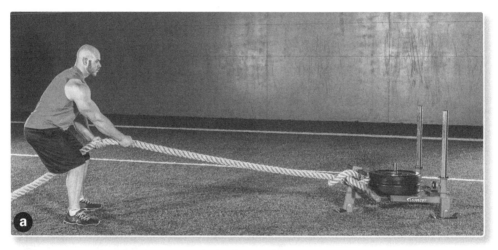

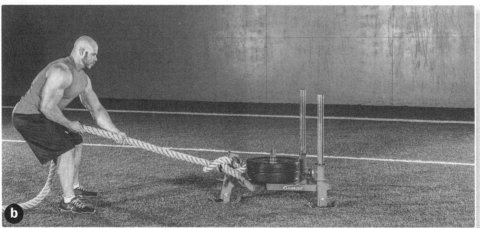

Sled Drag

Intended Uses

The sled drags improves muscular endurance of the lower body, especially the quadriceps muscles.

Prerequisites

- No preexisting lower-back, ankle, knee, or hip injuries.

Steps

- Begin by attaching a TRX suspension-training system to the training sled.
- Load the sled with a resistance approximately 20 to 30 percent of your body weight.
- While facing the sled, grab the handles, extend the arms, and assume an athletic position.
- Walk backward 20 to 30 meters while dragging the sled (*a-b*).

Key Points

- Maintain a rigid trunk throughout the exercise.
- Do not round the shoulders while dragging the sled forward.

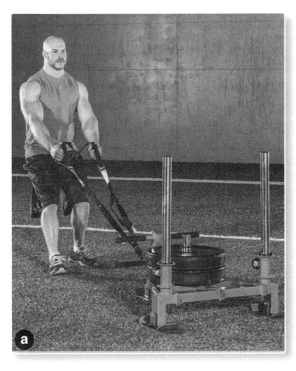
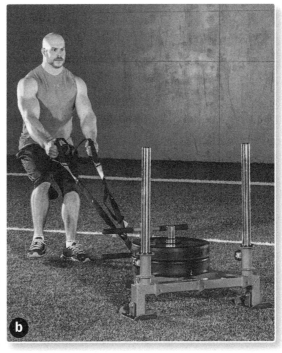

HEAVY BOXING BAGS

Boxing drills using a heavy bag can be extremely demanding physically and are an excellent way to improve overall agility, balance, stamina, and coordination. The following drills were selected based on their simplicity and their ability to be combined into a large number of movement combinations.

Heavy Boxing Bag Jab

Intended Uses

Jabs, along with other boxing drills, are excellent conditioning drills for improving aerobic and anaerobic fitness.

Prerequisites

- No preexisting hand, wrist, or elbow injuries.

Steps

- Put on a pair of boxing or speed gloves and position yourself a little less than an arm's reach from the heavy bag.
- Place your feet at approximately shoulder-width and stagger the feet using a basic toe-heel alignment.
- Keep the torso upright, the trunk braced, the front foot mostly forward, the back foot turned out, and the shoulders slightly turned toward the heavy bag.
- Relax the upper body, keep the elbows pointed down, and positon your back fist near your chin and the front fist about 1 foot (30 cm) in front of the back glove (a).
- Slightly bend the ankles, knees, and hips.
- In this position, lean the trunk slightly forward, hold the rear glove slightly higher than the front, and have the palms facing one another.
- Simultaneously shift your weight from the back foot (while keeping it on the ground) to the front foot while extending the lead arm.
- As you throw the jab, turn the palm downward.
- Connect with the bag, maintaining a slight bend in the elbow at contact (b).
- Quickly return to the starting positon and then proceed with another jab or the appropriate punch combination.

Key Points

- Do not hyperextend the elbow when punching.
- Focus on throwing the jab from the shoulder.
- Do not tuck your thumbs.
- Tighten up your fist only on impact to maximize speed of movement.

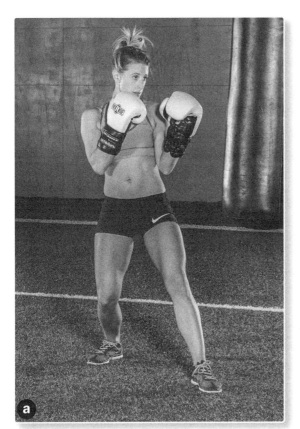

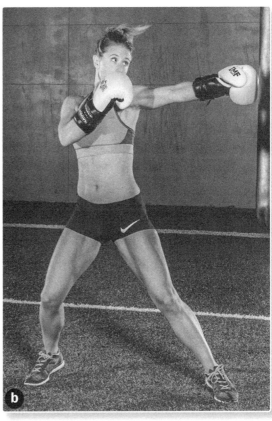

Heavy Boxing Bag Cross

Intended Uses

The cross is a more powerful punch than the jab. This punch can be used to create punch combinations that are effective for aerobic and anaerobic conditioning.

Prerequisites

- No preexisting hand, wrist, or elbow injuries.

Steps

- Put on a pair of boxing or speed gloves and position yourself a little less than an arm's reach from the heavy bag.
- Place your feet at approximately shoulder-width and stagger the feet using a basic toe-heel alignment.
- Keep the torso upright, the trunk braced, the front foot mostly forward, the back foot turned out, and the shoulders slightly turned toward the heavy bag.
- Relax the upper body, keep the elbows pointed down, and positon your back fist near your chin and the front fist about 1 foot (30 cm) in front of the back glove.
- Slightly bend the ankles, knees, and hips.
- In this position, lean the trunk slightly forward, hold the rear glove slightly higher than the front, and have the palms facing one another (a).
- Simultaneously shift your weight from the back foot (while keeping it on the ground) to the front foot, pull the lead hand back to protect the face, and throw the back hand at the target (b).
- Rotate the hips (counterclockwise for a right-hander and clockwise for a left-hander) to generate more power.
- Connect with the bag, maintaining a slight bend in the elbow at contact.
- Quickly return to the starting positon and then proceed with the next punch.

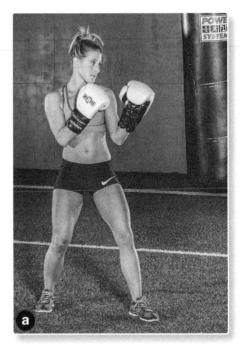

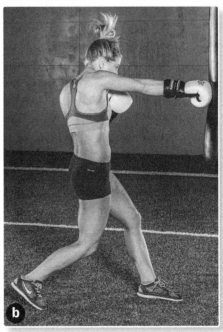

Key Points

- Do not hyperextend the elbow when punching.
- Focus on throwing the punch from the shoulder.
- Do not tuck your thumbs.
- Tighten up your fist only on impact to maximize speed of movement.

Heavy Boxing Bag Hook

Intended Uses

The hook is a more powerful punch than the jab. This punch can be used to create punch combinations that are effective for aerobic and anaerobic conditioning.

Prerequisites

- No preexisting hand, wrist, or elbow injuries.

Steps

- Put on a pair of boxing or speed gloves and position yourself a little less than an arm's reach from the heavy bag.
- Place your feet at approximately shoulder-width and stagger the feet using a basic toe-heel alignment.
- Keep the torso upright, the trunk braced, the front foot mostly forward, the back foot turned out, and the shoulders slightly turned toward the heavy bag.
- Relax the upper body, keep the elbows pointed down, and positon your back fist near your chin and the front fist about 1 foot (30 cm) in front of the back glove.
- Slightly bend the ankles, knees, and hips.
- In this position, lean the trunk slightly forward, hold the rear glove slightly higher than the front, and have the palms facing one another (*a*).
- While keeping the back foot planted, simultaneously rotate the hips inward by pivoting on the toes of the front foot and shifting the weight to the back foot.
- As you pivot, the lead arm should be bent at a 90-degree angle and the forearm should be parallel to the ground at the point of impact (*b*).
- Connect with the bag, maintaining the bend in the elbow at contact.
- Quickly return to the starting positon and then proceed with the next punch.

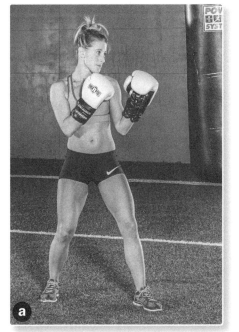

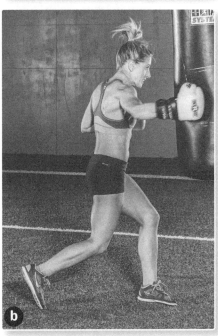

Key Points

- Do not elevate the elbow higher than the forearm when punching.
- Focus on throwing the punch from the shoulder.
- Do not tuck your thumbs.
- Tighten up your fist only on impact to maximize speed of movement.

Heavy Boxing Bag Walking Lunge

Intended Uses

The heavy bag walking lunge is a good exercise for improving trunk stability through use of an off-centered load.

Prerequisites

- Good trunk strength and stability.
- No preexisting lower-body or back injuries.

Steps

- While maintaining a good athletic positon, set the back, lift the heavy bag from the ground, and put it over one shoulder (*a*).
- Lunge forward with the opposite-side leg while keeping the bag in positon on the other shoulder (*b*).
- Drive off the front leg, come to a full standing positon, and then lunge out on the opposite leg.
- Continue lunging forward, alternating legs, for a given distance or set time.
- On subsequent sets, shift the load to the other shoulder so that you train both sides of the trunk equally.

Key Points

- Maintain a rigid torso throughout the duration of the exercise.
- Do not allow the knee of the lead foot to pass in front of the toes.
- Keep the pelvis locked and pointed forward during the entire exercise. Do not allow the pelvis to rotate.

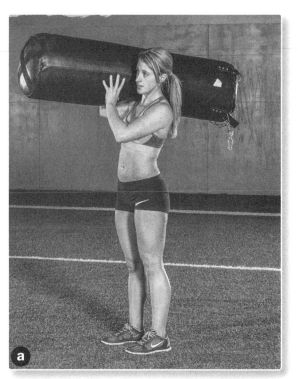

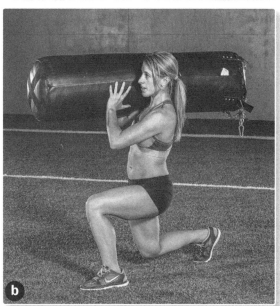

INTRODUCTORY ALTERNATIVE TRAINING PROGRAMS

The introductory program is meant to familiarize you with the various training exercises and modalities in this chapter. Some of the exercises are performed in a circuit fashion, whereas others may be performed over a specific distance. Table 10.1 covers a sample program for heavy resistance bands, table 10.2 shows a sample program for water-filled stability balls, table 10.3 displays a program for training sleds, and table 10.4 presents a program for heavy bags.

Table 10.1   Introductory Resistance Band Circuit-Training Program

Exercise	Repetitions
Heavy resistance band standing row, p. 186	15–20
Heavy resistance band standing chest press, p. 187	15–20
Heavy resistance band squat, p. 190	15–20
• Rest for 30 to 60 seconds and then repeat three or four times.	

Table 10.2   Introductory Water-Filled Stability Ball Program

Exercise	Repetitions
Water-filled stability ball lift, p. 192	10
Water-filled stability ball carry, p. 194	30 meters (15 down and back)
Water-filled stability ball squat, p. 193	10
• Rest for 30 to 60 seconds and then repeat three or four times.	

Table 10.3   Introductory Weighted Training Sled Program

Exercise	Repetitions
Sled push, p. 195	30 meters × 10
Sled drag, p. 197	30 meters × 10
Sled pull, p. 196	Using a 30- to 40-foot (9 to 12 m) rope × 10
• Perform as quickly as possible with good form and technique.	

Table 10.4 Introductory Heavy Boxing Bag Program

Exercise	Repetitions
ROUND 1	
Heavy boxing bag jab, p. 198	5
Heavy boxing bag cross, p. 200	5
Heavy boxing bag hook, p. 201	5

- Continue repeating these combinations for 3 minutes.
- Rest for 1 minute before moving to round 2.

Exercise	Repetitions
ROUND 2	
Heavy boxing bag jab, p. 198	3
Heavy boxing bag cross, p. 200	3
Heavy boxing bag hook , p. 201	3

- Continue repeating these combinations for 3 minutes.
- Rest for 1 minute before moving to round 3.

Exercise	Repetitions
ROUND 3	
Heavy boxing bag jab, p. 198	1
Heavy boxing bag cross, p. 200	1
Heavy boxing bag hook , p. 201	1

- Continue repeating these combinations for 3 minutes.
- Rest for 1 minute before moving to round 4.

ROUND 4 (FINAL ROUND)

- Perform any combination you wish for 1 minute at 90 to 100% effort.

PART III

Maximum Interval Program Design

CHAPTER 11

Testing Considerations and Variables

Testing is a critical step in the development of a training program. The first step in reaching your training goals is to figure out where you are. Think about how you use a GPS or other navigation system to get directions to a destination. If the GPS system can't establish where you are, it cannot tell you how to get where you want to go. Testing helps determine your current levels of health, fitness, and performance so that you can develop your roadmap to success.

Ideally, you would perform testing before, or within a few weeks of, beginning a training program to establish a baseline. Testing allows you to identify your strengths and weaknesses and determine the best way to maintain or improve physical abilities. Testing also allows you to reassess your fitness levels periodically to measure progress and gauge the effectiveness of your training program. In this chapter we discuss how to select the appropriate tests to measure these factors and how to ensure that you are getting the best information possible when performing each test.

TEST SELECTION

When determining what tests to select, the first thing to consider is the desired outcome of the training program. You can select from literally thousands of tests to measure health, fitness, and performance! But the feasibility of many of these tests, in terms of resources, time, and experience in performing and conducting them, is a key limiting factor. In chapter 12 we provide numerous examples of tests that measure both fitness and performance, are relatively easy to perform, and require minimal time, experience, and equipment to do well. Our aim is to present options to suit the goals of most readers, but we cannot possibly cover every possible test that might be applicable to a given sport or activity. Therefore, in this chapter we discuss in broad terms some of the factors to consider when selecting a test and ways to improve the results that you obtain from these measures.

Health- and Performance-Related Components of Fitness

Table 11.1 includes a list of the health- and performance-related components of fitness. Although the variables are often split into these two categories, understanding the distinction can be difficult, probably because most of these components are interrelated to some extent. For example, strength, speed, power, and mobility are all underpinning characteristics of agility. Therefore, a person who is deficient in one of these areas might also be hindered in terms of agility.

Table 11.1 Health- and Performance-Related Components of Fitness

HEALTH-RELATED COMPONENTS	
Muscular strength	Maximal amount of force that a muscle or muscle group can exert
Muscular endurance	Ability of a muscle or muscle group to sustain force over time
Mobility	Available range of motion around a joint
Cardiovascular fitness	Rate at which the body is able to oxidize available energy substrates (carbohydrate, protein, and fat) to sustain activity
Body composition	Total amount of lean mass compared with total mass, typically expressed as a percentage
PERFORMANCE-RELATED COMPONENTS	
Speed	Time required to move between two points
Agility	Ability to change direction rapidly and efficiently*
Balance	Ability to maintain or regain equilibrium over a fixed or moving base of support
Coordination	Ability to move fluidly and efficiently with good body control
Power	Ability to express force rapidly
Reaction time	Ability to process information rapidly and produce an appropriate moment response based on the stimuli

*True agility, versus change-of-direction speed, requires a stimulus to initiate the movement response.

Health Assessment

Health is the foundation of fitness and performance. Therefore, to attain optimal levels of fitness and performance, good health is essential. For this reason, some basic health assessments should be performed before testing or beginning an exercise program. At minimum, a basic health-risk appraisal should be performed before you begin an exercise program. The Physical Activity Readiness Questionnaire (PAR-Q) is a good tool for people who are participating in a self-guided exercise program (Spivey 2010). This questionnaire has been recognized as a good minimal prescreening for low- to moderate-level activity. If you answer yes to any of the questions listed in the PAR-Q, a more comprehensive evaluation by a qualified medical professional is warranted. To complete the questions listed in the PAR-Q, visit www.csep.ca/cmfiles/publications/parq/par-q.pdf.

Needs or Goals Analysis

When selecting tests, the best approach is to begin with the end in mind. In other words, what are the desired outcomes of your training program and how can you make certain that you have attained these goals? Generally, this process begins with performing a needs, or goals, analysis. Within this analysis, you should consider several factors, including the physiological, metabolic, and biomechanical demands of the activity in which you are seeking to make improvements. The following are a few questions that you should address before selecting which assessments to perform.

1. **What are the main muscles or muscle groups needed to perform the target activity, and what actions are they performing?**

    Are these muscles primarily used for strength and power movements in this activity (Type II fast-twitch muscle fibers) or endurance (Type I slow-twitch muscle fibers)? For instance, distance running uses predominately Type I muscle fibers, whereas sprinting uses predominately Type II muscle fibers. For this reason, strength and power tests would likely be better predictors of sprint performance than muscular endurance tests. Similarly, tests that assess muscular endurance of the trunk would likely be better predictors of potential injury for endurance athletes who must attempt to stabilize these muscles against gravity for long periods, especially under fatigue when mechanics may be compromised.

Generally, muscles produce force (muscle fibers shorten to accelerate), reduce force (muscle fibers elongate to decelerate the body or limbs), and stabilize the body (tension is developed in the muscle fibers, but no real change in the length of the fiber is realized).

2. **What range of motion and what type and duration of power are necessary for the activity?**

Most endurance activities, such as distance running, require smaller ranges of motion and require more sustained power over long distances for extended periods. In contrast, most explosive activities, such as sprinting and jumping, typically require greater ranges of motion and rapid force and power development over shorter distances.

Therefore, although ROM is important for both groups of athletes to improve performance and reduce injury risk, athletes who perform explosive actions are likely to have greater dynamic ROM at certain joints because they are required to move the body through these ranges more frequently. These athletes would benefit from this type of testing and training.

3. **What energy systems (phosphagen, glycolytic, aerobic) are used and in what amounts?**

During various activities, different energy systems are called on to help provide energy. The ATP–PCr system is essential for exercises that require short bursts of explosive activity lasting less than 15 seconds. When the fuel sources for this energy system have been exhausted, the glycolytic energy system can be used to help supply energy to the body from stored carbohydrate (glycogen). As these energy supplies become depleted, generally within two to three minutes of moderate- to high-intensity activity, the body begins to rely more on the aerobic, or oxidative, energy system to provide energy. This system becomes more active in the production of energy when energy needs to be sustained for greater than two or three minutes. Consequently, the intensity of the exercise is lower than it is during anaerobic activity.

But a tradeoff between intensity and time is at play here, meaning that the longer the duration of the activity is, the lower the intensity must be to sustain the activity. Thus, the primary energy system called on to provide energy is based largely on the intensity and duration of the activity. Table 11.2 shows the relationship between intensity and duration for the energy systems. Table 11.3 shows the approximate energy contribution by energy system for each activity.

To attain the desired training goals, a basic knowledge of which energy systems are needed for an activity or sport is essential. Using the concept of specificity, we know that we should train the energy system that we want to augment. For example, doing

Table 11.2 Energy Utilization by Intensity and Duration

Duration of event	Event intensity	Primary energy system
0–6 seconds	Extremely high	Phosphagen
6–30 seconds	Very high	Phosphagen and fast glycolytic
30–120 seconds	High	Fast glycolytic
2–3 minutes	Moderate	Fast glycolytic and oxidative
>3 minutes	Low	Oxidative

Reprinted, by permission, from J.T. Kramer, 2008, Bioenergetics of exercise and training. In *Essentials of strength training and conditioning*, 3rd ed., edited for the National Strength and Conditioning Association by T.R Baechle and R.W. Earle (Champaign, IL: Human Kinetics), 32.

Table 11.3 Primary Metabolic Demands of Various Sports

Sport	Phosphagen system	Anaerobic glycolysis	Aerobic metabolism
Baseball	High	Low	—
Basketball	High	Moderate to high	—
Boxing	High	High	Moderate
Field events	High	—	—
Field hockey	High	Moderate	Moderate
Football (American)	High	Moderate	Low
Ice hockey	High	Moderate	Moderate
Lacrosse	High	Moderate	Moderate
Marathon	Low	Low	High
Mixed martial arts	High	High	Moderate
Power lifting	High	Low	Low
Soccer	High	Moderate	High
Strength competitions	High	Moderate to high	Low
Swimming:			
• Short distance	High	Moderate	—
• Long distance	—	Moderate	High
Tennis	High	—	—
Track (athletics):			
• Short distance	High	Moderate	—
• Long distance	—	Moderate	High
Ultraendurance events	Low	Low	High
Volleyball	High	Moderate	—
Wrestling	High	High	Moderate
Weightlifting	High	Low	Low

Note: All types of metabolism are involved to some extent in all activities.

Adapted, by permission, from N.A. Ratamess, 2008, Adaptations to anaerobic training programs. In *Essentials of strength training and conditioning*, 3rd ed., edited for the National Strength and Conditioning Association by T.R Baechle and R.W. Earle (Champaign, IL: Human Kinetics), 95.

long, slow distance testing and training activities with a shot-putter would likely have no positive effect on performance because shot putting relies on the ATP–PCr energy system. In fact, excessive endurance training may actually impede performance in this sport because it may increase the athlete's risk of overtraining. Conversely, an endurance athlete may benefit form training the ATP–PCr and glycolytic energy systems. But if the aerobic system is neglected, performance would be hindered because this energy system is crucial for long-duration events.

4. **What are common injuries, or injury sites, related to this activity?**

With most activities, injury is always a risk. For instance, during long runs the muscles of the trunk may become fatigued and make it difficult to maintain good posture. Therefore, distance runners may be prone to lower back issues. Good muscular endurance in this area may help alleviate some of the postural changes caused by fatigue in this population. Thus, improving muscular endurance of the trunk would be of interest. Based on this notion, the front and side plank tests may be useful for measuring improvements in this area.

Testing may also help us identify potential injury issues to address. For example, Emma is a high school volleyball athlete who successfully passed a squat assessment, but she was unable to perform the box step-off without her knees collapsing inward (valgus collapse). Because volleyball requires repeated jumps within a match, the repetitive stress of her landing in this irregular positon over time could result in injury. Therefore, jumping activities were contraindicated for Emma in her training program until she built up the requisite strength to absorb the landing with proper technique.

This area of assessment can be tricky and may require a bit more experience and expertise to administer. Therefore, seeking the assistance of a certified strength and conditioning specialist with training in this area may be beneficial. Chapter 12 includes a few basic movement screenings that help identify poor movement patterns that could lead to injury or warrant referral to a medical professional.

Validity and Reliability

Validity and reliability are major concepts related to testing. Validity is the ability of a test to produce an accurate measurement of a specific outcome or attribute, and a reliable test is one that is repeatable. For a test to be valid, it must be reliable, but a test can be reliable without being valid. For example, if a person selected a vertical jump assessment to measure lower-body strength, the test would be reliable as long as the same protocols and procedures were followed for each trial. But the test may not be valid for measuring strength because this test is primarily used for measuring power. These two variables are related, because people with stronger lower bodies generally tend to jump higher, but a more valid test of lower body strength would be a 1–3RM squat. Another example would be the push-up versus the 1.5 mile (2.4 km) run to test endurance. Both are endurance tests, but the run measures endurance of the cardiovascular system using primarily the lower body, whereas the push-up test measures upper-body muscular endurance. Both measure endurance, but they test different body regions and different systems (cardiovascular versus muscular endurance).

FACTORS THAT AFFECT TEST PERFORMANCE

To get the best information possible, the following factors should be considered before testing. Thinking about these aspects of testing will not only ensure that you get accurate information but also enhance safety.

Testing Area

Before testing, make certain that the testing area promotes safe and efficient testing. For any speed or agility assessments, use an open area free of clutter and sharp objects. Additionally, the space around the perimeter of the testing area should be sufficient to allow people to exit the testing area safely. For instance, for a 30-meter dash, allow at least 15 to 20 meters after the finish line to allow the person to slow down and stop without worrying about running into anything.

Environmental Conditions

Environmental conditions may affect the accuracy and safety of certain tests. For example, performing an aerobic endurance test indoors in a climate-controlled facility will likely produce the most reliable results. When the test is performed outside, factors such as wind, humidity, and ambient temperature can affect the results (Harman 2008). Outdoor testing becomes even more problematic when it is performed in an area that has wide temperature fluctuations throughout the year. If an initial test and follow-up test are performed under different circumstances (e.g., one test during the summer under high ambient temperatures and the other during the winter under much lower temperatures), the results will not be comparable. Additionally, when testing outside, especially during the summer months, particular attention must be paid to heat and humidity. If testing outside, the tests should be performed early or late in the day to avoid peak temperatures and reduce the potential for heat-related illness. Maintaining proper hydration status should also be a priority. For all these reasons, testing indoors provides the most consistent and typically the safest conditions.

Testing Surface

All testing should be performed on resilient flooring that has a nonslip surface to reduce the risk of slipping and falling. Furthermore, for athletes, testing on a surface similar to what they play on is best.

Testing Order

Test should be ordered in a manner so that one test does not significantly affect the subsequent test. For instance, if the beep test was performed before an agility test, agility performance may be negatively affected because of fatigue. Performing the agility test first would likely have less effect on the beep test, so the order in which these are performed should be switched. Based on the recommendations of Harman (2008), the following would be considered the best testing sequence to use when doing multiple tests:

- Nonfatiguing tests: height, weight, body composition, grip strength, movement screens, vertical jump, standing long jump, medicine ball throws, and so on
- Agility tests: pro-agility test, 5-0-5, T-test
- Maximum power and strength tests: 1–6 repetition max (RM) testing, Olympic lifting movements (clean, snatch, and jerk)
- Sprint tests: 10-, 20-, and 30-meter sprints
- Local muscular endurance tests: push-ups, curl-ups, planks, pull-ups, one-minute squat test
- Anaerobic capacity tests: 300-meter run and 300-meter shuttle run
- Aerobic capacity tests: distance or time tests and beep test

Experience and Fitness Level

Many of the performance and fitness tests selected for this text can be performed relatively easily by both beginners and advanced athletes, assuming the absence of major orthopedic or cardiovascular limitations. But certain tests, such as a 1–6 RM bench press, may not be appropriate for a person who has performed only bodyweight exercises for the upper body (e.g., push-ups). In this case the person should be given a few weeks to become familiarized with this test using a lighter training load (e.g., 12–20 RM) before attempting to test using a heavier load.

Number of Trials and Rest Periods Between Tests

For most tests, two or three practice trials at one-half to three-quarters (50 to 75 percent) intensity should be allowed for familiarization purposes. After this, two or three test trials should generally be allowed, and the best of those trials should be recorded as the final score. But for exercises such as the bench press, people should attempt to get their max within five attempts; otherwise, fatigue may influence the amount of weight that they can lift as the number of sets progresses.

Adequate rest should be allowed between trials. In general, for nonfatiguing tests, additional tests can be performed within a minute of each other. For most tests, however, a rest of between three and five minutes between trials is needed to allow for energy system recovery.

Motivation

In many cases, accurate test scores come down to motivation. If a person is not motivated to perform a test with maximal effort or intensity, the results obtained are relatively useless. Many factors can influence motivation, including the testing environment, the importance of the test, and the perceived value of the test by the participant. For example, it may be difficult to motivate a baseball player to see the value in performing a 1.5-mile (2.4 km) run test, because baseball is a speed and acceleration game and not particularly dependent on aerobic endurance. But if the player is required to run this distance to make the team, he may be motivated to give a true effort, even though it may not be relevant to the sport. For that reason among others, test selection is critical. The greater the appearance is of direct carryover between a test and the attribute or skill we are trying to measure, the better the motivation is to give max effort to the activity.

Additionally, training partners, teammates, and onlookers may provide motivation to give greater effort during testing sessions. In some cases, however, this attention may increase anxiety and hinder individual performance. The best approach is to determine what motivational strategy works best for the person and attempt to replicate this strategy in future testing sessions.

Fatigue Level

Fatigue plays a major role in attaining a best performance. For this reason, participants should abstain from vigorous physical activity within the 48 to 72 hours before testing.

Nutritional Status and Hydration

Proper nutrition and fueling can play a significant role in energy levels. For example, the beep test is a measure of aerobic endurance. The aerobic energy system relies heavily on stored energy (glycogen, fat, and, though not ideal, protein) to sustain activity. If a person is not ingesting an appropriate amount of calories, fewer of these nutrients will be stored for utilization. A shortfall may affect a person's ability to sustain performance for the duration of such a test.

Hydration also plays a critical role in performance. Dehydration by as little as 2 percent of total body weight can impair exercise and cognitive performance (Murray 2007). For this reason, a person should strive to attain and maintain appropriate hydration status at all times.

TEST RELEVANCE

When selecting or developing a testing battery, we are typically interested in the tests' ability to measure improvement or help predict performance. The testing battery needs to be relevant to the person's needs and measure the variable of greatest interest. For example, it would make little sense to perform a 30-meter sprint test with a swimmer, unless it was performed in the water. Land speed is irrelevant to this athlete's sport-specific needs, will likely not be trained, and does not provide any usable information for improving performance in the water.

Sample Testing Batteries

Table 11.4 is an example of a testing battery advocated for law enforcement officers by the Cooper Fitness Institute . This battery of tests was created to predict performance in certain job tasks specific to this occupation (Research CIfA 2002).

The testing battery presented in table 11.5 is a sample testing battery for a Division II collegiate female volleyball team. The purpose of each test is included.

Finally, the last two sample testing batteries were designed for those who just want to measure their general fitness levels. Table 11.6 shows a testing battery for people who have access to a gym or gym equipment, whereas the sample featured in 11.7 can be performed practically anywhere using only body weight as resistance.

Adapting or Creating a Test

After doing your research, you may find that no specific standardized test meets your needs. In this case, you may have to develop your own test to measure your progress. When creating your own tests, you need to standardize the way in which you will test so that your results are reliable. For instance, let's say that an ice hockey coach wanted to develop a test to assess change-of-direction speed for ice hockey. Overall, the coach likes the basic running pattern for the pro-agility test, but in ice hockey touching the ground with the hand may be not only irrelevant but dangerous. The coach decides to modify this test by performing it on ice and allowing the players to touch the line with the skate blade rather than the hand. Based on these modifications the coach would not be able to compare the players' results to players who touch the line with the hand or perform these tests on a different surface (e.g., turf, grass, basketball court, and so on). But as long as the testing procedures remain

Table 11.4   Sample Law Enforcement Testing Battery

Job task	Predictive factor	Recommended test(s)
Sustained pursuit	Aerobic power	1.5-mile (2.4 km) run
Sprint	Anaerobic power	300 m run
Dodging	Aerobic power, anaerobic power, flexibility	1.5-mile (2.4 km) run, sit-and-reach test
Lifting and carrying	Muscular strength, muscular endurance, anaerobic power	1RM bench press, one-minute push-up test, vertical jump
Dragging and pulling	Muscular strength, muscular endurance, anaerobic power	1RM bench press, one-minute push-up test, vertical jump
Pushing	Muscular strength, muscular endurance, anaerobic power	1RM bench press, one-minute push-up test, vertical jump
Jumping and vaulting	Anaerobic power, leg power and strength	Vertical jump
Crawling	Flexibility, muscular endurance, body fat composition	Sit-and-reach test, one-minute push-up test, one-minute sit-up test, body fat testing (caliper, underwater weighing, impedance)
Use of force for less than two minutes	Anaerobic power, muscular strength, muscular endurance	Vertical jump, 1RM bench press, sit-and-reach test, one-minute push-up test, one-minute sit-up test
Use of force for greater than two minutes	Aerobic power, muscular strength, muscular endurance	1.5-mile (2.4 km) run

Adapted with permission from The Cooper Institute, Dallas, Texas. From *Physical Fitness Assessments and Norms for Adults and Law Enforcement.* Available at www.CooperInstitute.org.

Table 11.5 Sample Testing Battery for a Division II Collegiate Female Volleyball Team

Test	Purpose
Movement screens: hip hinge, squat, lunge, drop landing	To assess general movement ability and mobility and to identify poor movement patterns that could potentially lead to injury
Vertical jump	To measure lower-body power
5-0-5 agility	To measure change-of-direction speed
3RM back squat	To measure lower-body muscular strength
Front or side plank	To measure muscular endurance of the trunk
Push-up	To measure upper-body endurance and general upper-body fitness

Table 11.6 Sample General Fitness Testing Battery I—With Equipment

Test	Purpose
Movement screens: hip hinge, squat, lunge	To assess general movement ability and mobility and to identify poor movement patterns that could potentially lead to injury
8–10 RM squat	To measure lower-body muscular fitness
8–10 RM bench press	To measure fitness of the upper-body pressing muscles (chest, shoulders, triceps)
Pull-up	To measure fitness of the upper-body pulling muscles (back, biceps)
Curl-up	To measure muscular endurance of the abdominal muscles
12-minute run on treadmill	To measure aerobic endurance

Table 11.7 Sample General Fitness Testing Battery II—No Equipment

Test	Purpose
Movement screens: hip hinge, squat, lunge	To assess general movement ability and mobility and to identify poor movement patterns that could potentially lead to injury
1-minute squat	To measure lower-body muscular fitness
1-minute push-up	To measure fitness of the upper-body pressing muscles (chest, shoulders, triceps)
Front plank	To measure muscular endurance of the abdominal muscles
1.5 mile run	To measure aerobic endurance

consistent, the coach can compare results for current and future athletes on the team and measure improvement. This test would be relevant based on the needs of the coach, and it seems to have good face validity because it appears to measure what it is intended to.

SUMMARY

Testing is an essential part of a comprehensive training program. Selecting valid and reliable fitness and performance tests that are relevant to the person's goals will produce the most meaningful results and allow a person to evaluate his or her current fitness level, set appropriate training goals, and determine whether the current training program is working or needs to be adjusted.

CHAPTER 12

Protocols for Measuring Fitness and Performance Parameters

This chapter discusses a variety of field tests aimed at measuring fitness and performance. These tests have been selected because they address several key aspects of fitness and performance and are relatively easy to perform with minimal equipment. Performing each of these tests is unnecessary; rather, the test battery selected should be tailored to meet each person's specific needs and goals.

MOVEMENT ASSESSMENTS

Before beginning an exercise program, people need to know whether they have the requisite skills to perform certain exercises without an increased risk of injury. The following assessments have been selected to help gauge movement proficiency. Other tests found in this chapter, such as the push-up, front plank, and side plank, can also be used as basic movement screens to assess trunk stability. Additionally, a number of inexpensive applications (apps) are available online for use with electronic tablets and cell phones. These apps allow basic biomechanical assessments to be saved, analyzed, and used later for comparison purposes.

Hip Hinge Assessment

Equipment Needed

Dowel rod and a mirror or testing partner.

Purpose

The hip hinge is a basic foundational movement pattern that is necessary for safe performance of many movements in sport and daily life. The ability to perform this assessment with good form and technique should be a prerequisite to performing exercises such as the bent-over row or Romanian deadlift.

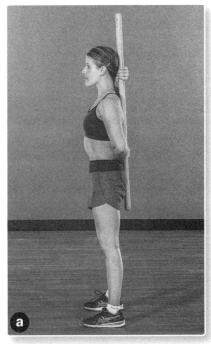

Steps

- Hold a dowel rod vertically along the spine so that it makes contact with the back of the head, upper back, and sacrum (three points of contact). The top hand should be placed at the top of the dowel just behind the neck, and the other hand should be placed toward the bottom of the dowel near the lumbar spine (*a*).
- Push the hips back and bend forward at the waist until the torso is as close to parallel to the ground as possible (*b*).
- The dowel should remain in contact with the three points of contact previously discussed.
- This is a pass–fail test. If you are able to maintain these three points of contact, you pass the test.

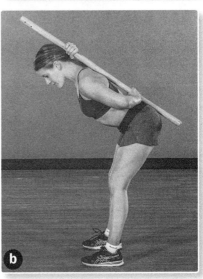

Squat Assessment

Equipment Needed

Mirror or testing partner.

Purpose

The squat is a cornerstone movement for many activities. The ability to perform this movement with skill and efficiency sets the foundation for many complex athletic movements, such as jumping. The checklist for this assessment has been adapted based on the work of Kritz, Cronin, and Hume (2009a).

Steps

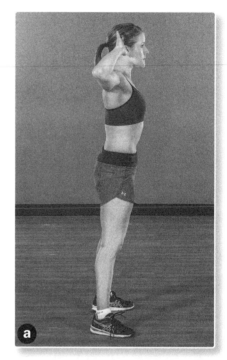

- With a partner or in front of a mirror, place the hands just behind the ears, push the elbows back, and perform a bodyweight squat (*a-b*).
- Use the following checklist to assess this movement:
    - **Head:** Held straight in line with the shoulders; gaze is straight ahead or slightly up.
    - **Thoracic spine:** Shoulder blades pulled back and together, slightly extended or neutral, and held stable.
    - **Lumbar spine:** Neutral and stable throughout movement.
    - **Hip joint:** Stable with no significant medial or lateral movement and no dropping of the hips; hips should also stay aligned with knees.
    - **Knees:** Aligned with the hips and feet, stable, no excessive movement inside or out, forward or back.
    - **Feet and ankles:** Feet flat and stable, heels in contact with the ground at all times.
- This is a pass–fail test. If you are able to meet these criteria, you pass the test.

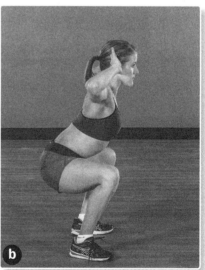

Lunge Assessment

Equipment Needed

Mirror or testing partner.

Purpose

In many sports and daily activities, such as walking and running, we are required to move the legs in an alternated, staggered, or reciprocating fashion. Inability to maintain good body position and alignment during these movements may lead to inefficient movement as well as increased risk of injury. The checklist for this assessment has been adapted based on the work of Kritz, Cronin, and Hume (2009b).

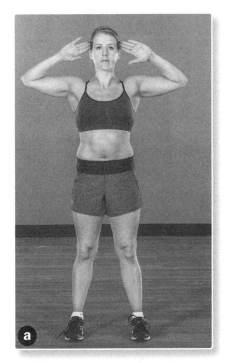

- With a partner or in front of a mirror, place the hands just behind the ears, push the elbows back, and perform a bodyweight lunge (*a-b*).

- Use the following checklist to assess this movement:

  - **Head:** Held straight in line with the shoulders; gaze is straight ahead or slightly up.

  - **Thoracic spine:** Shoulder blades pulled back and together, slightly extended or neutral and held stable, and above the hips.

  - **Lumbar spine:** Neutral and stable throughout movement.

  - **Hip joint:** Aligned with the lead knee and ankle, hips horizontally aligned (one side not higher than the other).

  - **Knees:** Front knee over the lead ankle.

  - **Feet and ankles:** Aligned with the knee; front foot flat, back foot on the ball of the foot with toes flexed; both feet aligned and balanced.

- This is a pass–fail test. If you are able to meet these criteria, you pass the test.

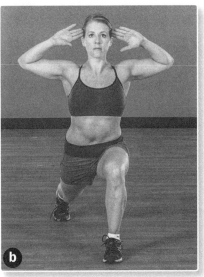

Drop Landing Assessment

Equipment Needed

Plyometric box or step aerobics step 12 to 16 inches (30 to 40 cm) tall, mirror or testing partner.

Purpose

This assessment is used to determine how well a person is able to control body alignment and posture under high eccentric landing forces. This assessment should be performed before any plyometric training is done to determine the person's readiness to perform plyometric and other jumping exercises. If the person is unable to maintain good posture and alignment during this assessment, other tests, such as the vertical jump and broad jump, should not be performed until the person is able to perform this exercise successfully.

Steps

- While standing on top of a 12- to 16-inch (30 to 40 cm) box, assume a comfortable, upright stance with the feet approximately hip-width apart.

- Step off the box (do not jump off) (*a*) and land in the athletic position (chest up, shoulders back, feet approximately shoulder-width apart, and knees in alignment with the second toes) and in a balanced position (*b*). Additionally, the feet should land at the same time, rather than one followed by the other. A correct landing will not only be seen but also heard because the feet will make a single sound as they contact the ground.

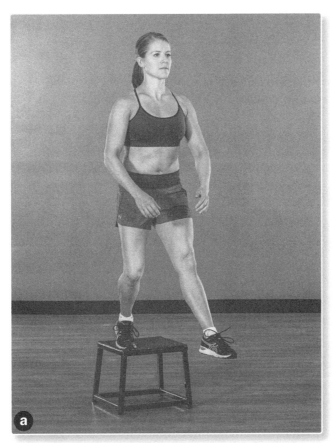

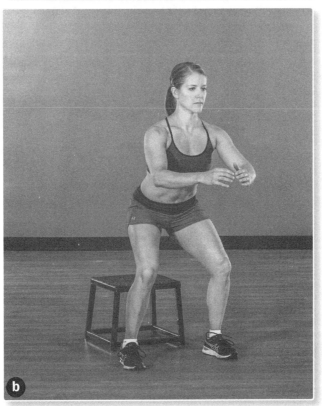

LINEAR AND CHANGE-OF-DIRECTION SPEED ASSESSMENTS

In most sports, speed is essential for success. But straight-ahead running speed is not the only attribute that makes the difference between winning and losing. The ability to accelerate, decelerate, and change direction rapidly and efficiently with minimal loss in speed is crucial. This section features several linear and change-of-direction speed tests. Again, not every one of these tests should be performed. The speed and agility tests that replicate the specific needs of the sport, in terms of specific movement patterns and distances traveled, should be used.

10-, 20-, and 30-Meter Sprint Tests

Equipment Needed

Stopwatch and testing partner or a laser timer, a measuring tape, track or large open area, and markers or cones.

Purpose

The purpose of these tests is to measure both linear speed and acceleration. To measure the ability to accelerate, the 10- or 20-meter test should be selected. To measure top-end speed, the 30-meter dash is appropriate. These tests would be appropriate for most field-sport athletes, such as soccer and lacrosse players. Although stopwatches can be used to measure the distance traveled, the use of a laser timer can significantly improve the validity and reliability of these tests. Additionally, a laser timer that has built-in timing gates allows the user to collect information about both acceleration (10 meters) and top-end speed (30 meters) in a single run. Ideally, this test should be performed on the same surface and in the same footwear that the athlete would use for the specific sport. For example, for a soccer or lacrosse player, these tests would be performed on grass or artificial turf, wearing cleats or turf shoes. Conversely, for a basketball player, the tests would be performed on a hardwood court.

Steps

- Begin by marking the starting line with a cone.
- Place another cone directly in line with the starting cone at the selected distance (10, 20, or 30 meters).
- Stand behind the starting line in a two-point athletic stance or a traditional three-point stance.
- If using a stopwatch, a partner will be needed to time the run. When pressing the button on the stopwatch, the timer should use the index finger rather than the thumb to improve the accuracy of the measure.
- On the "Go" command or on first movement, the timer starts the stopwatch. The timer then stops the stopwatch when the sprinter crosses the finish line.
- Time to the nearest 0.10 second should be recorded.
- Allow up to three sprints with a minimum of 3 to 5 minutes of rest between sprints to allow recovery and minimize the effects of fatigue.
- The fastest time achieved should be recorded as the person's final score.

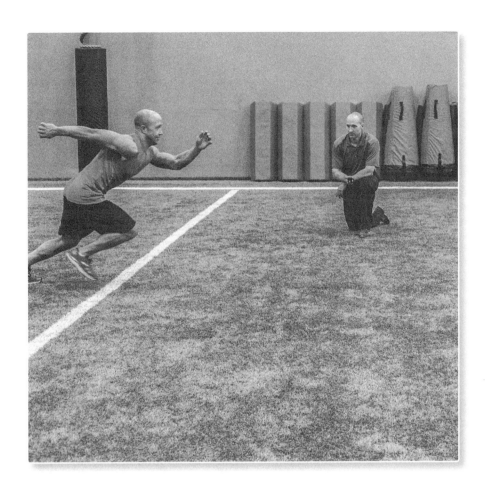

Pro-Agility Test

Equipment Needed

Stopwatch and testing partner, a measuring tape, track or large open area, and three markers or cones.

Purpose

The pro-agility test, often referred to as the 5-10-5 or the 20-yard shuttle, is frequently used to measure change-of-direction speed for American football players. In fact, it is one of the primary tests used in the NFL combine (Jones 2012).

Steps

- Set up three cones 5 yards (4.6 m) apart in a straight line.
- Assume an athletic stance (two or three point depending on the sport) just behind the center cone.
- On the "Go" command or on first movement, the timer starts the stopwatch. When pressing the button on the stopwatch, the timer should use the index finger rather than the thumb to improve the accuracy of the measure.
- The runner sprints 5 yards to the cone on the right, touches the ground with the right hand, makes a 180-degree turn, sprints 10 yards to the farthest cone, touches the ground with the left hand, turns 180 degrees again, and sprints 5 yards back to the center cone.
- The stopwatch should be stopped when the person passes the center cone for the last time.
- Time to the nearest 0.10 second should be recorded.
- Allow up to three trials with a minimum of 3 to 5 minutes of rest between sprints to allow recovery and minimize the effects of fatigue.
- The fastest time achieved should be recorded as the person's final score.

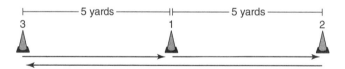

5-0-5 Test

Equipment Needed

Stopwatch and testing partner or a laser timer, a measuring tape, track or large open area, and three markers or cones.

Purpose

This test is commonly used to assess an athlete's change-of-direction speed. This test is popular among rugby, soccer, handball, and volleyball players (Jones 2012).

Steps

- Set up three cones—one for the starting line, one at 10 meters, and one at 15 meters.
- Begin behind the starting line. When ready, jog toward the 10-meter cone.
- When the runner reaches the 10-meter cone, the timer starts the stopwatch.
- The runner should sprint as fast as possible between the 10- and 15-meter cones.
- At the 15-meter cone, the runner turns 180 degrees and sprints back toward the starting line.
- The timer stops the stopwatch when the person crosses the 10-meter cone on the way back to the starting line.
- The total time taken to cover the 5 meters up and back (10 meters total) should be recorded to the nearest 0.10 second.
- This test should be performed with the runner changing direction off both the right and left legs.
- The fastest time of two or three trials should be recorded as the final score for each leg.

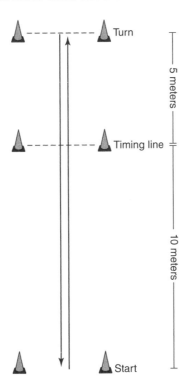

T-Test

Equipment Needed

Stopwatch and testing partner or a laser timer, a measuring tape, large open area, and four cones.

Purpose

The T-test is a change-of-direction speed test that incorporates several discrete movement tasks (forward acceleration, lateral shuffle, and backpedal) into one test (Jones 2012).

Steps

- Set up four cones in the shape of a T.
- Sprint 10 yards (9.14 m) forward to the center cone and touch it with the right hand. Then immediately shuffle 5 yards (4.57 m) toward the cone on the far left and touch it with the left hand. Then shuffle 10 yards to the cone on the far right and touch it with the right hand. Shuffle back to the center cone and then backpedal though the starting line.
- The stopwatch is started on the "Go" command or the first movement by the runner, and the stopwatch is stopped when the runner crosses the starting line on the way back.
- The total time taken to cover the distance should be recorded to the nearest 0.10 second.
- The fastest time of two or three trials should be recorded.

Variations

For sports like volleyball, these distances may be cut in half to increase sport specificity because less distance would typically be traveled.

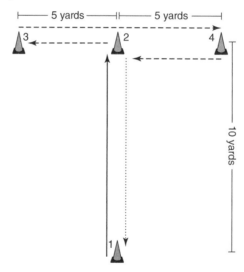

POWER ASSESSMENTS

Power is the optimal combination of strength and speed. Power is an essential element in sport, especially during running, jumping, and changing direction. Powerful athletes tend to be more successful than their less powerful counterparts. In this section several well-known power tests are discussed. In chapter 13 we learn how to look at the measurements generated by these tests and how to determine relative power (power in relation to body weight).

Countermovement Vertical Jump Test

Equipment Needed

Lifting chalk, a wall, and measuring tape.

Purpose

The countermovement vertical jump is likely the most widely used test for determining lower-body power. This test is appropriate for almost every type of athlete because it is generally considered a good overall indicator of athleticism. A variety of portable field-based measurements can be used to measure vertical jump. These include devices that require the person to jump and displace as many plastic fins as possible (e.g., Vertec) to switch mats that estimate height, or vertical displacement, based on flight time. But for this assessment, all that is needed is some lifting chalk and a tape measure.

Steps

- Chalk the fingertips of the preferred-side hand.
- Then, while standing next to a wall, reach as high as possible while keeping both feet flat on the ground. Make a mark on the wall with the chalked fingers.
- Without moving your feet and keeping the arm closer to the wall extended overhead, rapidly lower your center of mass by allowing the ankle, knees, and hips to bend (countermovement) to a self-selected depth (approximately 90 to 110 degrees of knee bend).
- Without pausing, jump vertically as high as possible and make a second chalk mark on the wall.
- The distance between the first chalk mark and the highest mark should be measured to the nearest 1/2 inch (1 centimeter).
- Allow 30 to 60 seconds of rest between jumps.
- The best of three attempts should be recorded. If the final jump is the highest jump, a fourth jump can be made to ensure that maximal height is attained.

Variations

The countermovement vertical jump allows a person to take advantage of stored elastic energy by rapidly preloading the lower body before jumping. By quickly bending the ankles, knees, and hips, the person is able to harness the elastic properties of the muscles to jump higher. The squat jump does not allow the person to preload the lower-body, so this test isolates the concentric force production of the lower body. This test would be appropriate for athletes who are required to produce a large amount of force without always having the benefit of a preload, such as a swimmer jumping into the water from the blocks or a lineman in American football.

Squat Jump Assessment

Equipment Needed

Lifting chalk, a wall, and measuring tape.

Purpose

The squat jump is similar to the traditional vertical jump, but it is designed to minimize the contribution of the stored elastic energy created by a countermovement before jumping. Therefore, this test is a good measure of lower-body concentric force production.

Procedure

- Chalk the fingertips of the preferred-side hand.
- Then, while standing next to a wall, reach as high as possible while keeping both feet flat on the ground. Make a mark on the wall with the chalked fingers.
- Without moving your feet and keeping the arm closer to the wall extended, lower your center of mass by allowing the ankle, knees, and hips to bend until the upper portion of the thigh is parallel to the ground.
- Hold this position for two to three seconds and then jump vertically as high as possible and make a second chalk mark on the wall.
- The distance between the first chalk mark and the highest mark should be measured to the nearest 1/2 inch (1 cm).
- Allow 30 to 60 seconds of rest between jumps.
- The best of three attempts should be recorded. If the final jump is the highest jump, a fourth jump can be made to ensure that maximal height is attained.

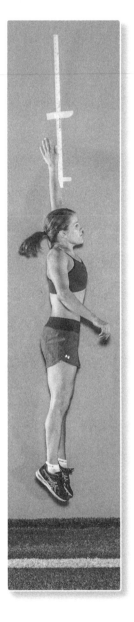

Standing Long Jump Test

Equipment Needed

Measuring tape and a cone.

Purpose

The standing long jump, or broad jump, is a commonly used test to measure horizontal force production and power. This test is relatively easy to perform, requiring only a marker and a taped line.

Steps

- Begin by standing with the feet approximately hip-width apart and the toes on the starting line (e.g., taped line or line between two cones).
- Perform a countermovement arm swing while simultaneously bending the ankles, knees, and hips (a).
- Swing the arms forward while jumping up and out as far as possible (b).
- Land on both feet.
- Hold this position until a measurement can be taken.
- The distance should be measured from the starting line to the base of the rear-most heel (ideally, the heels will be side by side).
- Allow 30 to 60 seconds of rest between jumps.
- Record the best distance of three trials.

Variations

To measure leg power rather than total-body power, simply place the hands on the hips.

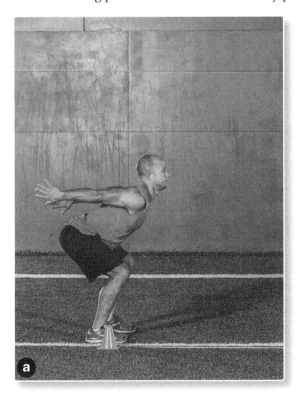
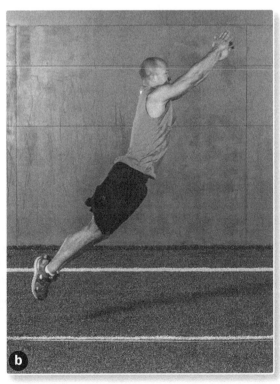

Medicine Ball Pass Test

Equipment Needed

Medicine balls, measuring tape, and a cone.

Purpose

This test to measure upper-body power is easy and inexpensive to administer. It is appropriate for people who must generate force quickly, such as combative and tactical athletes.

Steps

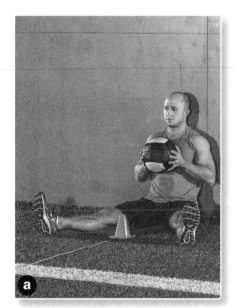

- Select a medicine ball that is approximately 5 percent of your total body weight. For example, a 200-pound (90.7 kg) person would use a 10-pound (4.5 kg) ball, whereas a 100-pound (45.4 kg) person would use a 5-pound (2.3 kg) ball.
- While sitting on the floor with the lower back, head, and shoulders against a wall and the legs extended, hold the medicine ball with both hands against the chest (*a*).
- Extend the arms out straight and place a cone to the side of the body to mark your maximal reach. Extend a taped line out from this point.
- Reposition the ball back on the chest, forcefully extend the arms, and pass the medicine ball as far as possible forward (*b*).
- Measure the distance the ball travels from the maximal reach distance to where the ball first hits the ground.
- Allow 30 to 60 seconds of rest between trials.
- Allow up to three trials and record the greatest distance achieved.

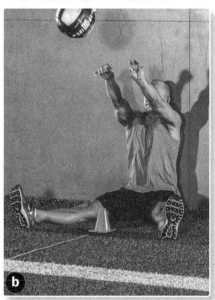

Variations

- This test can be performed in a standing position to add a more sport-specific element.
- This test can be administered without a partner by using a sand pit or beach volleyball court. From a standing position, extend the arms and drop the ball in the sand to get your maximal reach. Then pass the ball forward as far as possible and measure the distance between the impact points in the sand.
- From a standing position, other traditional upper-body plyometric exercises can be used, such as a side toss, backward overhead medicine ball (BOMB) toss, a forward throw, or scoop toss.

MUSCULAR STRENGTH AND ENDURANCE TESTS

Muscular strength and endurance are essential in most sports and in many activities of daily living. Although maximal interval training is more suited to developing muscular endurance, some people may see some strength improvements as well. This progress will be largely based on the person's current training status; novices will see greater improvements than those who have more experience with resistance training.

Repetition Max Testing

To measure muscular strength and endurance, repetition max (RM) testing using traditional free weights and machine-based exercises can be used. A RM can be defined as the greatest number of repetitions that can be lifted at a given load. For instance, if a person can bench press 200 pounds (90.7 kg) for no more than 12 repetitions, then 200 pounds would be his or her 12RM. A resistance that will allow a person to perform up to 6 repetitions would be considered a good strength measure. A weight that will allow the user to lift a resistance for 12 repetitions or more would be considered a good measure of muscular endurance.

Certain exercises are more suited than others to measuring strength. The bench press, squat, and leg press are all examples of good exercises for measuring strength. These exercises can also be used to measure endurance when performed for greater than a 12RM. In addition, free-weight exercises such as the squat are highly related to athletic performance based on their biomechanical similarity to many explosive athletic movements, such as the vertical jump.

Exercises that are single-joint in nature, such as biceps curls, leg curls, and leg extensions should be performed only with a weight that would allow a minimum of an 8RM to be performed. Thus, these exercises may work well to measure muscular endurance and general fitness in isolated muscle groups but would be poor for measuring true strength or athletic performance.

For those with experience with resistance training, a conservative estimate of their RM can be used to determine their initial testing load. For example, after performing a light warm-up at 135 pounds (61.2 kg) on the bench press, the lifter selects a training load within 10 or 20 pounds (4.5 or 9.1 kg) of his or her estimated 1RM. The person should be able to perform two or three repetitions at this load (i.e., a 2 or 3RM). Although this method would adequately measure strength, if the goal is to determine the 1RM, after three to five minutes of rest the person would add an additional 10 to 20 pounds and attempt to lift the heavier weight. Ideally, the 1RM should be found within five attempts. Otherwise, cumulative fatigue may produce invalid results. Another option is to perform multiple RMs and estimate the 1RM based on the number of reps completed at a given load (table 12.1). For instance, if April was able to squat 170 pounds (77.1 kg) for 6 reps, her estimated 1RM would be 200 pounds (90.7 kg). Although these charts provide a good conservative estimate of the 1RM, they are only estimates. Some people will be able to lift more or less than what is estimated. But these charts serve as a good starting point for less experienced lifters to set initial volume and training load goals without performing a max or near max lift. Also, note that these charts may be less accurate for any exercises other than the squat, bench press, and deadlift.

Table 12.1 Estimating 1RM and Training Loads

Max reps (RM)	1	2	3	4	5	6	7	8	9	10	12	15
%1RM	100	95	93	90	87	85	83	80	77	75	67	65
Load (pounds or kg)	10	10	9	9	9	9	8	8	8	8	7	7
	20	19	19	18	17	17	17	16	15	15	13	13
	30	29	28	27	26	26	25	24	23	23	20	20
	40	38	37	36	35	34	33	32	31	30	27	26
	50	48	47	45	44	43	42	40	39	38	34	33
	60	57	56	54	52	51	50	48	46	45	40	39
	70	67	65	63	61	60	58	56	54	53	47	46
	80	76	74	72	70	68	66	64	62	60	54	52
	90	86	84	81	78	77	75	72	69	68	60	59
	100	95	93	90	87	85	83	80	77	75	67	65
	110	105	102	99	96	94	91	88	85	83	74	72
	120	114	112	108	104	102	100	96	92	90	80	78
	130	124	121	117	113	111	108	104	100	98	87	85
	140	133	130	126	122	119	116	112	108	105	94	91
	150	143	140	135	131	128	125	120	116	113	101	98
	160	152	149	144	139	136	133	128	123	120	107	104
	170	162	158	153	148	145	141	136	131	128	114	111
	180	171	167	162	157	153	149	144	139	135	121	117
	190	181	177	171	165	162	158	152	146	143	127	124
	200	190	186	180	174	170	166	160	154	150	134	130
	210	200	195	189	183	179	174	168	162	158	141	137
	220	209	205	198	191	187	183	176	169	165	147	143
	230	219	214	207	200	196	191	184	177	173	154	150
	240	228	223	216	209	204	199	192	185	180	161	156
	250	238	233	225	218	213	208	200	193	188	168	163
	260	247	242	234	226	221	206	208	200	195	174	169
	270	257	251	243	235	230	224	216	208	203	181	176
	280	266	260	252	244	238	232	224	216	210	188	182
	290	276	270	261	252	247	241	232	223	218	194	189
	300	285	279	270	261	255	249	240	231	225	201	195

Max reps (RM)	1	2	3	4	5	6	7	8	9	10	12	15
%1RM	100	95	93	90	87	85	83	80	77	75	67	65
Load (pounds or kg)	310	295	288	279	270	264	257	248	239	233	208	202
	320	304	298	288	278	272	266	256	246	240	214	208
	330	314	307	297	287	281	274	264	254	248	221	215
	340	323	316	306	296	289	282	272	262	255	228	221
	350	333	326	315	305	298	291	280	270	263	235	228
	360	342	335	324	313	306	299	288	277	270	241	234
	370	352	344	333	322	315	307	296	285	278	248	241
	380	361	353	342	331	323	315	304	293	285	255	247
	390	371	363	351	339	332	324	312	300	293	261	254
	400	380	372	360	348	340	332	320	308	300	268	260
	410	390	381	369	357	349	340	328	316	308	274	267
	420	399	391	378	365	357	349	336	323	315	281	273
	430	409	400	387	374	366	357	344	331	323	288	280
	440	418	409	396	383	374	365	352	339	330	295	286
	450	428	419	405	392	383	374	360	347	338	302	293
	460	437	428	414	400	391	382	368	354	345	308	299
	470	447	437	423	409	400	390	376	362	353	315	306
	480	456	446	432	418	408	398	384	370	360	322	312
	490	466	456	441	426	417	407	392	377	368	328	319
	500	475	465	450	435	425	415	400	385	375	335	325
	510	485	474	459	444	434	423	408	393	383	342	332
	520	494	484	468	452	442	432	416	400	390	348	338
	530	504	493	477	461	451	440	424	408	398	355	345
	540	513	502	486	470	459	448	432	416	405	362	351
	550	523	512	495	479	468	457	440	424	413	369	358
	560	532	521	504	487	476	465	448	431	420	375	364
	570	542	530	513	496	485	473	456	439	428	382	371
	580	551	539	522	505	493	481	464	447	435	389	377
	590	561	549	531	513	502	490	472	454	443	395	384
	600	570	558	540	522	510	498	480	462	450	402	390

Reprinted, by permission, from T.R. Baechle, R.W. Earle, and D. Wathen, 2008, Resistance training. In *Essentials of strength training and conditioning*, 3rd ed., edited for the National Strength and Conditioning Association by T.R. Baechle and R.W. Earle (Champaign, IL: Human Kinetics), 397-398.

Back Squat Assessment

Equipment Needed

Barbell, weight plates, squat rack.

Purpose

The back squat may be the single most used strength assessment among athletes. This multijoint, structural exercise is often selected based on its biomechanical specificity to many sporting actions (e.g., jumping) and muscle groups used (e.g., gluteus maximus, quadriceps, hamstrings).

Steps

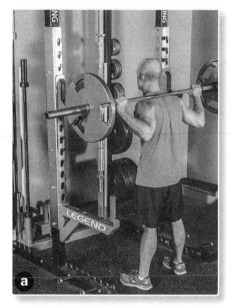

- Begin by adjusting the pins on the squat rack so that the bar is approximately chest height.
- Adjust the stops on the weight rack so that they are just below shoulder level at the lowest point of the movement.
- Using an overhand, common grip, grasp the barbell.
- Duck under the bar and position it on top of the shoulder blades. Stick the chest out and upward while simultaneously pulling the shoulder blades together, creating a shelf for the bar to rest on, and brace the trunk by contracting the abdominals.
- The ankle, knees, and hips should be slightly bent, and the feet should be positioned approximately shoulder-width apart.
- Extend the hips, knees, and ankles to unrack the bar (*a*).
- Take a small step backward.

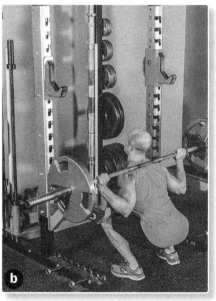

- While keeping the trunk braced, chest up, and shoulder blades together, allow the hips, knees, and ankles to flex and sit down as if you are dropping your center of mass between your feet (*b*).
- When the top of the thighs are parallel to the ground, extend the hips, knees, and ankles and drive the barbell back to the starting position.

Spotting

- While standing directly behind the lifter, the spotter assumes a shoulder-width stance. The hips, knees, and ankles are slightly flexed, and the arms are extended outward so that they are to the sides of the lifter.
- As the lifter unracks the weight and steps back, the spotter simultaneously steps back. When the lifter begins the descent, the spotter squats downward in unison with the lifter and has the arms still outstretched.
- Should the lifter be unable to complete a lift, the spotter wraps his or her arms around the lifter's torso, extends the ankles, knees, and hips while keeping the back in a neutral position, and helps the lifter return to the starting position.

Deadlift Test

Equipment Needed
Barbell and weight plates.

Purpose
The deadlift is a good measure of overall strength, because it requires a strong grip as well as good lower-body strength. This test is excellent for tactical athletes and first responders because it is biomechanically similar to many of their essential job tasks, such as dragging a victim or lifting a stretcher.

Steps
■ Address the bar by squatting down and grasping the barbell with an alternated grip and hands positioned at approximately shoulder-width.

■ With the both feet flat on the ground and turned slightly outward, set the back and brace the trunk.

■ Roll the bar back toward the shins so that the bar is directly over the center of the feet and sit back, as if performing a squat (*a*).

■ While keeping the arms fully extended, keep the back set and trunk braced and stand up until the knees, hips, and torso are fully extended (*b*).

■ Make certain that the hips and shoulder rise at the same rate.

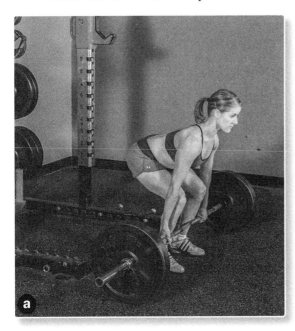 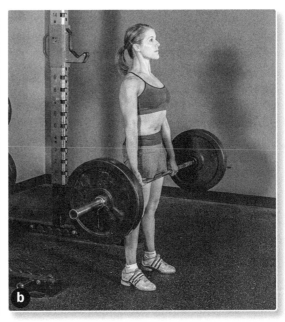

Bench Press Assessment

Equipment Needed

Weight bench, barbell, weight plates.

Purpose

Although the specificity of this exercise to sport performance is often questioned, the bench press is an excellent overall assessment of upper-body strength. It measures the strength of the chest, shoulders, and triceps muscles.

Steps

- The person begins on a flat bench using a standard five-point contact (head, shoulders, and glutes in contact with the bench and both feet on the floor).
- Position the hands with a grip slightly wider than shoulder-width and grab the bar with an overhand grip.
- Lift the bar off the rack until it is positioned directly over the chest (*a*).
- In a controlled manner, lower the bar to the chest.
- Touch the bar against the chest and push the bar back to the starting position (*b*).

Spotting

- Because this exercise is performed over the face, a spotter is recommended for safety purposes.
- The spotter assumes an athletic stance behind the lifter. Using an alternated grip on the bar, the spotter helps the lifter remove the bar from the rack.
- The spotter keeps contact with the bar during the entire exercise movement.

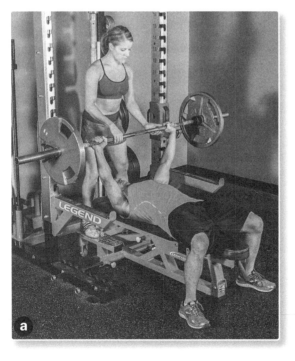
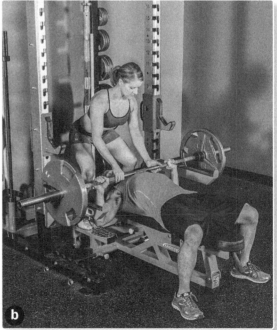

Curl-Up Test

Equipment Needed

Stopwatch, exercise mat.

Purpose

The curl-up exercise is a general measure of endurance for the abdominal muscles. In most cases, this test is preferred over the sit-up test because it is a more accurate measure of abdominal muscle endurance. When performing the full sit-up, the hip flexors must also be used to accomplish the full range of motion.

Steps

- While lying on the back, bend the knees until they are at a 90-degreee angle. The feet are completely flat on the ground, and the arms are positioned across the chest (*a*).
- Lift the shoulder blades up until the trunk is flexed at approximately 30 degrees. Maintain a neutral head position (*b*).
- Lower the shoulder blades in a controlled manner until they are back in full contact with the ground.
- You are not allowed to rest during this exercise.
- The test is over when you decide to end it.
- The final score is the maximum number of curl-ups completed consecutively with good technique and form.

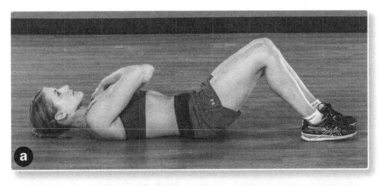

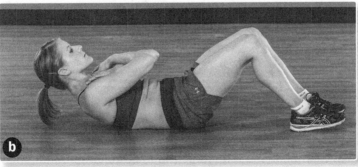

Pull-Up Test

Equipment Needed

Pull-up bar.

Purpose

The pull-up test can be used to measure upper-body pulling strength or endurance, depending on current fitness status. As previously mentioned, if a person is able to perform six or fewer repetitions on this test, it would be considered a strength assessment. If the person can perform more than six repetitions, it would be considered a general fitness and endurance test.

Steps

- Begin by hanging from pull-up bar with the arms straight and the hands wrapped around the bar in an overhand position (*a*).
- Bend the arms and pull the body upward until the chin is above the bar (*b*).
- After each pull-up, return to the starting position before performing the next repetition.
- You are allowed to rest in the downward phase.
- The test is over when you decide to end it, your technique is poor, or you let go of the bar.
- The final score is the maximum number of pull-ups you can complete consecutively with good technique and form.

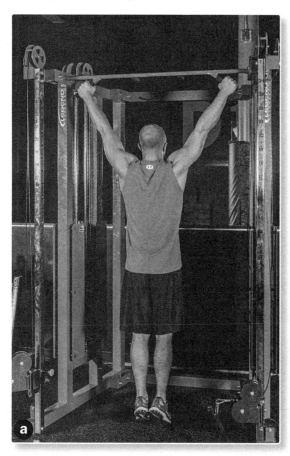
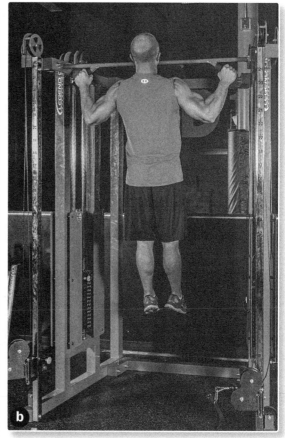

Push-Up Test

Equipment Needed

■ Stopwatch, yoga block.

Purpose

The push-up may be the most popular bodyweight exercise of all time. This test is most often used as general measure of muscular endurance for the upper body, specifically the chest, shoulders, and triceps. As with the pull-up exercise, if a person is unable to perform more than six repetitions, it would be considered a strength assessment.

Steps

■ Place the hands approximately shoulder-width apart with the arms fully extended, toes in contact with the floor, torso held rigid, and head in neutral position (*a*).

■ Lower the trunk to the floor (keeping your torso flat and rigid) by allowing the arms to bend until the upper arm is just below parallel to the ground (*b*). To improve the reliability of this test, a yoga block can be placed under the chest to provide a landmark to ensure that the appropriate depth of each repetition is achieved.

■ Extend the elbows and push the body back to the starting position.

■ Perform as many push-ups as possible in one to two minutes or until you decide to end the test.

■ You are allowed to rest only in the up position. Repetitions that are performed with poor technique (e.g., hips lift or sag) or that do not use the entire exercise range of motion should not be counted.

Variations

This test can also be performed from a bent-knee, or modified, position.

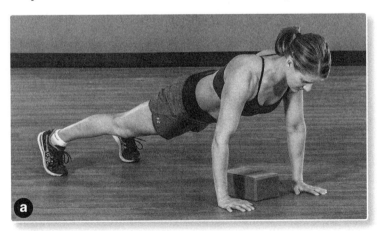

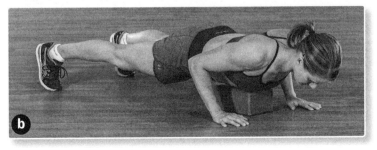

Front Plank Assessment

Equipment Needed

- Stopwatch, exercise mat.

Purpose

The front plank is used to measure isometric endurance of the trunk. This test can also be used as a basic movement screen to identify weakness in the trunk musculature. Isometric endurance of the trunk is essential for reducing the risk of injury and transferring forces efficiently during the latter stages of a competition.

Steps

- Begin by lying on the belly with the elbows positioned directly under the shoulders and the forearms in full contact with the ground.
- Lift the trunk upward so that a straight line can be drawn through the center of the ankles, knees, hips, and shoulders. Only the forearms and toes remain in contact with the ground.
- As soon as you reach this position, the stopwatch should start.
- The test is over when you can no longer maintain proper form (e.g., hips sag, bottom is pushed up, and the trunk is no longer aligned) or you decide to end the test.

Variations

This test can also be performed with the arms fully extended, such as when performing a push-up. This variation may be more specific to law enforcement personnel who are required to use defensive tactics when trying to control a person who is resisting arrest.

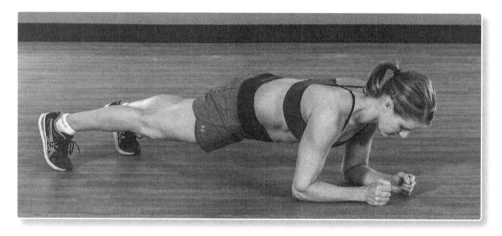

Side Plank Assessment

Equipment Needed

■ Stopwatch, exercise mat.

Purpose

The side plank, similar to the font plank, measures isometric endurance of the trunk, but this exercise puts greater emphasis on the oblique muscles to stabilize.

Steps

■ Begin by lying on the side with the left elbow positioned directly under the left shoulder and the left forearm in full contact with the ground.

■ Place the right foot on top of the left foot and then lift the hips and trunk upward until the torso is aligned.

■ As soon as you reach this position, the stopwatch should start.

■ The test is over when you can no longer maintain proper form (e.g., hips sag, bottom is pushed up, and the trunk is no longer aligned) or you decide to end the test.

■ Repeat this test on the right side.

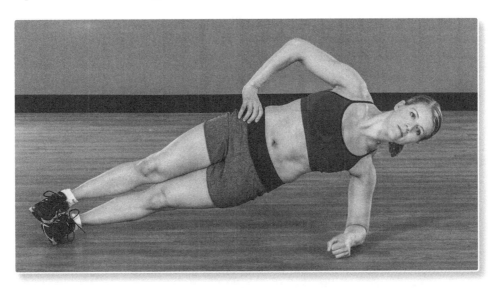

One-Minute Squat Test

Equipment Needed

Chair, aerobic steps, or plyo box.

Purpose

The purpose of this test is to measure lower-body muscular endurance. This test can be used as a baseline measure of muscular endurance for the fitness enthusiast.

Steps

- Find a chair or plyo box that allows the upper portion of the thighs to be parallel to the ground when you are sitting on it. An alternative is to use a step aerobics box, which may be easier to adjust to your height.
- Using the chair as a landmark, squat down until the buttocks contact the chair and then stand back up.
- Perform as many squats as possible in one minute using proper form and technique.
- You may rest in the standing position for this test, but the clock should remain running.
- The number of completed squats performed should be recorded as the final score for this test.

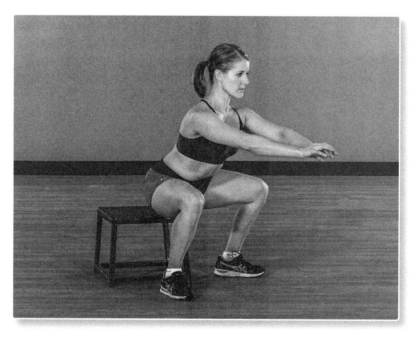

ANAEROBIC ENDURANCE TESTS

The purpose of anaerobic endurance testing is to assess sustained anaerobic power and the efficiency of the glycolytic energy system during activities that last between 30 seconds and 2 minutes. These rigorous tests are considered advanced exercises. Thus, these assessments should be performed only after the participant has developed a good base of conditioning.

300-Meter Run Test

Equipment Needed
Stopwatch, a partner to time and record the test, 400-meter track.

Purpose
The purpose of this test is to measure sustained anaerobic power and the efficiency of the glycolytic energy system. This test is frequently used in law enforcement communities to predict performance in a sustained pursuit situation.

Steps
- Using the inside lane of a 400-meter track, measure 300 meters.
- A partner is needed to time the run. When pressing the button on the stopwatch, the timer should use the index finger rather than the thumb to improve the accuracy of the measure.
- On the "Go" command, the timer starts the stopwatch. Generally, the timer simply raises a hand overhead and drops it to signal the start of the run because the distance between the timer and runner often makes it difficult to hear. The timer stops the stopwatch when the runner crosses the 300-meter line.
- Time to the nearest 0.10 second should be recorded as the final score.

300-Meter Shuttle Run Test

Equipment Needed

Stopwatch, a partner to time and record the test, 400-meter track or open field, heart rate monitor if available.

Purpose

The purpose of this test is to measure sustained anaerobic power and the efficiency of the glycolytic energy system while incorporating changes of direction. This test can also be used to measure fatigue by looking at the person's recovery heart rate, as well as the percentage of change between tests. These tests replicate many of the demands faced by athletes who are engaged in intermittent-type sports such as soccer, ice hockey, and lacrosse.

Steps

- Place two cones 25 yards (22.9 m) apart.
- To perform this test, you run between these cones six times.
- The time taken to cover this distance should be collected and recorded to the nearest 0.10 second.
- Rest for 5 minutes. At the first and third minute during the recovery phase, record heart rate. Heart rate can be taken manually by palpating the carotid artery and using the index and forefingers. Take the pulse for 10 seconds and multiply the count by six to get the estimated 1-minute heart rate (10-second HR × 6 = estimated 1-minute HR). If available, a heart rate monitor will provide an instantaneous measurement of heart rate and is typically more accurate and easy to use.
- After the 5-minute rest period, repeat the test.
- Time and heart rate should be taken for each trial.

AEROBIC ENDURANCE TESTS

The job of the aerobic energy system is to deliver oxygen and nutrients to the body. Aerobic endurance tests are also frequently used as an overall measure of cardiovascular health, fitness, and performance. The following tests can be used to measure the efficiency of the aerobic system.

Distance and time tests can be used to measure improvement in aerobic fitness. The benefit of these tests is that they can be used with practically any piece of cardiovascular equipment or with no equipment at all. For these tests, people simply set a target time to perform aerobic activity and record how far they are able to go in the allotted time. For example, using a stationary rower, they record the distance traveled in meters over a 5-minute period. They might exercise on a step mill for 10 minutes and then record the number of steps they take in that time.

One negative aspect of these assessments is that many do not have norms or standards associated with them. Some, however, not only have estimated standards but also provide estimates of aerobic capacity. Examples include the 1.5-mile (2.4 km) run test and the 12-minute run test, which will be discussed in this section. Scores for interpreting the results of these tests will be featured in chapter 13.

1.5-Mile Run Test

Equipment Needed
Treadmill or a stopwatch and track.

Purpose
The 1.5-mile (2.4 km) run is a field test commonly used to predict aerobic capacity, or $\dot{V}O_2max$ (Reiman and Manske 2009).

Steps
- Using a treadmill or track, run 1.5 miles as fast as possible.
- Time to the nearest 0.10 sec should be recorded as the final score.

12-Minute Run Test

Equipment Needed
Treadmill.

Purpose
Similar to the 1.5-mile run test, the 12-minute run test is a field test often used to predict aerobic capacity, or $\dot{V}O_2max$.

Steps
- Using a treadmill, run for 12 minutes and attempt to cover as much distance as possible.
- The exact distance traveled should be recorded as the final score.

Beep Test

Equipment Needed

Large open area, two markers (lines or cones) placed 20 meters apart, and an audio recording of the beep test protocol.

Purpose

The beep test, or multistage fitness test, is frequently used by athletes in intermittent-type sports to measure aerobic fitness and estimate $\dot{V}O_2max$ (Reiman and Manske, 2009). This test is popular among these athletes because it is more sport specific than traditional aerobic endurance tests that focus on repetitive, long-duration, linear movement. Additionally, this assessment can be used in a large-group setting, so it is useful when working with teams.

Steps

- Two lines set up 20 meters apart should be used for this test.
- As they listen to a prerecorded audio tape, participants attempt to keep cadence with a sound signal, or beep, until they are no longer physically able to maintain the set pace.
- The starting signal for this test corresponds to a speed of 8.5 kilometers per hour (5.3 mph) and increases by .5 kilometers per hour (.3 mph) for each minute of the test.
- The test ends when the subject is no longer able to maintain the pace set by the recording.
- A participant who fails to touch the line before the beep has an opportunity to speed up and reach the other line to avoid missing another beep.
- If a participant misses two lines in a row, the test ends.
- The last completed stage is recorded as the person's final score.

CHAPTER 13

Interpreting Results and Setting Goals

After conducting tests to measure fitness and performance, the next step is to understand how to use the information obtained during testing. Many options are available for interpreting test results from fitness and performance measures. The best method to use depends on the purpose of the testing. Some people test to see whether they are improving, others want to see how they stack up, and some may want to explore advanced methods of evaluation to improve specific aspects of performance. In this chapter, we present several commonly used methods of interpreting individual test results and some tips on how to set training goals based on those results.

RAW DATA ASSESSMENT

For people who simply want to make sure that they are progressing in their training program, a variety of options are available. In this section, we look at several methods of evaluating raw data obtained from fitness and performance tests.

Personal Best

One of the simplest techniques for measuring improvement is to keep track of when you achieve a personal best or personal record (PR). For example, once a week as part of your training routine, you may choose to do a five-minute distance and time test. Figure 13.1 shows an example of how this could be charted using a stair climber as the primary training modality. In this example, you would have set a PR in week 6.

Amount of Change

Another option for measuring performance is to look at the amount and percentage of change from a pretest to a posttest. To calculate the amount of change, simply subtract the old value from the new value. For instance, if A.J. was able to perform 20 push-ups during his posttest and then 6 weeks later was able to perform 30 push-ups, the net change would be 10 push-ups. We could also measure this in terms of percentage of change. To calculate percentage of change, perform the following calculation:

Step 1: Subtract the old values from the new value.

Pretest (20 push-ups) – posttest (30 push-ups) = 10 push-ups

Step 2: Divide the amount of change by the old value.

10 push-ups / 20 push-ups = .50

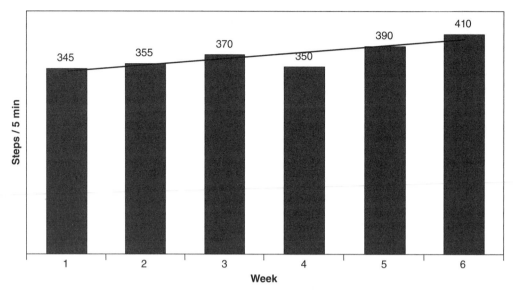

Figure 13.1 Number of steps for five-minute time trial on stair stepper.

Step 3: Convert to a percentage by multiplying the decimal number by 100.

.50 × 100 = 50% increase

These measurements are also valuable when determining the amount of improvement within a group. Table 13.1 shows the vertical jump scores after 10 weeks of resistance training and conditioning. One factor to consider about using percentage of change is that people who are more fit will tend to see smaller changes in the amount of improvement and percentage of change. This is because they are likely closer to their genetic ceiling. Essentially, they have less room for improvement than someone who is less fit. For this reason, norms and percentile rankings may also be used for assessment purposes.

Table 13.1 Division II Girls Basketball Vertical Jump Height in Inches (cm)

Name	Pretest	Posttest	Difference	% change
Mia	15.0 (38.1)	17.0 (43.2)	2.0 (5.1)	13.33
Emma	15.5 (39.4)	16.5 (41.9)	1.0 (2.5)	6.45
Olivia	14.0 (35.6)	16.5 (41.9)	2.5 (6.3)	17.85
Gabrielle	15.0 (38.1)	16.0 (40.6)	1.0 (2.5)	6.66
Addison	17.0 (43.2)	18.5 (47.0)	1.5 (3.8)	8.82
April	18.0 (45.7)	19.0 (48.3)	1.0 (2.5)	5.55
Joncee	15.0 (38.1)	16.5 (41.9)	1.5 (3.8)	10.00
Mary	16.5 (41.9)	17.0 (43.2)	0.5 (1.3)	3.03
Lea	17.0 (43.2)	17.5 (44.5)	0.5 (1.3)	2.94
Christa	20.0 (50.8)	20.5 (52.1)	0.5 (1.3)	2.50
Rachel	16.0 (40.6)	17.5 (44.5)	1.5 (3.8)	9.38
Paige	17.5 (44.5)	18.0 (45.7)	0.5 (1.3)	2.86
Lauren	18.0 (45.7)	18.0 (45.7)	0.0 (0.0)	0.00
Becky	15.0 (38.1)	16.5 (41.9)	1.5 (3.8)	10.00
Michelle	17.5 (44.5)	19.0 (48.3)	1.5 (3.8)	8.57

Note: Posttest was conducted after 10 weeks of resistance-training conditioning.

NORMATIVE COMPARISON AND PERCENTILE RANKING

In most cases, the first question asked after a test is, Was that good? Normative data allows us to compare our performance against that of others. Norms can be used for a variety of fitness and performance tests, but two questions are key when using norms as references to assess your performance.

1. **Are the norms that you are using based on data collected from a similar population?** Norms allow us to measure our individual performance if they are based on a representative group. For instance, using vertical jump norms developed from data collected on Division 1 collegiate male basketball players would be appropriate for evaluating vertical jump performance of Division I male basketball players. But these data would have little relevance in interpreting the vertical jump scores for a group of junior high basketball players because of the differences in skill and physical maturation. As a result, the comparison would hardly be fair.

2. **Was the same testing protocol used?** People often modify a testing protocol based on their situation or needs, but if the test used is not performed in the same manner as the test that the norms were developed from, they cannot be compared. For example, the standing long jump can be performed with the hands on the hips or with a counter-movement arm swing. The technique used can have a profound effect on the results of the test. In fact, in our labs we have found anywhere from a 16 to 22 percent increases in the distance that can be traveled if an arm swing is used. Consequently, if these numbers were to be compared with norms that derived their data from a standing long jump that did not use an arm swing, the person's overall rating would be inflated and give the appearance of a better performance on this assessment than what actually happened.

Norms for several of the assessments described in chapter 12 are provided at the end of this chapter.

Percentile rankings are also another way to measure how an individual score compares within a group. The percentile ranking simply tells us what percentage of scores fall above or below a certain mark. Percentile ranks, like percentages, fall on a continuum scale ranging from 0 to 100. So, for example, someone who has a percentile ranking of 90 percent performed better than 90 percent of the people who performed the same test.

QUALITATIVE EVALUATION

Sometimes the subjective improvements gained from a training program cannot be overlooked. An athlete who simply feels faster, a person who can walk a flight of stairs without being winded at the top, or someone who feels that she or he has more energy has experienced a significant change, although it is not easily quantifiable. Keeping a fitness journal or just making small notes at the end of your training log on a daily basis can serve as a great motivational tool, especially when changes in the quantitative testing data are less noticeable.

ABSOLUTE VERSUS RELATIVE STRENGTH

Strength, or the ability to exert force, can be measured in several ways. Absolute strength is determined simply by tallying the total amount of weight lifted. An example of this would be performing a one-repetition max (1RM) test on the squat or bench press. But this single piece of information does not tell us the full story. Although bench-pressing 300 pounds (136 kg) is impressive for anyone, it is more impressive for a person who weighs

150 pounds (68 kg) than for someone who weighs 220 pounds (100 kg). This comparison of strength in relation to body weight is known as relative strength. Using a simple equation we can calculate a ratio of strength to body weight:

Relative strength ratio (RSR) = weight lifted / body weight

Here is an example using the lifters mentioned previously:

Lifter 1: 1.36 RSR = 300 pounds weight lifted / 220 pounds body weight
(136 kg / 100 kg)

Lifter 2: 2.0 RSR = 300 pounds weight lifted / 150 pounds body weight
(136 kg / 68 kg)

A higher RSR reflects higher relative strength. In this example, we can see that although both people have the same absolute strength, the second lifter can produce more force per unit of body weight than the first lifter. Therefore, in relative terms the second lifter is stronger.

ABSOLUTE VERSUS RELATIVE POWER

We can also measure power in both absolute and relative terms. For example, let's say that a 220-pound (100 kg) athlete and a 150-pound (68 kg) athlete were both able to jump 20 inches (50.8 cm). The jump height would be equal. We can convert the jump height for each to peak power in watts using the following equation (Sayers et al. 1999):

Peak power (W) = 60.7 × (jump height in cm) + 45.3 × (body mass in kg) – 2,055

The first step in this equation is to convert pounds to kilograms and inches to centimeters, which can be done using the following equations:

Kilograms = weight in pounds / 2.2

Centimeters = inches jumped × 2.54

Both athletes jumped 50.8 centimeters. The athlete weighing 220 pounds weighs 100 kilograms, and the athlete weighing 150 pounds weighs approximately 68 kilograms.
Plugging this data into the equation yields the peak power in watts:
220-pound (100 kg) person:

[60.7 × (50.8 cm)] + [45.3 × (100 kg)] – 2,055 = 5,558.56 watts

150-pound (68 kg) person:

[60.7 × (50.8 cm)] + [45.3 × (68 kg)] – 2,055 = 4,108.96 watts

By comparing the wattage, we can see that the heavier athlete produced more power because he or she had to move a greater mass.

In figure 13.2 a leg power nomogram in watts based on the Sayers equation is presented. This chart offers a method of measuring power without use of a calculation. It can also assess power in terms of weight. This measure is known as the power-to-weight ratio, which can be determined by using the following equation:

Power / kilograms = power in watts / weight in kilograms

Therefore, the athlete who weighs 220 pounds (100 kg) would produce 55.59 watts per kilogram of body weight, whereas the 150-pound (68 kg) athlete would produce 60.42 watts per kilogram. Therefore, in relative terms the 150-pound athlete is more powerful, whereas in absolute terms the 220-pound athlete would produce more power.

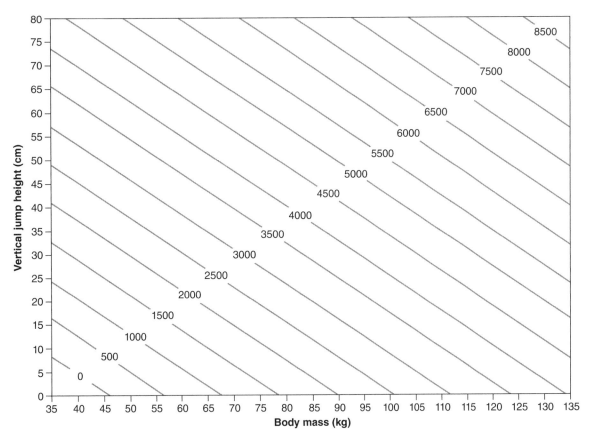

Figure 13.2 Leg power nomogram in watts.

From P.J. Kier, V.K. Jamnik, and N. Gledhill, 2003, "Technical-methodological report: A nomogram for peak leg power output in the vertical jump," *Journal of Strength and Conditioning Research* 17(4): 701-703. Reprinted by permission of the National Strength and Conditioning Association.

ECCENTRIC UTILIZATION RATIO

The eccentric utilization ratio, or EUR, is a calculation that can be used to measure use of the stretch-shortening cycle (SSC) (McGuigan et al. 2006). The SSC is essential for sports that require explosive movements like sprinting and jumping. The SSC is activated when the muscles are rapidly stretched. This quick stretch sends a message to the brain to contract the muscles forcefully to protect the tissue from overstretching and subsequent damage. When used for performance, this rapid prestretch before an explosive movement can produce a more forceful contraction, which results in greater power output.

The squat jump (SJ) emphasizes concentric force production of the lower extremities, whereas the countermovement phase of the countermovement jump (CMJ) activates the SSC and rapid eccentric loading. By using both the SJ and CMJ, the EUR can be calculated to determine the relative contribution of the SSC during different stages of training. This formula is expressed mathematically as the following:

$$EUR = CMJ / SJ$$

Table 13.2 illustrates the EUR for a group of Division II collegiate male soccer players just before the beginning of the spring season compiled over a period of years. The higher the EUR is, the greater the contribution of the SSC is to performance and the greater is the potential power that the athlete can produce

Generally, during preseason, greater emphasis is placed on plyometric and sprint training. These forms of training rely heavily on the use of the SSC. Therefore, this type of training

Table 13.2 EUR for a Group of Division II Collegiate Male Soccer Players

Name	SJ	CMJ	EUR
James	21.8	23.4	1.07
Rob	21.2	24.0	1.13
Reid	20.6	23.2	1.13
Doug	20.4	23.2	1.14
Kurt	27.2	28.1	1.03
Allen	22.4	25.0	1.12
Brian	17.6	18.6	1.06
Jason	20.6	19.7	0.96
Keiren	18.1	18.5	1.02
Asher	20.8	23.4	1.13
Cooper	25.9	25.5	0.98
Eli	23.8	24.2	1.02
Teddy	21.1	22.0	1.04
Henry	17.8	20.2	1.13
Charlie	20.5	22.2	1.08
Andy	22.8	24.6	1.08

Data were collected using a Just Jump mat.

places a greater emphasis on the SSC than on the higher-volume, slower-speed type of training typically emphasized in the off-season. Thus, the EUR calculated during the off-season would likely be lower than that calculated in the preseason if this traditional model was followed.

MAXIMAL OXYGEN UPTAKE

Aerobic fitness is generally measured in term of $\dot{V}O_2$max. $\dot{V}O_2$max is defined as "the greatest amount of oxygen a person can use while performing dynamic exercise involving a large part of total muscle mass" (Fletcher et al. 1990). More commonly referred to as maximal oxygen uptake, $\dot{V}O_2$max can be estimated using the 1.5-mile (2.4 km) run test, 12-minute run test, and beep test. The following equations provided by Reiman and Manske (2009) can be used to estimate $\dot{V}O_2$max from each of the following tests.

12-minute run test

$$\dot{V}O_2\text{max (ml} \cdot \text{kg}^{-1} \cdot \text{min}^{-1}) = 0.0268 \text{ (distance covered in meters)} - 11.3$$

1.5-mile (2.4 km) run test

$$\dot{V}O_2\text{max (ml} \cdot \text{kg}^{-1} \cdot \text{min}^{-1}) = 483 / \text{ time to run 1.5 miles}$$
(in minutes and fractions of minutes instead of seconds) + 3.5

Beep test

$$\dot{V}O_2\text{max (ml} \cdot \text{kg}^{-1} \cdot \text{min}^{-1}) = 3.46 \times \{1 \times \text{level} + [\text{shuttles} (\div \text{level} \times .4325 + 7.0048)]\} + 12.2$$

Figure 13.3 provides cardiorespiratory fitness classifications based for $\dot{V}O_2$max (ml · kg^{-1} · min^{-1}) based on age and gender.

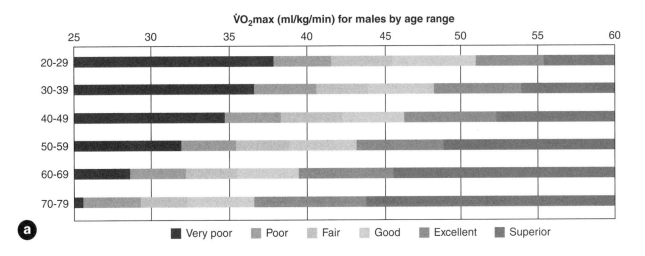

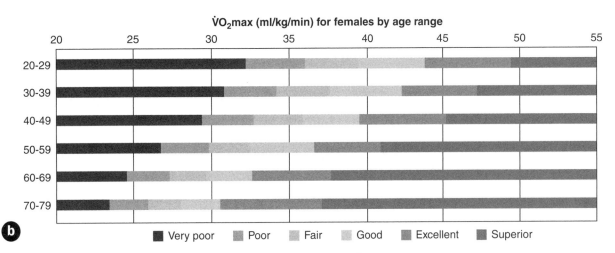

Figure 13.3 Cardiorespiratory fitness classifications based for $\dot{V}O_2$max.

Source: *Physical Fitness Assessments and Norms for Adults and Law Enforcement,* by The Cooper Institute, Dallas, Texas. Available at www.CooperInstitute.org.

EASE OF RECOVERY

Another method of measuring fitness is how quickly a person can recover from the stress created by exercise. A few of these methods are discussed in the following section.

Heart Rate Recovery

Heart rate recovery (HRR) is the speed at which the heart rate returns to normal values after exercise. A rapid HRR response to exercise can be used as a marker of physical fitness (Sayers et al. 1999). According to a review by Dimkpa (2009), a faster HRR is associated with a higher $\dot{V}O_2$max and greater endurance capacity. HRR can be calculated by taking heart rate at specific time points, usually one and two minutes after peak exercise heart rate has been achieved. Typically, in healthy people HRR will be approximately 15 to 20 beats per minute immediately postexercise (Dimkpa 2009).

This evaluation can be used after any of the aerobic or anaerobic endurance tests featured in chapter 12. Using a heart rate monitor is recommended whenever possible.

Speed Decrement and Fatigue Index

Speed drop-off can be determined by performing a series of repeated sprints with minimal rest after each. Figure 13.4 displays the results from a 20-meter repeat sprint ability test in which a recovery of only 15 seconds was allowed between sprints. This means that the person performing this test had a work-to-rest ratio between 1:3 and 1:4.

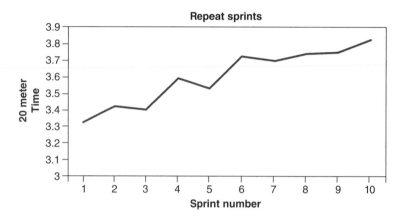

Figure 13.4 Repeated sprint test results illustrate the drop in speed that takes place when recovery time is limited.

With this information, the speed (or performance) decrement can be calculated using the following equations provided by Turner and Stewart (2013):

$$\text{Speed decrement} = ([\text{sprint 1} + \text{sprint 2} + \text{sprint 2} + \text{final sprint}] / \text{sprint 1} \times \text{number of sprints}) - 1 \times 100$$

Using the example from figure 13.3, the speed decrement would be calculated as follows:

$$\text{Speed decrement} = ([3.33 + 3.42 + 3.41 + 3.59 + 3.54 + 3.72 + 3.71 + 3.74 + 3.76 + 3.83] / 3.33 \times 10) - 1 \times 100$$

$$\text{Speed decrement} = (36.05 / 33.3) - 1 \times 100$$

$$\text{Speed decrement} = (1.08) - 1 \times 100$$

$$.08 \times 100 = 8\%$$

The overall performance speed decrement for the 10 sprints was approximately 8 percent.

The fatigue index is another measure that can be used with our repeat sprint example (figure 13.4. This measure is a bit more sensitive to extreme scores because only the fastest and slowest sprint times are used. To calculate the fatigue index, the following equation by Turner and Stewart (2013) can be used:

$$\text{Fatigue index \%} = ([\text{slowest sprint} - \text{fastest sprint}]) / \text{fastest sprint} \times 100$$

$$\text{Fatigue index \%} = ([3.83 - 3.33]) / 3.33) \times 100$$

$$15\% = (0.50 / 3.33) \times 100$$

When using either of these measurements, speed decrement or fatigue index, the lower the percentage is, the more fatigue resistant the individual is and the better his or her anaerobic capacity is.

GOAL SETTING

Goal setting is an important part of developing a training program. Training on a daily basis is difficult without a goal to strive toward and focus on. Having goals provides motivation and direction and helps provide meaning to training. In this section we review various types of goals and ways of setting effective long-term and short-term training goals to maximize your chances of success.

Subjective and Objective Goals

Goals can be subjective or objective. Subjective goals are typically general statements of intent, such as having fun, improving energy level and quality of life, or becoming more healthy and fit. Although these endeavors are all worthy, knowing when we achieve these goals is difficult. For instance, how do we know when we become fit? For this reason, setting objective goals as well as subjective goals helps us know when we have achieved these desired outcomes. Objective goals are focused on achieving a certain result, usually in a specified time frame. For example, a person may set a goal of losing 10 pounds (4.5 kg) in 20 weeks. This goal is objective because it can be easily measured. No question will arise about when or if this goal has been attained.

Both subjective and objective goals have a place in a training program. Subjective goals help frame the overall feeling that we want to achieve. For instance, in our previous example, losing 10 pounds is not about weight; it is about what that weight represents. By losing this weight, how is this person's quality of life improved? Will this person be a better athlete, be able to play with her or his children more easily, or feel more confident? When we can tie our objective goals back to a subjective feeling, our outcome motivation tends to be higher. Therefore, when goal setting, the first question we should ask is, "Why do we want to achieve this goal?" After answering this question, we can link the subjective goals to objective goals to make certain that we are moving toward the desired outcome.

Objective goals include two broad categories: outcome goals and performance goals. Outcome goals focus on what our intended result will look like. Examples include winning a state championship, beating an opponent, and running a half marathon. These goals provide motivation, but they don't tell us much about how to achieve our goals.

Performance goals are aimed at achieving some standard or level of performance, generally based on our previous performances or experience. Some of the techniques discussed earlier in this chapter, such as measuring percentage and amount of change, can be useful here.

Process goals are the little things that we must do on a consistent basis to help us achieve our performance goals. To achieve outcome goals, we have to set several performance and process goals along the way.

The examples provided in this section illustrate the funneling concept that occurs in goal setting, from the long-term subjective and objective goals to the short-term performance and process goals. Focusing the majority of energy and effort on performance and process goals should inevitably lead to achieving the desired long-term goal.

SMART Goals

People often tend to express their goals in general terms, such as, "I would like to be more athletic," or "I want to get fit." But without knowing what this means for the person, setting appropriate training goals is difficult. To address this problem, the acronym SMART can be helpful in guiding you through the goal-setting process. The acronym SMART stands for specific, measureable, attainable, relevant, and time bound.

Specific: Specific goals state in clear, concise, and unambiguous terms what the purpose of training is. For example, Rich may want to improve his cardiovascular fitness. This aspiration is a good subjective goal, but is it is not quite specific enough. Setting a goal of improving his $\dot{V}O_2$max to 45 ml $\cdot$ min^{-1} $\cdot$ kg^{-1} is a better goal because it is specific and no question will come up about whether it has been attained.

Measureable: As previously stated, although some qualitative goals are good motivators, having tangible measurements helps us determine whether we are on the right track when pushing toward our goals. Our previous example of achieving a $\dot{V}O_2$max of 45 ml $\cdot$ min^{-1} $\cdot$ kg^{-1} is a good, measureable performance goal. Success can be measured by using the 1.5-mile (2.4 km) run outlined in chapter 12. A good process goal to make certain that Rich is moving toward his performance goal would be to perform maximal interval training two times per week in addition to running three times per week.

Attainable: The goals set should be realistic and attainable. A good rule of thumb is that goals should be just out of reach. For example, if Rich had current $\dot{V}O_2$max of 41 ml $\cdot$ min^{-1} $\cdot$ kg^{-1}, which would place him in the fair fitness category, aiming for 55 ml $\cdot$ min^{-1} $\cdot$ kg^{-1} would likely lead to frustration because a $\dot{V}O_2$max at that level would put him in the superior category. For this reason, a prudent strategy for Rich would be to aim for the next classification level up, the good category. After he attains that goal, he can set another training goal.

Relevant: The goals set must be relevant to the person's needs, interests, and goals. Using our example, how is improving $\dot{V}O_2$max relevant to Rich's goals? In this case, he eventually wants to be fit enough to run recreationally and possibly compete in some 5K races. Based on this aspiration, his goal of improving his $\dot{V}O_2$max to reach the good classification category appears relevant.

Time bound: Providing timelines for achieving goals helps reduce procrastination and maintain motivation to train. For example, Rich may set an initial training goal of improving his $\dot{V}O_2$max by 10 percent in three months. Referring back to our $\dot{V}O_2$max equation, he would need to shave approximately 1:10 (from 12:50 to 11:40) off his initial 1.5-mile run time to achieve his goal in the three-month period.

SUMMARY

A variety of ways to interpret test results have been presented in this chapter. These methods provide you with several options for measuring performance so that you can set effective and efficient long-term and short-term training goals. Furthermore, adhering to the SMART goal-setting strategy will help you develop specific training goals to ensure success.

ADDITIONAL NORMATIVE DATA

Using the following tables, an athlete can see how he or she compares to various groups of individuals. However, please use this information with caution. It is not necessarily wise to compare a high-school athlete with a collegiate or even professional athlete's level of performance because of differences in developmental age, training experience, and status. While this information can be useful to help provide a frame of reference for performance, the more specific the information is to the competition level, the age group, and the athlete's sex, the more accurate this information will be.

Table 13.3 Normative Values for the Squat Among Various Athletic Populations

Reference	Population	Gender	Score (mean ± *SD*, pounds)
BASKETBALL			
Latin et al. 1994	NCAA DI	M	334 ± 81
	G		332 ± 79
	F		356 ± 84
	C		304 ± 70
FOOTBALL			
Garstecki et al. 2004	NCAA DI	M	510 ± 90
	QB		440 ± 99
	RB		513 ± 73
	WR		453 ± 88
	OL		552 ± 75
	TE		510 ± 81
	DL		543 ± 77
	LB		530 ± 81
	DB		458 ± 88
SOCCER			
Wisloff et al. 1998	Norwegian elite	M	330 ± 42
VOLLEYBALL			
Fry et al. 1991	NCAA DI	F	180 ± 26

G = guard; F = forward; C = center; QB = quarterback; RB = running back; WR = wide receiver; OL = offensive lineman; TE = tight end; DL = defensive lineman; LB = linebacker; DB = defensive back.

Reprinted, by permission, from M.P. Reiman and R.C. Manske, 2009, *Functional testing in human performance* (Champaign, IL: Human Kinetics), 169.

Table 13.4   Pro Agility Times for college Football Players Participating in the NFL Combine

	PRO AGILITY (S)							
% rank	DL	LB	DB	OL	QB	RB	TE	WR
90	4.22	4.07	3.89	4.45	4.07	4.02	4.18	3.97
80	4.32	4.13	3.96	4.53	4.12	4.14	4.21	4.03
70	4.38	4.16	4.05	4.57	4.16	4.18	4.26	4.07
60	4.41	4.21	4.07	4.61	4.20	4.22	4.31	4.10
50	4.46	4.24	4.12	4.69	4.25	4.25	4.35	4.15
40	4.52	4.28	4.18	4.77	4.33	4.31	4.39	4.20
30	4.58	4.31	4.19	4.83	4.36	4.34	4.42	4.24
20	4.68	4.41	4.21	4.93	4.38	4.38	4.46	4.26
10	4.75	4.53	4.27	5.06	4.41	4.49	4.56	4.33
X_	4.48	4.26	4.11	4.74	4.26	4.26	4.35	4.15
SD	0.22	0.17	0.15	0.39	0.15	0.16	0.13	0.15
n	89	38	76	125	38	58	39	85

Data collected from 1999 NFL combine.
DL = defensive lineman; LB = linebacker; DB = defensive back; OL = offensive lineman; QB = quarterback; RB = running back; TE = tight end; WR = wide receiver.

Reprinted, by permission, from J. Hoffman, 2006, *Norms for fitness, performance, and health* (Champaign, IL, Human Kinetics), 114.

Table 13.5   Fitness Categories by Age Groups and Sex for Push-Ups

	AGE AND SEX									
	20-29		30-39		40-49		50-59		60-69	
Category	M	F	M	F	M	F	M	F	M	F
Excellent	36	30	30	27	25	24	21	21	18	17
Very good	35	29	29	26	24	23	20	20	17	16
	29	21	22	20	17	15	13	11	11	12
Good	28	20	21	19	16	14	12	10	10	11
	22	15	17	13	13	11	10	7	8	5
Fair	21	14	16	12	12	10	9	6	7	4
	17	10	12	8	10	5	7	2	5	2
Needs improvement	16	9	11	7	9	4	6	1	4	1

Source: Canadian Physical Activity, Fitness & Lifestyle Approach: CSEP-Health & Fitness Program's Appraisal and Counselling Strategy, 3rd edition, © 2003. Reprinted with permission from the Canadian Society for Exercise Physiology.

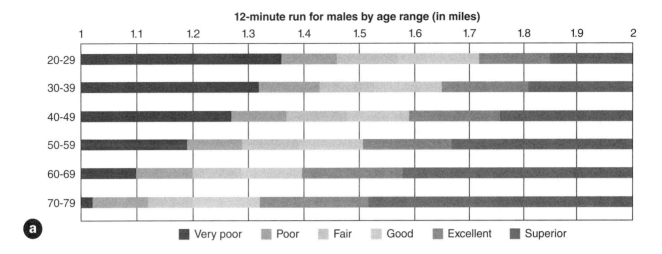

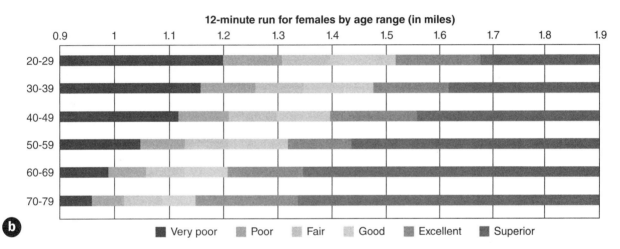

Figure 13.5 Aerobic fitness norms for a 12-minute run.

Source: *Physical Fitness Assessments and Norms for Adults and Law Enforcement,* by The Cooper Institute, Dallas, Texas. Available at www.CooperInstitute.org.

CHAPTER 14

Creating a Personalized Program

Designing a training program can be a challenge even for experienced strength and conditioning coaches. It involves finding the right balance of key variables and adhering to established principles of exercise and program organization. A great deal of background information is required to develop effective strength and conditioning programs for athletes as well as for people who just want to become more fit. A strength and conditioning program, regardless of what tools it uses, will only work if it is a good fit for you. Although some benefits may be gained from doing a canned training program, optimal benefits will be achieved only if the program takes your personal background, goals, and preferences into account. The information in this chapter provides a foundation for successfully adapting or designing a training program to suit your needs.

PROGRAM VARIABLES

Several key training variables must be addressed, manipulated, and successfully integrated to create an effective, comprehensive training program. The interplay of these variables can have a profound impact on the results you get. The variables must be balanced according to your needs, whether the primary goal is reducing fat, improving health and fitness, or enhancing sport performance. These concepts must be fully understood to optimize training results.

Five major variables must be considered when designing a training program:

1. Intensity
2. Volume
3. Rest
4. Recovery
5. Muscle balance

Intensity

Intensity refers to the quality and difficulty of the exercise. An inverse relationship exists between the intensity of an exercise and its volume (sets × repetitions). Intense exercise sessions are stressful and can be extremely fatiguing, so you must reduce the volume of training because fatigue will limit the number of quality repetitions that you will be able to perform. You will also need more rest and recovery after intense training sessions when compared with less intense sessions.

In a traditional strength-training workout, intensity is prescribed according to a percentage of the maximum weight (a percentage of one-repetition maximum, or 1RM) or maximum number of repetitions that you can lift at a certain weight (called a repetition maximum, or RM). For example, if you can squat 300 pounds (136 kg), then training at 70 percent of the 1RM would mean working out with 210 pounds (95 kg). On the other hand, if you wanted to train at your 10RM, you would work with a weight that you could lift a maximum of 10 times.

People are typically instructed to perform plyometric, speed, and agility drills at maximal intensity. In other words, with these types of training, athletes train at or close to their maximum speed and power. The intent of these exercises is to teach athletes how to be more explosive, so training at less than maximal intensity doesn't develop this ability.

With maximum interval training, intensity is calibrated a little differently. Here the focus is on helping you become resistant to the effects of fatigue. This type of training is not the most effective training approach to increase strength, power, or maximal speed. The selected intensity should allow you to complete the desired volume of exercise with good form and technique.

Volume

The volume is the quantity of the work that is being done. With strength training it is usually the number of repetitions multiplied by the number of sets. For example, performing three sets of 10 repetitions produces a volume of 30. But when performing maximum interval training, volume can be expressed in a number of ways. It can also be expressed in terms of time, distance, number of jumps, number of throws, and so on. For example, when performing kettlebell swings for 30 seconds, volume can be quantified by time. Volume can also be expressed in terms of distance, such as sprinting for 40 meters. Or it can reflect the number of repetitions, such as performing 20 crunches.

The greater the volume is, the lower the training intensity should be. Besides having an inverse relationship with intensity, volume is a powerful stimulus for various types of adaptations from training. For example, low volume is appropriate for activities that require a great deal of technique, speed, and power. Moderate volumes are good for developing hypertrophy. Higher volumes help enhance resistance to fatigue.

Rest

Rest refers to the time taken after each set of an exercise. Longer rest periods allow you to achieve greater training intensity. For example, if you train with heavy weights, you should allow at least three to five minutes of rest after each set to recover. You could then lift a greater amount of weight each set. Rest can also be important for the transferability of training. For instance, if you play a sport that typically has 10 to 20 seconds of rest after each play, you can design your training program to mimic those work and rest periods.

With maximum interval-training workouts, rest periods have a large effect on the difficulty of the training. Consider the sample workouts in table 14.1. Both workouts involve the same exercises, the same number of times through the circuit, and the same volume of training. The difference is that the athlete rests for 15 seconds after each exercise in workout A but does not rest after each exercise in workout B. As a result, the athlete can handle more weight on the kettlebells and will feel less fatigued when performing workout A than when performing workout B. **Note: The italicized exercises are in part II. Refer to the exercise finder for more information.**

Recovery

Recovery refers to the time between exercise sessions. This period is important because it is when all the adaptations that we are training for occur. Failure to allow adequate recovery can eventually lead to a state of overtraining and injury. Although training every day is

Table 14.1 Effect of Rest Between Exercises

	Workout A	Workout B
Exercises in circuit (kettlebell weight)	Kettlebell two-handed swing (25 kg) Bodyweight plank Kettlebell one-handed swing (right) (15 kg) Bodyweight plank Kettlebell one-handed swing (left) (15 kg) Bodyweight plank Kettlebell goblet squat (25 kg) Bodyweight plank Kettlebell deadlift (25 kg) Bodyweight plank Kettlebell push-up Bodyweight plank Kettlebell prone row (right) (15 kg) Bodyweight plank Kettlebell prone row (left) (15 kg)	Kettlebell two-handed swing (20 kg) Bodyweight plank Kettlebell one-handed swing (right) (10kg) Bodyweight plank Kettlebell one-handed swing (left) (10 kg) Bodyweight plank Kettlebell goblet squat (20 kg) Bodyweight plank Kettlebell deadlift (20 kg) Bodyweight plank Kettlebell push-up Bodyweight plank Kettlebell prone row (right) (10 kg) Bodyweight plank Kettlebell prone row (left) (10 kg)
Duration of each exercise (seconds)	30	30
Rest after each exercise (seconds)	15	0
Number of circuits	3	3

possible, special care must be taken to ensure that the activities are organized so that the same muscles, physical abilities, and qualities are not trained on successive days.

Table 14.2 shows two sample weeks of workouts. In the figure, workout A involves lower-body strength training and the power clean on Monday, sprints on Tuesday, plyometrics on Wednesday, lower-body strength training and the power snatch on Thursday, and sprint-based conditioning on Friday. On the surface this plan looks like an appropriate distribution of the workload across the week. The reality is that workout A involves a great deal of lower-body work Monday through Friday, so the schedule does not optimize recovery.

Workout B in table 14.2 takes a different approach. Monday involves total-body strength training with very heavy weights. Tuesday is focused on power training. Wednesday is a day off. Thursday involves lower-body strength training combined with sprints. Friday uses upper-body strength training, kettlebells, and core exercises for conditioning. In workout B the training sessions are distributed to allow the body a chance to recover.

Training needs to be organized so that the muscles and energy systems get a chance to recover. In general, the 48-hour rule (i.e., rest a muscle group 48 hours before training it again) is a good one to follow. To help conceptualize the concept of recovery, table 14.3 describes the relationship between energy systems, qualities, and training. The table shows that certain types of training essentially train the same energy systems and require the same qualities. For example, strength, power, acceleration, maximum velocity, and even agility training all link up well and are considered compatible. On the other hand, hypertrophy training, speed endurance, and conditioning all link up. Using this example, strength and acceleration work would complement each other if they were done on the same day, but strength and speed endurance would not. This table provides some guidance on how to organize training so that the body has a chance to recover.

Muscle Balance

Several important concepts are related to muscle balance. First, you should train all the muscles around a joint, whatever the type or purpose of your training. Failing to do this

Table 14.2 Workouts With Insufficient (A) and Sufficient (B) Recovery

Individual exercises are followed by sets × reps × intensity or weight, as applicable. Sprints are listed in repetitions × distance format.

	Monday	**Tuesday**	**Wednesday**
Workout A	Power clean, 3 × 3–6 × 60–70% Back squat, 3 × 8–12 × 70–80% Lunge, 3 × 12–15 each leg Romanian deadlift, 3 × 8–12 Glute ham raise, 3 × 12–15	Sprints, 5 × 5 meters Sprints, 5 × 20 meters Bounds, 5 × 20 meters	Vertical jump, 10 × Box jumps, 10 × Standing long jump, 10 × Hurdle hop, 3 × 10 meters
	Thursday	**Friday**	
	Power snatch, 3 × 3–6 × 60–70% Front squat, 3 × 4–6 × 70–80% Split squat, 3 × 12–15 each leg Good morning, 3 × 8–12 Back raise, 3 × 12–15	Sprint conditioning (seconds from start until the next sprint begins): *1 × 10 (5)* *1 × 20 (10)* *1 × 40 (20)* *1 × 60 (30)* *1 × 100 (40)* *1 × 100 (40)* *1 × 60 (30)* *1 × 40 (20)* *1 × 20 (10)* *1 × 10*	

	Monday	**Tuesday**	**Wednesday**
Workout B	Back squat, 3 × 3 × 6 × 80–90% Romanian deadlift, 3 × 3–6 Bench press, 3 × 3–6 × 80–90% Bent-over row, 3 × 3–6 Military press, 3 × 3–6	Power snatch, 3 × 3–6 × 60–70% Power clean, 3 × 3–6 × 60–70% Clean pull, 3 × 3–6 × 60–70% Vertical jump, 10× Box jumps, 10× Standing long jump, 10× Hurdle hop, 3 × 10 meters	Off
	Thursday	**Friday**	
	Front squat, 3 × 4–6 × 70–80% Split squat, 3 × 12–15 each leg Good morning, 3 × 8–12 Back raise, 3 × 12–15 Sprints, 5 × 5 meters Sprints, 5 × 20 meters Bounds, 5 × 20 meters	Dumbbell bench press, 3 × 12–15 Pull-up, 3 × max Dumbbell shoulder press, 3 × 12–15 Biceps and triceps, 3 × 12–15 each Circuit (30 sec on, 15 sec rest; repeat three times): *Kettlebell two-handed swing* *Bodyweight plank* *Kettlebell one-handed swing (right)* *Bodyweight plank* *Kettlebell one-handed swing (left)* *Bodyweight plank* *Kettlebell goblet squat* *Bodyweight plank* *Kettlebell deadlift* *Bodyweight plank* *Kettlebell push-up* *Bodyweight plank* *Kettlebell prone row (right)* *Bodyweight plank* *Kettlebell prone row (left)*	

creates strength imbalances around the joint that can set you up for injury in the long term. For example, if you perform a pushing exercise like a chest press on a suspension trainer, you should balance that out with a pulling exercise like the suspension trainer row. Similarly, a number of total-body, kettlebell, heavy ropes, sprinting, and medicine ball exercises should be incorporated over time into a program to help ensure that you achieve muscle balance.

Table 14.3 Characteristics of Various Training Types

Quality	Volume	Intensity	Energy system	Comments
Strength	Low	High	Phosphagen	All-out effort
Power	Low	High	Phosphagen	All-out effort, speed of movement important
Hypertrophy	Moderate	Moderate	Phosphagen, glycolytic	Incomplete recovery between sets
Conditioning	Moderate to high	Moderate to low	Glycolytic, oxidative	Incomplete recovery between sets
Speed (acceleration)	Low	High	Phosphagen	Technique, all-out effort
Speed (maximum velocity)	Moderate	High	Phosphagen, glycolytic	Technique, all-out effort
Speed (speed endurance)	High	Moderate to high	Glycolytic	Incomplete recovery between sets
Agility	Low to high	Moderate	Phosphagen, glycolytic	Technique, all-out effort

Second, you should perform an equivalent amount of work on opposite movements. For example, if you perform three sets of pushing movements, you should perform three sets of pulling movements. This approach prevents one side of the body from being overdeveloped.

Third, these concepts apply to nontraditional examples as well. They are not limited to weight room exercises. For example, if you are pushing a weighted sled as part of your workout, you would also want to spend some time walking backward and pulling it.

PRINCIPLES OF EXERCISE

The principles of individualization, specificity, overload, and progression should form the foundation of any successful strength and conditioning program. Regardless of the training goal or equipment used, these basic training principles should be applied to ensure the safety and effectiveness of a program. Failing to adhere to these principles can lead not only to injury but also to inadequate or haphazard training gains.

Individualization

Everyone is different, and those differences must be considered in creating and evaluating a training program. No two people have the same objectives, start in the same state, or develop identically from the same program.

Incorporating the principle of individualization starts with determining the reason for training. This reason has a tremendous influence on program development. It should drive every decision you make regarding the program. It determines your intensity, volume, training frequency, and even the exercises and modes of exercise. Unfortunately, most people don't stop to consider this important first step and just jump into a workout program. Failing to identify the primary reason for training can lead to haphazard programming, which may ultimately lead to suboptimal results and frustration.

The next important bit of information to uncover is what your current strengths are and how much improvement you want to make. To map out the best way to reach a destination, you must first know where you are. After you have established the specific training goals, the next step is to consider where you are beginning your fitness journey in relation to where you want to go. This information drives the pace at which you can proceed.

Specificity

The principle of specificity says that you get what you train for. In other words, the body adapts to the demands placed on it. If you don't perform certain exercises or you avoid training certain attributes, performance in those areas will not improve. For example, performing a lot of sprints in training will likely improve your 40-yard dash time, but it won't increase your bench press strength. Specificity calls for taking into account several factors, such as the muscles and motions being used, the energy systems that produce energy for the activity, and, in many cases, the speed of movement required to perform the activity.

For example, let's say that you want to improve your bench press. This activity involves the muscles of the chest, shoulders, and triceps. Training to increase how much you can bench press involves increasing maximal strength. As the amount of weight that you must move increases, the speed of movement goes down. Table 14.4 shows that during the bench press, many of the issues that result in a failed attempt are related to pectoralis major and deltoid strength (getting the bar off the chest) or triceps strength (arm extension, sticking at the midpoint).

Table 14.5 shows examples of how to address each typical problem area in the bench press. Note that each of the problem areas is addressed by focusing on the specific movement patterns and muscle groups used for this exercise. For example, although many exercises strengthen the triceps, we still need to select exercises that address the specific pressing motion needed to perform the bench press.

Table 14.6 is an example of a training program that applies the principle of specificity. For this example, an athlete wants to improve his or her bench press but is having trouble

Table 14.4 Bench Press Muscle Involvement and Common Reasons for Failure

	Descent phase	**Press phase**
Prime mover muscles involved	Latissimus dorsi, posterior deltoids, biceps brachii	Pectoralis major, anterior deltoid, triceps brachii
Antagonist muscles involved	Pectoralis major, anterior deltoid, triceps brachii	Latissimus dorsi, posterior deltoids, biceps brachii
Stabilizer muscles involved	Medial deltoids, rotator cuff	Medial deltoids, rotator cuff
Speed of movement	Slow and controlled	Slow and controlled
Typical problem areas	Bar is out of groove Descent is too fast	Cannot get bar off chest Uneven arm extension Stick at midpoint of press

Table 14.5 Solutions to Common Bench Press Problems

Typical problem area	**Solution**
Bar is out of groove during descent.	Strengthen lats and posterior deltoids using seated rows with a bench press grip and reverse band bench presses. Strengthen descent motion using eccentric bench presses.
Descent is too fast.	Strengthen descent motion using eccentric bench presses or reverse band bench presses.
Cannot get bar off chest during press.	Strengthen pectoralis major and anterior deltoid using dumbbell bench presses, decline presses, and military presses.
Uneven arm extension during press.	Strengthen each arm independently using dumbbell bench presses and dumbbell floor presses.
Stick at midpoint of press.	Strengthen triceps using dips, close-grip bench presses, floor presses, and towel bench presses.

Table 14.6 Program Using the Specificity Principle to Improve Bench Press

Individual exercises are followed by sets × reps and (intensity or weight), as applicable.

Monday	Thursday
Bench press, 3–5 × 4–8 (75–85%)	Floor press, 3–5 × 8–12 (80–90%)
Dumbbell floor press, 3 × 4–8	Dip, 3 × 8–12
Seated row, bench press grip, 3–5 × 4–8	Bent-over row, bench press grip, 3 × 8–12
Military press, 3 × 4–8	Dumbbell shoulder press, 3 × 8–12

at the midpoint of the press. This program is meant to be done twice a week (Monday and Thursday in this example). On Monday the bench press is trained, followed by dumbbell floor presses to work on the elbow extension, seated rows to work on keeping control of the bar during the descent, and the military press to strengthen the deltoids. Note that the training is fairly heavy with a low to moderate number of repetitions.

The Thursday session is focused on the triceps. The floor press is the first exercise, performed at a percentage of the bench press. This is followed by weighted dips. Bent-over rows help strengthen the descent, and the dumbbell shoulder press strengthens the deltoids. Note that a moderate number of repetitions are used for each set on this day to allow the joints to recover.

Overload

The overload principle states that to keep making gains, the body must be continually challenged by training. The body adapts, which is why everyone exercises. One of the great ironies with exercise is that the process of adapting, which is what produces gains in strength, speed, muscle size, and so on, also leads to plateaus. After the body adapts, we have to find ways to make the workouts more difficult over time or we stop making progress.

The overload principle is normally applied by changing one of four variables. We can change the intensity, volume, kind of exercise, or amount of rest (i.e., rest between sets, rest within sets, and rest between training sessions). Any one of these variables can have a big effect on the difficulty of a training session, and all these variables are interrelated.

The intensity is the difficulty of the work that is being done. With strength training, intensity is expressed as a percentage of either how much weight you can lift one time (one-repetition maximum, or 1RM) or how much weight you can lift for a number of repetitions. For example, an 8RM lift is how much weight you can lift eight times. Intensity can also be expressed as speed, power output, height, distance, and so on.

The rest is the amount of time between sets, circuits, and workouts. When more rest is allowed, more recovery occurs, which means that work can be done at a higher intensity. When less rest is allowed, less time is available to recover, which means that the intensity cannot be sustained.

The exercises selected can also have an effect on the difficulty of the training session. Many exercises train the same muscles and the same joints, using similar movement patterns. But changing an exercise to one that is similar but stresses the body slightly differently may be sufficient to keep the body adapting. An example would be performing a one-handed kettlebell swing instead of a two-handed swing.

Table 14.7 shows examples of changing each of the preceding variables. The first column shows the base workout. The columns to the right of the base workout show the new workout after changing one of the variables (so the second column shows changing the intensity, the third shows changing the volume, and so on). Notice how all the variables are interrelated; when one variable changes, others must also change. Changing the intensity has an effect

Table 14.7 Effect of Changing Workout Variables

Individual exercises are followed by sets × reps × intensity or weight, as applicable.

Base workout	Change intensity	Change volume	Change rest	Change exercises
Back squat, 3 × 12 × 240 lb (109 kg) Lunge, 3 × 12 × 95 lb (43 kg) each leg Romanian deadlift, 3 × 12 × 225 lb (102 kg) Glute ham raise, 3 × 15 Seated calf raise, 3 × 15 × 90 lb (41 kg)	Back squat, 3 × 12 × 245 lb (111 kg) Lunge, 3 × 10 × 105 lb (48 kg) Romanian deadlift, 3 × 10 × 235 lb (107 kg) Glute ham raise, 3 × 12 × 10 lb (4.5 kg) Seated calf raise, 3 × 12 × 100 lb (45 kg)	Back squat, 3 × 15 × 225 lb (102 kg) Lunge, 3 × 15 × 80 lb (36 kg) Romanian deadlift, 3 × 15 × 200 lb (91 kg) Glute ham raise, 3 × 18 Seated calf raise, 3 × 18 × 75 lb (34 kg)	Back squat, 3 × 12 × 185 lb (84 kg) Lunge, 3 × 12 × 65 lb (29 kg) each leg Romanian deadlift, 3 × 12 × 165 lb (75 kg) Glute ham raise, 3 × 15 Seated calf raise, 3 × 15 × 65 lb (29 kg)	Front squat, 3 × 8 × 185 lb (84 kg) Split squat, 3 × 12 × 95 lb (43 kg) each leg Good morning, 3 × 12 × 95 lb (43 kg) Reverse hyperextension, 3 × 15 Standing calf raise, 3 × 15 × 180 lb (82 kg)
Rest 2 minutes after each set	Rest 2 minutes after each set	Rest 2 minutes after each set	Rest 30 seconds after each set	Rest 2 minutes after each set

on the volume (increasing the amount of weight to be lifted means that it cannot be lifted as many times). Changing the volume has an effect on intensity (performing more repetitions per set means that less weight can be lifted). Decreasing the amount of resting between sets also reduces the amount of weight that can be lifted.

Table 14.8 shows how to apply the overload principle to a maximum interval-training session. In the figure, the base workout is shown. Performed as described, the base workout will take an athlete approximately 18 minutes. The next column shows the session with a change in the weight of the kettlebell as well as an increase in the weight used when performing the squats and lunges. An example of changing the volume (each exercise is performed for

Table 14.8 Applying the Overload Principle to an MIT Circuit

Base session	Change intensity	Change volume	Change rest	Change exercises
Kettlebell two-handed swing, 30 lb (14 kg) Bodyweight plank Bodyweight jumping jacks Kettlebell two-handed swing, 30 lb (14 kg) Bodyweight plank Bodyweight squat Kettlebell two-handed swing, 30 lb (14 kg) Bodyweight plank Bodyweight walking lunge Kettlebell two-handed swing, 30 lb (14 kg) Bodyweight plank Bodyweight inchworm Perform each exercise for 20 seconds, rest 10 seconds after each exercise, and perform circuit three times.	Kettlebell two-handed swing, 40 lb (18 kg) Bodyweight plank Bodyweight jumping jacks Kettlebell two-handed swing, 40 lb (18 kg) Bodyweight plank Squat, 20 lb (9 kg) dumbbells in each hand Kettlebell two-handed swing, 40 lb (18 kg) Bodyweight plank Walking lunge, 20 lb (9 kg) dumbbells in each hand Kettlebell two-handed swing, 40 lb (18 kg) Bodyweight plank Bodyweight inchworm Perform each exercise for 20 seconds, rest 10 seconds after each exercise, and perform circuit three times.	Kettlebell two-handed swing, 30 lb (14 kg) Bodyweight plank Bodyweight jumping jacks Kettlebell two-handed swing, 30 lb (14 kg) Bodyweight plank Bodyweight squat Kettlebell two-handed swing, 30 lb (14 kg) Bodyweight plank Bodyweight walking lunge Kettlebell two-handed swing, 30 lb (14 kg) Bodyweight plank Bodyweight inchworm Perform each exercise for 30 seconds, rest 10 seconds after each exercise, and perform circuit three times.	Kettlebell two-handed swing, 30 lb (14 kg) Bodyweight plank Bodyweight jumping jacks Kettlebell two-handed swing, 30 lb (14 kg) Bodyweight plank Bodyweight squat Kettlebell two-handed swing, 30 lb (14 kg) Bodyweight plank Bodyweight walking lunge Kettlebell two-handed swing, 30 lb (14 kg) Bodyweight plank Bodyweight inchworm Perform each exercise for 20 seconds, take no rest after each exercise, and perform circuit three times.	Kettlebell one-handed swing, 20 lb (9 kg) Bodyweight plank Heavy ropes slam Kettlebell two-handed swing, 20 lb (9 kg) Bodyweight plank Kettlebell goblet squat, 20 lb (9 kg) Kettlebell one-handed swing, 20 lb (9 kg) Bodyweight plank Heavy ropes shuffle slam Kettlebell two-handed swing, 20 lb (9 kg) Bodyweight plank Bodyweight inchworm Perform each exercise for 20 seconds, rest 10 seconds after each exercise, and perform circuit three times.

a longer time) is also provided. The rest after each exercise can be reduced or eliminated. Finally, an example of changing the exercises is included. For each modification, the workout will still take 18 minutes.

When applying the overload principle, keep the principle of specificity in mind. Failing to do this can mean that you will develop the wrong qualities and energy systems, which may conflict with your training goals. For example, performing a set of 100 bodyweight squats may be challenging because lactic acid will build up and cause a burning sensation in the legs. This type of activity primarily trains the glycolytic energy system, so it improves muscular endurance. In contrast, performing a set of squats that would allow you to perform only four repetitions before you fatigue would primarily work the ATP–PCr energy system and would emphasize muscular strength rather than endurance. So if your goal is to increase maximum squat strength, performing the set of four to near muscular fatigue will be more conducive to producing this training outcome.

Progression

According to the overload principle, to continue making gains over time, you have to find a way to make the workouts more challenging. The principle of progression tells us that this overload should be added using a steady, sequential approach to maximize safety and effectiveness. This goal is accomplished in two parts.

First, you need to build a fitness foundation. Building a solid fitness foundation prepares the joints, skeleton, and muscles for the rigors of advanced exercises and workout programs. This preparation reduces the chances of developing an injury from the workout program.

The second part of the principle of progression is developing a technical foundation before attempting advanced exercises. Correct technique ensures that the exercise is effective and that the joints are being loaded appropriately. Learning correct technique is important because when you become fatigued, technique typically suffers. When this happens, you not only gain less benefit from the exercise but also increase the likelihood of becoming injured.

Whether we're talking about fitness or technique, progression can be thought of as a series of steps. Each step builds on what came before. Adding the steps one by one and taking the time to ensure that each is solid before adding more ensures that you'll have a stable structure.

Most long-term training programs for athletes evolve from an extended period that is focused on all-around fitness to a period when that fitness is applied to the needs of the sport and finally to a period when the athlete is peaking for the sport. This process helps athletes follow an appropriate training progression. These concepts can also be applied to those who are reaching for any type of training goal. Creating a fitness foundation and a technical foundation and building on the foundations in a measured, steady manner is critical for success!

SEQUENCING AND PRIORITIZING YOUR TRAINING

The principles of training described earlier help to determine whether an exercise is going to be effective in achieving your goals. At some point, all the various types of exercise and workout sessions have to fit together into a larger, unified whole, or program. This part of the chapter presents suggestions to simplify the complex process of achieving the right mix of modes of exercise and program design variables.

When putting together your training program and determining the order in which you proceed, two important considerations have to be balanced.

First, although there are always exceptions, you normally perform the exercises in a natural sequence in which you tackle those that call for more energy early and save the lighter, less taxing work for the end. In general, exercises that require speed and power should be performed at the beginning of a training session (sprinting, plyometrics, or the Olympic lifts). Total-body exercises like kettlebell swings should follow. Next should come multijoint exercises like the squat or press. Exercises that are more isolated in nature should be performed last.

Second, while keeping the first point in mind, you need to put your training program together in a way that allows you to prioritize your goals. You should do the aspect of training that you believe is most important first and give it the most attention. A list of physical qualities that you might want to train is included in the left column of table 14.8.

The right column of table 14.9 shows how you would arrange your workouts if you decide to focus on conditioning work. Conditioning is trained three times a week, which is the most of any of the qualities. Strength, power, speed, and agility are trained once per week. Hypertrophy, which aligns well with conditioning work, is trained twice a week. Mobility is always important, so it is emphasized twice a week. If you decide at some point to prioritize agility training instead, then the frequency would need to be reworked with that in mind.

Table 14.9 Sample of Prioritizing Training to Focus on Conditioning

Quality	Frequency per week
Strength	1
Power	1
Hypertrophy	2
Speed	1
Agility	1
Conditioning	3
Mobility	2

CHAPTER 15

Using Periodization to Push Performance to the Next Level

Up to this point, the concept of program design has been concerned with the short term—with this workout, this week, this month. To get the kind of adaptations that you want from your training, it has to take place consistently over a long time. When planning your training, you still need to keep in mind the principles of chapter 14. But you need to train in such a way that it doesn't result in boredom, overtraining, injury, or ineffectiveness. You can accomplish this by periodizing the workouts.

Periodization is an approach to training used by strength and conditioning coaches and athletes that involves breaking down training into carefully planned blocks of time. These blocks systematically manipulate all the exercise variables to maximize performance while minimizing the risk of injury and overtraining.

To the uninitiated, periodization can seem confusing. This chapter demystifies the concept of periodization and provides a systematic explanation of how to create a periodized training program.

The process of planning a periodized workout program can be made easier by addressing one step at a time. Here are the steps for developing a periodized training program:

- Organize the training program.
- Decide on goals for each phase.
- Plan the first mesocycle in detail.

ORGANIZING A PERIODIZED TRAINING PROGRAM

Periodization has its own language, which can be difficult to wade through. On top of that, the various periodization systems use different terminology, which can add a layer of confusion. The largest block of training in periodization is called a macrocycle. This block is typically 12 months long, but it can be longer or shorter depending on the athlete and the sport. Usually it represents a peak for training. For example, we want American football players to peak during their season, which runs during the fall and winter. In other sports, like track and field, athletes may have more than one season and therefore have more than one peak, so they may have multiple macrocycles in a training year.

The macrocycle is divided into three main phases of training:

1. Preparatory phase
2. Competition phase
3. Recovery phase

The preparatory phase develops the athlete's physical foundation. It can be viewed as a time for the athlete to get in shape for her or his sport. The competition phase involves peaking for the sport, and it occurs when games or competitions are taking place. The recovery phase is the time after the last competition, when the athlete is still physically active but is also getting rest and recovery to heal and regain mental focus. Note that some macrocycles may include all the phases described or only one or two of them

The three main phases of training are broken down into periods. The preparatory phase of training is typically divided into two types of periods—general preparation and special preparation. The general preparation period (GPP) usually makes up two-thirds of the preparatory phase. This is the get-in-shape period of training when all the physical qualities are developed. The special preparation period (SPP) makes up the remainder of the preparatory phase. This period applies the fitness developed in the GPP to the needs of the sport. Note that these descriptions aren't absolutes. Advanced athletes have longer SPPs, and some preparatory phases may even be 100 percent SPP.

The competition phase is also divided into two types of periods. The first is the precompetition period, which is a transitional period between the SPP and the first competition. The second is the competition period, which is the time during which games or competitions are occurring.

The recovery phase of training is normally only a few weeks long, so there isn't a need to divide it into different types of recovery periods.

Periods of training are broken down into more manageable blocks of time called mesocycles. Mesocycles normally last four weeks. Again, this definition is not an absolute; mesocycles can be longer or shorter depending on the athlete's sport calendar. Mesocycles are broken down into smaller subdivisions called microcycles, which typically last a week but can also be longer or shorter.

Figure 15.1 shows a sample of what periodized training would look like for an American football player. The figure shows how the months fall into the phases and periods of training. The roman numerals in the figure represent mesocycles, so mesocycle I is in January, mesocycle II is in February, and so on. Note that May is divided into two shorter mesocycles. January is divided into microcycles a, b, and c. The assumption is that the athlete is going to take a lot of time off around the end-of-year holidays, so the training year starts on January 6.

Year-long macrocycle											
Recovery phase	Preparatory phase							Competition phase			
Recovery period	General prep period				Special prep period			Precomp period	Competition period		
Jan	Feb	Mar	Apr	May		Jun	Jul	Aug	Sep	Oct	Nov	Dec
I	II	III	IV	V	VI	VII	VIII	IX	X	XI	XII	XIII

Week	Microcycle
Week 1	I:a
Week 2	I:b
Week 3	I:c

Figure 15.1 Periodized training for an American football player.

When dividing the training year into blocks of time, we normally begin by determining when the competitive season phase falls and by extension when the recovery and preparation phases take place. For example, as illustrated in figure 15.1, competitions run from September through December. Add in the high-intensity two-a-day practices in August and, depending on the level, camp and preseason games, and we have a competition phase that runs from August through December.

After the competition phase, athletes should take time to recover from the stress of training and competition. If there are no bowl games or playoff games, the month of January is a recovery phase for football players. The rest of the year (February through July) is the preparatory phase.

After the calendar is divided into phases, each phase is subdivided into periods, beginning with the competition phase. We know that September through December is when the regular-season games take place, so this makes up the competition period. August, which includes gamelike workouts and scrimmages designed to prepare players for the real thing, is the precompetition period.

February through July makes up a six-month preparatory phase. The bulk of that should be allotted for GPP, so February through the middle of May (three and a half months) would be GPP, and the rest would be SPP. Spending slightly more time in GPP means we have time to improve the athlete's base before the high-intensity training that will occur during both SPP and competition. The SPP then applies that physical base directly to the needs of the sport.

This type of approach can be taken for any sport or goal situation. The important thing is to begin the process with the big picture in mind rather than jump into the tiny details. Dividing up the training year, as described in this section, provides a road map for reaching your training goals.

DECIDING ON GOALS FOR EACH PERIOD

With periodization, the various periods (GPP, SPP, precompetition, and so on) have different characteristics and different goals. These different characteristics require that the strength and conditioning program use different exercises, modes of exercises, intensity, and volume in each period. To complicate matters further, everything has to be done while balancing the athlete's sport commitments (practice, travel, and competitions). Table 15.1 provides an overview of the characteristics and goals for the periods of training that would apply to most team sports. Table 15.2 provides a similar overview for an endurance-based sport such as the marathon. Note that these are examples only; you are always free to select your own goals for each phase of training!

Despite differences in the type of exercises and the role of maximum interval training within the overall training picture, the training approaches for team athletes and endurance athletes have some similarities. For example, during the GPP the team-sport athlete who is following the type of program outlined in figure 15.1 performs higher-volume training with a great deal of variety. In contrast, during the GPP the endurance athlete who is following the type of program outlined in figure 15.2 performs higher-volume training and more cross-training (i.e., more general training) while working to develop an endurance base. In both cases, however, training becomes more intense and more specific as the athlete progresses through the macrocycle.

After the goals and characteristics of each period of training have been determined, the next step is to select the types of exercises that will be used, frequency of training, and general trends for manipulating volume and intensity. These choices set the parameters for the workouts to be used in the detailed program design. Table 15.3 provides an example of this using our American football player.

Table 15.1 Common Goals and Characteristics by Period for a Team-Sport Athlete

Period	Goals	Characteristics
General preparation	Physical foundation for injury prevention Fitness base Technique base	Higher volume Low to moderate intensity General training (not sport-specific)
Special preparation	Maintenance of fitness base Maintenance of technical base Increase in speed, agility, strength, and power Application of physical fitness to the sport	Moderate to low volume Moderate to high intensity Some general training, focus on sport-specific training Increased complexity in terms of exercises and drills
Precompetition	Maintenance of fitness base Maintenance of technical base Increase in speed, agility, strength, and power Sport-specific training	Low volume High intensity Sport-specific training Increased complexity in terms of exercises and drills Addressing athlete's deficiencies relative to performance
Competition	Maintenance of fitness base Maintenance of technical base Maintenance or increase in speed, agility, strength, and power Sport-specific training	Low volume High intensity Sport-specific training Increased complexity in terms of exercises and drills Addressing athlete's deficiencies relative to performance Training frequency decreases because of demands of competition
Recovery	Rest and recovery Maintenance of fitness base	Higher volume Low intensity Unstructured training More variety than in previous periods

Table 15.2 Common Goals and Characteristics by Period for an Endurance-Sport Athlete

Period	Goals	Characteristics
General preparation	Physical foundation for injury prevention Fitness base Technique base	Higher volume Low to moderate intensity Long, slow distance training Cross-training
Special preparation	Maintenance of fitness base Maintenance of technical base Increase in speed, agility, strength, and power Application of physical fitness to the sport	Moderate to high volume Moderate to high intensity Some interval training Maximal strength and power training Sport-specific training Addressing athlete's deficiencies relative to performance
Precompetition	Maintenance of fitness base Maintenance of technical base Increase in speed, agility, strength, and power Sport-specific training	Moderate to high volume High intensity Interval training Sport-specific training Addressing athlete's deficiencies relative to performance
Competition	Maintenance of fitness base Maintenance of technical base Maintenance or increase in speed, agility, strength, and power Sport-specific training	Moderate volume High intensity Sport-specific training Increased complexity in terms of exercises and drills Addressing athlete's deficiencies relative to performance Training frequency decreases because of demands of competition
Recovery	Rest and recovery Maintenance of fitness base	Moderate to low volume Low intensity Cross-training More variety than in previous periods

Table 15.3 Sample Workout Overview by Period and Training Objective for an American Football Player

Period	Strength	Speed	Agility	Power	Conditioning
General preparation	3–4 times per week 3–5 × 12–15 × 60–70% Squat Hip extension Press Row	1–2 times per week 3–5 × 10–40 meters Technique drills	1–2 times per week Technique drills	1–2 times per week 3 × 4–6 × 60–70% Olympic lifts: Hang power clean, pull, push jerk 10–20 foot contacts for vertical jumps, standing long jumps, and hops	2 times per week 15–20 minutes each session *Kettlebells* *Heavy ropes* *Bodyweight* *Suspension trainer*
Special preparation	4–5 times per week 3–5 × 4–12 × 70–90% Squat Hip extension Press Row	1–2 times per week 3–5 × 10–60 meters Technique drills Stride length drills	1–2 times per week Technique drills Position-specific drills	1–2 times per week 3 × 4–6 × 60–70% Olympic lifts: Hang power clean, pull, push jerk 20–30 foot contacts for vertical jumps, standing long jumps, box jumps, and hops	2 times per week 15–20 minutes each session *Kettlebells* *Heavy ropes* *Bodyweight* *Suspension trainer*
Precompetition	3 times per week 3–5 × 4–12 × 70–90% Squat Hip extension Press Row	1–2 times per week 3–5 × 10–60 meters Technique drills Stride length drills Resisted starts	2–3 times per week Technique drills Position-specific drills	1–2 times per week 3 × 4–6 × 60–70% Olympic lifts: Hang power clean, pull, push jerk 20–30 foot contacts for vertical jumps, standing long jumps, box jumps, and hops	2 times per week 15–20 minutes each session *Kettlebells* *Heavy ropes* *Bodyweight* *Suspension trainer*
Competition	3 times per week 3–5 × 4–12 × 70–90% Squat Hip extension Press Row	1 time per week 3–5 × 10–60 meters Technique drills Stride frequency drills Resisted starts	2–3 times per week Technique drills Position-specific drills	1 time per week 3 × 4–6 × 60–70% Olympic lifts: Hang power clean, pull, push jerk 20–30 foot contacts for vertical jumps, standing long jumps, box jumps, and hops	As needed
Recovery		1–2 times per week Technique drills	1–2 times per week Technique drills		3–5 times per week 15–20 minutes each session *Kettlebells* *Heavy ropes* *Bodyweight* *Suspension trainer*

During the GPP, strength training is focused on building the athlete's foundation. This means lighter weights, higher volume, and fundamental exercises. In the SPP, the number of strength-training sessions per week increases, as does the intensity. The lean muscle developed in the SPP is put to use to become a stronger, more explosive football player. In precompetition and competition, the goal is to perform three strength-training sessions per week to maintain strength and muscle size.

Speed and agility training sessions are performed one to two times per week during the GPP and SPP. The volume starts low as the athlete learns the movements and gets in shape, and then increases as the athlete progresses through the SPP. As the year progresses, the exercises become more complicated and more position specific.

Power training focuses on a combination of the Olympic-style lifts and plyometrics. Because the focus of power training is to move quickly, the volume and intensity don't really change with the Olympic lifts. On the other hand, the volume (number of foot contacts) and variety of the plyometric exercises change as the training year progresses.

Conditioning is conducted twice a week through the precompetition period. It is not conducted during the season, unless the athlete is deficient in this area. Notice that conditioning becomes the primary training tool during the recovery phase.

This example illustrates how to organize the year, determine goals for each part of the year, and use those goals to focus the training. Planning the main components ahead of time ensures that a balanced approach is achieved. Establishing a solid structure allows adjustments to be made should unforeseen complications or injuries occur, while keeping the big picture in mind.

PLANNING THE FIRST MESOCYCLE IN DETAIL

Organizing the training program and developing the goals for each block of time creates the roadmap for your periodized program. At this point, you may be tempting to sit down and write out the workouts for the entire macrocycle. Although this might be a creative exercise, it would be a mistake. People are not spreadsheets. People respond to exercise in unique ways, and even the most well-planned program components are influenced by real-life factors that can't be predicted or controlled. The smartest thing to do is to sit down and plan only the first mesocycle in detail, bearing in mind that the rest are already planned in principle because of the first two steps that you performed.

For example, figure 15.2 shows an example using the training year that was developed in the figures and tables presented earlier in this chapter. This represents the first microcycle of the general preparation phase of training, so the intent is to get the athlete used to training and develop a physical foundation. Strength training is performed four times a week for brief sessions. The intensity is low (around 60 percent), and the volume is moderate to high. Speed, agility, and power training are meant to introduce the movements and get the athlete familiar with them. Conditioning is performed twice a week.

Figure 15.3 shows how the training would progress throughout this mesocycle (mesocycle II). The workouts are organized to progress in difficulty over the first three weeks. The fourth week is a testing week. Week 5 is meant to be a week of reduced intensity to aid in recovery. The figure shows how strength, speed, agility, power, and conditioning change over the course of the mesocycle. From that point, it's easy enough to plug everything into the workouts.

When the athlete is halfway through this mesocycle, it is time to sit down and plan the next mesocycle in the same detail. This process should be repeated as the year progresses.

Year-long macrocycle												
Recovery phase	Preparatory phase							Competition phase				
Recovery period	General prep period					Special prep period		Precomp period	Competition period			
Jan	Feb	Mar	Apr	May	Jun	Jul		Aug	Sep	Oct	Nov	Dec
I	II	III	IV	V	VI	VII	VIII	IX	X	XI	XII	XIII

Week	Microcycle
Week 1	I:a
Week 2	I:b
Week 3	I:c
Week 4	I:d
Week 5	I:e

I:a	Monday	Tuesday	Wednesday	Thursday	Friday	Saturday	Sunday
Strength	Back squats, 3×15×60% Romanian deadlifts, 3×15 Bench press, 3×15×60% Bent-over rows, 3×15 Standing military press, 3×15	Power clean, hang, above the knee, 3×6×60% Clean pull, hang, above the knee, 3×6×60% Push jerk, 3×6×60%	Off	Front squats, 3×12×60% Split squats, 3×12 each leg Good mornings, 3×12 Reverse hyperextensions, 3×12	Incline press, 3×12 Pull-ups, 3×max Side/rear deltoid raise superset, 3×12 each Biceps/triceps superset, 3×12 each	Off	Off
Speed	Technique drills, 10 minutes Standing starts, 3×10 meters	Off	Off	Technique drills, 10 minutes Standing starts, 3×40 meters	Off	Off	Off
Agility	Technique drills, 10 minutes	Off	Off	Technique drills, 10 minutes	Off	Off	Off
Power	Off	Vertical jump, 10× Standing long jump, 10×	Off	Off	Off	Off	Off
Conditioning	Off	Off	Kettelbell/heavy rope circuit, 15-20 minutes	Off	Off	Bodyweight/suspension trainer/sprint circuit, 15-20 minutes	Off

Figure 15.2 A sample year-long macrocycle.

	II:a				II:b				II:c				II:d				II:e			
Strength	M	T	R	F	M	T	R	F	M	T	R	F	M	T	R	F	M	T	R	F
	3×15 60%	3×6 60%	3×12 60%	3×12	3×15 60%	3×6 60%	3×12 60%	3×12	3×12 70%	3×6 60%	3×15 60%	3×15	Max	Max	Max	Max	3×15 60%	3×6 60%	3×15 60%	3×15
Speed	M		R		M		R		M		R		M		R		M		R	
	3×10 m		3×40 m		4×10 m		4×40 m		5×10 m		5×40 m		Test 20 m		Test 60 m		5×10 m		5×40 m	
Agility	No change				No change				No change				No change				No change			
Power	20 contacts				25 contacts				30 contacts				Test: VJ, SLJ				30 contacts			
Conditioning	No change				No change				No change				No change				No change			

Figure 15.3 Training progression for mesocycle II.

276

PART IV

Maximum Interval Performance Programs

CHAPTER 16

Strength and Power

Strength refers to the ability to exert force. The stronger you are, the more force you can exert. Strength is an important component of abilities that are essential for sport performance, like sprinting, agility, throwing, hitting, and kicking.

Power can be thought of as the ability to exert force quickly. It's not just how much force you can exert; it is how quickly you can do it. For example, you need strong legs and a strong core to hit a baseball, but if you cannot swing the bat quickly enough to connect with the pitch, then all the strength in the world won't help your performance.

Strength and power are foundational abilities for athletics and life in general. Strength represents a person's ceiling in terms of force production. It is a quality that allows people to move an opponent or object, to maintain their posture, to sprint, to jump, to throw, to change direction, to react to a changing environment, and to perform everyday tasks. Power, or exerting force quickly, is highly dependent on strength. To a point, stronger athletes have the potential to be more powerful. Many of the explosive maneuvers used in various sports are a product of both strength and power. Some types of power training are more effective as an athlete becomes stronger. In other words, strength and power work hand in hand.

HOW STRENGTH AND POWER ARE TRAINED

A number of tools can be used to train for strength, such as barbells, dumbbells, kettlebells, and strongman implements like stones, logs, tires, and so on. When training for strength, the focus is on multijoint exercises, heavy weights, low volume, and complete recovery between sets. Normally, when training for strength we perform three to five sets per exercise, for fewer than eight repetitions per set, with at least 80 percent of maximum weight, and allowing two to three minutes of recovery after each set.

Training for strength is normally organized in one of two ways. First, it can be trained around the idea of improving specific lifts. Table 16.1 shows an example of a week of strength workouts designed to improve three standard exercises: the squat, bench press, and deadlift. Within this program, two days are focused on training the bench press and squat, and one day is geared toward the deadlift. Each of the exercises included in the workouts is meant to help enhance the lift that is being trained that day. Powerlifters and people who are training but not playing a sport use this kind of workout. **Note: The italicized exercises are found in part II. Refer to the exercise finder for more information.**

Strength can also be developed using a total-body approach to training. Table 16.2 shows a sample workout that would accomplish this. This type of workout is commonly seen in the training of athletes, and it too makes use of standard strength exercises. Almost every muscle of the body is trained in this session. This approach is used with athletes because they are attempting to improve several attributes with their training, so the amount of time devoted to any one aspect of training is limited.

Power is trained using the Olympic lifts and their variations, plyometrics, and explosive variations of free-weight exercises like jumping squats and speed squats. With power training,

Table 16.1 Sample Week of Workouts to Improve Specific Lifts

Day 1	Day 2	Day 3	Day 4	Day 5	Day 6
Back squat, 3 × 4–8 × 80–90% Quarter squat, 3 × 2–6 × 100–120% Good morning, 3 × 4–8 Back raise, 3 × 8–12 Calf raise, 3 × 12–15	Bench press, 3 × 4–8 × 80–90% Dumbbell bench press, 3 × 4–8 Floor press, 3 × 4–8 × 90–110% Seated row, bench-press grip, 3 × 4–8	Deadlift, 3 × 2–6 × 80–90% Deadlift, above the knees, 3 × 2–6 × 100–120% Romanian deadlift, 3 × 4–8 Reverse hyperextension, 3 × 12–15	Off	Front squat, 3 × 4–8 × 70–80% Eccentric squat, 3 × 2–6 × 60–70% Back raise, 3 × 8–12 Calf raise, 3 × 12–15	Board press, 3 × 4–8 × 80–90% Floor dumbbell press, 3 × 4–8 Dip, 3 × 4–8 Bent-over row, bench-press grip, 3 × 4–8

Table 16.2 Sample Total-Body Strength Workout

Exercise or lift	Sets/repetitions	Intensity
Back squat	3 × 4–8	80–90%
Romanian deadlift	3 × 4–8	n/a
Bench press	3 × 4–8	80–90%
Bent-over row	3 × 4–8	n/a
Military press	3 × 4–8	n/a

the focus is on correct technique and speed of movement. For that reason, fatigue is not a good thing because it tends to result in slow and sloppy training, which is counterproductive. To train for power, three to five sets of an exercise with up to six repetitions per set are typically performed. Two to three minutes of recovery after each set is normal. The amount of weight used for these types of exercises is around 50 to 70 percent of maximum.

Power training can be organized in a number of ways. One way is to integrate it into a strength-training workout. When this is done, the power exercises should be performed at the beginning of the training session. They can also be used as stand-alone workouts organized by exercise type (for example, an Olympic lifting workout or a plyometric workout). Any of these approaches can be effective. Table 16.3 provides examples of the various ways to organize power training.

In the training of athletes, it is not unusual to see some power training in the form of Olympic lifts integrated with strength training and to see stand-alone sessions of plyometrics. It is also common to see training focused on a single quality. Table 16.4 shows examples of how both approaches could be executed using exercises commonly performed for these purposes. Both of these extreme approaches to power training are effective. Because these two physical qualities are interrelated and key to successful sport performance, athletes need to focus on both strength and power to be successful.

Table 16.3 Sample Power-Training Workouts

Approach	Integrated power training workout	Olympic lifting workout	Plyometric workout
Workout	Power clean, 3 × 4–6 × 60–70% Clean pull, 3 × 4–6 × 70–80% Back squat, 3 × 4–8 × 80–90% Romanian deadlift, 3 × 4–8 Calf raise, 3 × 12–15	Power snatch, 3 × 2–4 × 60–70% Power clean + split jerk, 3 × 3 + 2 × 70–80% Clean pull, 3 × 4–6 × 70–80%	Squat jump, 10× Box jump, 10× Standing long jump, 10× Hurdle hop, 3 × 5 yards

Table 16.4   Sample Integrated and Stand-Alone Plyometric Power Training Workouts

	Monday	Tuesday	Wednesday	Thursday	Friday
Integrated training example	Power clean, 3 × 4–6 × 60–70% Clean pull, 3 × 4–6 × 70–80% Back squat, 3 × 4–8 × 80–90% Romanian deadlift, 3 × 4–8	Medicine ball throw, 10× *Medicine ball chest pass*, 10× Bench press, 3 × 4–8 × 80–90% Bent-over row, 3 × 4–8 Military press, 3 × 4–8	Off	Power snatch, 3 × 3–4 × 60–70% Box jump, 10× Hurdle hop, 3 × 5 yards Front squat, 3 × 4–8 × 70–80% Good morning, 3 × 4–8	Push jerk, 3 × 4–6 × 60–70% Floor press, 3 × 4–8 × 70–80% Pull-up, 3 × 4–8 Military press, 3 × 4–8
Stand-alone training example	Back squat, 3 × 4–8 × 80–90% Romanian deadlift, 3 × 4–8 Bench press, 3 × 4–8 × 80–90% Bent-over row, 3 × 4–8 Military press, 3 × 4–8	Power snatch, 3 × 3–4 × 60–70% Power clean + split jerk, 3 × 3 + 2 × 60–70% Clean pull, 3 × 4–6 × 70–80%	Off	Front squat, 3 × 4–8 × 70–80% Good morning, 3 × 4–8 Incline press, 3 × 4–8 Pull-up, 3 × 4–8 Military press, 3 × 4–8	Squat jump, 10× Box jump, 10× Standing long jump, 10× Hurdle hop, 3 × 5 yards

LIMITATIONS OF STRENGTH AND POWER TRAINING

Although strength and power training are essential for athletic success, important for activities of everyday life, and a fun method of training, several associated concerns should be considered before using it. These include wear and tear on the joints, diminishing returns, and the risk of injury.

Wear and Tear on the Joints   Any time people lift heavy weights or attempt to move quickly, they place the joints under an increased amount of stress. The joints are often the weak link with this type of training. Injuries to the lower back, knee, elbow, and shoulder can occur as a result of strength and power training. To reduce the risk of these issues, participants need to emphasize good technique and spend time developing a good physical foundation before moving to heavy and explosive training.

Diminishing Returns   As people get closer to reaching their genetic potential for strength and power, making gains becomes increasingly difficult. We have to spend more time and more energy to see increases in strength and power. If we're closer to our genetic potential, the likelihood of an injury from the training increases because we are pushing our physical limits. Ironically, in the training of athletes, there is a point in terms of strength development where more gains will not translate to improved performance. After an athlete has reached a high level of achievement in these attributes, it may be more beneficial to focus on the weak links in physical development, such as mobility or agility. In summary, although strength and power training are highly beneficial, they have to be balanced with other forms of training and kept in perspective.

Mistakes Can Lead to Injury   Power exercises must be performed quickly. For example, a power clean or power snatch is performed within a few seconds, meaning that no time is available to make adjustments and correct technical mistakes. As a result, mistakes can lead to injuries. For that reason, avoiding fatigue when performing these exercises is important. Thus, power exercises should be done at the beginning of a workout, before the muscles become significantly fatigued.

GUIDELINES FOR INTEGRATING MAXIMUM INTERVAL TRAINING

The potential benefits and various methods of strength and power training described must be evaluated alongside their limitations. The following are a few things to keep in mind when trying to integrate maximum interval training into a strength- and power-training program.

Avoid Adding to the Wear and Tear on the Joints Because strength and power training can be stressful to the joints, maximum interval training should balance this out so that it does not contribute to stress. The best way to do this is to avoid exercise modes that provide similar stresses. For example, strongman training, weighted sleds, and kettlebells provide similar joint stresses, so they should be avoided as maximum interval training during strength and power training. Instead, bodyweight exercises, suspension training, medicine balls, heavy ropes, and sandbags would be appropriate.

Avoid Using Strength and Power Exercises for Maximum Interval Training As described earlier, many of these exercises are not forgiving of mistakes, so extreme fatigue must be avoided. But the ability to withstand fatigue is the purpose of maximum interval training. Therefore, the Olympic lifts and plyometrics do not make good maximum interval-training exercises.

Avoid Confusing Different Training Qualities Strength and power both represent maximum, short-duration, all-out efforts. Maximum interval training represents a training approach that is submaximal and is done over a long duration with minimal rest and recovery. In other words, it focuses on training a quality entirely different from strength and power. As a result, it should not be trained on the same days as strength and power.

Maximum Interval Training Is a Conditioning and Recovery Tool Why incorporate maximum interval training into a strength and power program? First, maximum interval training is a powerful conditioning tool. It prepares the body to function at a high level in the presence of fatigue. This quality is not trained in strength and power training. Second, it burns a lot of calories. Finally, it can be used as a way to recover from the rigors of strength and power training.

SAMPLE PROGRAMS

For reasons described earlier, maximum interval-training programs used in conjunction with speed and power training will largely be focused on suspension training, bodyweight exercises, medicine balls, heavy ropes, and sandbags. Unlike strength and power training, maximum interval training consists of long durations, high volumes, and short rest periods. This part of the chapter presents examples of foundational programs that use each of those modes of training, advanced programs that integrate them all, and ways in which those programs should be integrated with speed and power training.

Table 16.5 shows three foundational programs. Each program centers on bodyweight exercises, suspension-training exercises, or heavy ropes exercises. These programs involve 20 seconds of exercise alternated with 10 seconds of recovery. In each program, the exercises are performed in sequence. For example, in the heavy ropes program you perform heavy ropes jumping jacks for 20 seconds, rest for 10 seconds, and then perform the next exercise, heavy ropes slam, for 20 seconds. You perform the circuit three times, allowing two minutes of rest between rounds

Table 16.6 offers three advanced programs. Each program integrates bodyweight training, suspension training, and heavy ropes training. These programs involve 30 to 45 seconds of exercise with no rest between exercises. The exercises are performed in sequence. The circuit should be performed three to five times, with two minutes of rest between rounds. The advanced exercises in this program should be attempted only after their prerequisites have been mastered. In addition, you should give yourself at least three months with the foundational program to establish a solid training base before moving to the advanced one.

The maximum interval-training sessions should take place on days when strength and power training is not performed. Table 16.7 shows an example of how to integrate this training into strength and power training. This works regardless of how you structure your strength and power training (the table provides examples from each extreme).

Table 16.5 Foundational Maximum Interval Training Strength and Power Programs

Foundational MIT bodyweight program	Foundational MIT suspension trainer program	Foundational MIT heavy ropes program
Bodyweight jumping jacks	Suspension squat	Heavy ropes jumping jacks
Bodyweight groiner	Suspension one-legged squat, right	Heavy ropes two-handed slam
Bodyweight speed squat	Suspension one-legged squat, left	Heavy ropes one-handed slam
Bodyweight reverse lunge	Suspension hip up	Heavy ropes wave
Bodyweight inchworm	Suspension leg curl	Heavy ropes woodchopper
Bodyweight bear crawl	Suspension row	Heavy ropes one-legged woodchopper, left
Bodyweight pull-up	Suspension chest press	Heavy ropes one-legged woodchopper, right
Bodyweight dip	Suspension reverse fly	Heavy ropes twist
Bodyweight push-up	Suspension biceps curl	Heavy ropes clockwise arm circle
	Suspension triceps extension	Heavy ropes counterclockwise arm circle

Table 16.6 Advanced Maximum Interval Training Integrated Strength and Power Programs

Advanced MIT integrated strength and power program 1	Advanced MIT integrated strength and power program 2	Advanced MIT integrated strength and power program 3
Heavy ropes slam	Heavy ropes jumping jack	Suspension squat
Bodyweight groiner	Suspension squat	Suspension one-legged squat, right
Suspension reverse lunge, right	Heavy ropes one-handed slam	Suspension one-legged squat, left
Suspension reverse lunge, left	Bodyweight walking lunge	Suspension hip up
Suspension leg curl	Bodyweight inchworm	Bodyweight inchworm
Bodyweight pull-up	Bodyweight bear crawl	Suspension chest press
Suspension chest press	Suspension row	Heavy ropes wave
Heavy ropes clockwise arm circle	Bodyweight dip	Heavy ropes twist
Heavy ropes counterclockwise arm circle	Heavy ropes woodchopper, right	Suspension biceps curl
	Heavy ropes woodchopper, left	Suspension triceps extension

Table 16.7 Sample Maximum Interval-Training Strength and Power Programs

	Monday	**Tuesday**	**Wednesday**
Integrated training	Power clean, 3 × 4–6 × 60–70% Clean pull, 3 × 4–6 × 70–80% Back squat, 3 × 4–8 × 80–90% Romanian deadlift, 3 × 4–8	Medicine ball behind-the-back throw, 10× *Medicine ball chest pass*, 10× Bench press, 3 × 4–8 × 80–90% Bent-over row, 3 × 4–8 Military press, 3 × 4–8	Advanced MIT integrated strength and power program 1
	Thursday	**Friday**	**Saturday**
	Power snatch, 3 × 3–4 × 60–70% Box jump, 10× Hurdle hop, 3 × 5 yards Front squat, 3 × 4–8 × 70–80% Good morning, 3 × 4–8	Push jerk, 3 × 4–6 × 60–70% Floor press, 3 × 4–8 × 70–80% Pull-up, 3 × 4–8 Military press, 3 × 4–8	Advanced MIT integrated strength and power program 2
	Monday	**Tuesday**	**Wednesday**
Stand-alone training	Back squat, 3 × 4–8 × 80–90% Romanian deadlift, 3 × 4–8 Bench press, 3 × 4–8 × 80–90% Bent-over row, 3 × 4–8 Military press, 3 × 4–8	Power snatch, 3 × 3–4 × 60–70% Power clean + Split jerk, 3 × 3 + 2 × 60–70% Clean pull, 3 × 4–6 × 70–80%	Advanced MIT integrated strength and power program 1
	Thursday	**Friday**	**Saturday**
	Front squats, 3 × 4–8 × 70–80% Good morning, 3 × 4–8 Incline press, 3 × 4–8 Pull–up, 3 × 4–8 Military press, 3 × 4–8	Squat jump, 10× Box jump, 10× Standing long jump, 10× Hurdle hop, 3 × 5 yards	Advanced MIT integrated strength and power program 2

LONG-TERM PROGRAMS

The rest of this chapter explains how to periodize a strength and power program that includes maximum interval training as a component, using the American football player described in chapter 15 as an example. This athlete's training year is shown in figure 16.1. The competition season runs from August through December. January is a recovery phase, and the months of February through July are a preparatory phase.

The athlete we are focusing on is an offensive lineman. To be successful at this position, he needs to be strong, explosive, and able to move quickly over short distances. Plays generally last a few seconds, and 20 to 30 seconds is available for recovery after each play. With that in mind, a strength and conditioning program for this athlete should focus on enhancing maximal strength, improving power, increasing short-distance speed and agility, and developing the ability to maintain those qualities during plays from the start of the game through the fourth quarter.

Table 16.8 shows the goals of each period of training and describes what tools will be used to achieve those goals. The general preparation period is primarily focused on developing

Year-long macrocycle											
Recovery phase	Preparatory phase							Competition phase			
Recovery period	General prep period					Special prep period		Precomp period	Competition period		
Jan	Feb	Mar	Apr	May		Jun	Jul	Aug	Sep	Oct	Nov	Dec
I	II	III	IV	V	VI	VII	VIII	IX	X	XI	XII	XIII

Figure 16.1 An example year-long training macrocycle for an American football player.

Table 16.8 Goals and Tools for Each Period in the Training Year

Period	Goals	Tools
General preparation	Increase muscle mass	Multijoint exercises
	Increase strength	Multijoint exercises
	Increase power	Olympic lifts
	Speed and agility fundamentals	Technique drills Short sprints
	Conditioning base	*Bodyweight exercises* *Suspension-training exercises* *Medicine ball exercises* *Sandbag exercises* *Heavy ropes exercises*
Special preparation	Maintain muscle mass	Multijoint exercises
	Increase strength	Multijoint exercises *Resistance bands and chains*
	Increase power	Olympic lifts Plyometrics
	Position-specific speed and agility	Technique drills Short sprints Pattern drills
	Sport-specific conditioning	*Bodyweight exercises* *Suspension-training exercises* *Medicine ball exercises* *Sandbag exercises* *Heavy ropes exercises*
Precompetition	Maintain muscle mass	Multijoint exercises
	Maintain or increase strength	Multijoint exercises *Resistance bands and chains*
	Increase power	Olympic lifts Plyometrics
	Position-specific speed and agility	Technique drills Short sprints Pattern drills
	Maintain conditioning	*Bodyweight exercises* *Suspension-training exercises* *Medicine ball exercises* *Sandbag exercises* *Heavy ropes exercises*
Competition	Maintain muscle mass	Multijoint exercises
	Maintain strength	Complex training
	Maintain power	Complex training
	Position-specific speed and agility	Pattern drills
	Maintain conditioning	As needed
Recovery	Conditioning	*Bodyweight exercises* *Suspension-training exercises* *Medicine ball exercises* *Sandbag exercises* *Kettlebell exercises* *Heavy ropes exercises*

the athlete's base. This means doing multijoint exercises, the Olympic lifts, technique drills, and conditioning. The special preparation period continues those exercises and incorporates the use of bands and chains into the strength-training portion of the program, plyometrics as a method of developing power, and position-specific pattern drills for speed and agility. During the competition period, strength and power training is maintained through complex training (the combining of strength and power training), and position-specific speed and agility is emphasized. The recovery period has a great deal of variety and is made up mostly of conditioning work using many of the available tools.

Table 16.9 shows the trends for the volume and intensity for each mode of exercise during each period of training. The changes in the volume and intensity for the different modes of training reflect the different focus of the periods. Note that speed, agility, and plyometric training are always performed at high intensity.

Now that the broad program is established, the rest of this chapter examines detailed sample workouts from each period to demonstrate how to integrate maximum interval training into a periodized strength and power program.

General Preparation Period

Table 16.10 shows a microcycle in the general preparation period for our football player. The athlete's training is organized for all seven days of the week. Because this microcycle is early in the off-season, no football practice is taking place. On Monday the athlete focuses on improving his maximal strength. This day will be the heaviest session of training each week throughout the entire preparatory period. Because the workout in table 16.10 is early in the general preparation period, the strength and power training intensity is only in the

Table 16.9 Volume and Intensity for Each Mode and Period of the Maximal Interval-Training Program

Period	Mode of training	Volume, intensity
General preparation	Multijoint exercises Olympic lifts Speed and agility Conditioning	M, M L, M L, H M, M
Special preparation	Multijoint exercises Olympic lifts Plyometrics Speed and agility Conditioning	L, H L, M L, H L, H M, M
Precompetition	Multijoint exercises Olympic lifts Plyometrics Speed and agility Conditioning	L, H L, M L, H M, H L, M
Competition	Multijoint exercises Olympic lifts Plyometrics Speed and agility Conditioning	L, H L, H L, H H, H n/a
Recovery	Multijoint exercises Olympic lifts Plyometrics Speed and agility Conditioning	n/a n/a n/a n/a H, M

Table 16.10 Sample Microcycle in Preparation Period for American Football Player

	Monday	Tuesday	Wednesday	Thursday
Strength	Back squat, 3 × 6–10 × 70–80% Romanian deadlift, 3 × 6–10 Bench press, 3 × 6–10 × 70–80% Bent-over row, 3 × 6–10 Military press, 3 × 6–10	n/a	n/a	Front squat, 3 × 6–10 × 60–70%
Hypertrophy	n/a	n/a	n/a	Lunge, 3 × 12–15 each leg Good morning, 3 × 12–15 Back raise, 3 × 12–15
Power	n/a	Power clean, hang, AK, 3 × 4–6 × 60% Clean pull, hang, AK, 3 × 4–6 × 70% Push jerk, 3 × 4–6 × 60%	n/a	n/a
Speed and agility	Technique drills Standing starts, 3 × 10 meters	n/a	n/a	Technique drills Standing starts, 3 × 40 meters
Conditioning	n/a	n/a	*Bodyweight and suspension trainer circuit,* 10–15 exercises, performed for 20 seconds each with 10 seconds of recovery after each exercise	n/a

	Friday	Saturday	Sunday
Strength	n/a	n/a	n/a
Hypertrophy	Dumbbell bench press, 3 × 12–15 Superset: dip and pull-up, 3 × max each One-arm dumbbell row, 3 × 12–15 Superset: side raise and rear deltoid raise, 3 × 12–15 Superset: biceps and triceps, 3 × 12–15	n/a	n/a
Power	n/a	n/a	n/a
Speed and agility	n/a	n/a	n/a
Conditioning	*Medicine ball and heavy ropes circuit,* 10–15 exercises, performed for 20 seconds each with 10 seconds of recovery after each exercise	n/a	*Bodyweight, medicine ball, heavy ropes circuit,* 10–15 exercises performed for 45 seconds with 15 seconds of recovery after each exercise

70 to 80 percent range. Speed and agility work is also included on Monday; the focus is on short distances and maximal intensity.

Tuesday is focused on power training. Early in the general preparation period, the only power-training work being done involves variations of the Olympic lifts. The intensity is kept relatively low (60 percent) so that the athlete can focus on technique and speed of movement. As the training year progresses, the athlete will begin integrating plyometrics on this day, but we're not there yet.

Wednesday is almost a day off, consisting only of a 20-minute conditioning workout. The selected exercises are meant to minimize stress on the joints. This workout helps improve the athlete's metabolic conditioning and serves as an active recovery workout.

On Thursday the athlete is training to increase his lower-body strength using front squats. In addition, several multijoint exercises are incorporated to focus on lower-body hypertrophy. Speed and agility work is also conducted on this day. The focus is on longer sprints and drills performed at maximal intensity.

Friday includes a strength-training workout focused on developing upper-body hypertrophy. In addition, this is the second conditioning workout of the week. This conditioning session involves medicine ball and heavy ropes exercises.

Saturday is a complete rest day. No training is performed. Sunday is the third conditioning workout of the week and incorporates many of the tools that the athlete is using for conditioning. This is both a conditioning workout and an active recovery workout.

Viewing all these workouts together, you can see that the focus is on the broad development of the athlete. At the end of the general preparation period, the athlete will be larger, stronger, more explosive, faster, and more agile, and he will have a solid technical foundation. Note that the focus (three sessions per week) is on using maximal interval training for conditioning.

Special Preparation Period

Table 16.11 shows a sample microcycle of the special preparation period. In some ways, the training is organized in a manner similar to that used in the general preparation period. Monday is a heavy strength day. The speed and agility work is expanded to include more tools than were used in the previous period. Tuesday continues to focus on power, but plyometrics have now been incorporated.

Wednesday is still a conditioning day. The major difference is that the maximum interval-training session has become more difficult than it was in the general preparation period. The time spent on each exercise has increased, the rest periods have been essentially eliminated, and the athlete repeats the session several times.

The first major change from the general preparation session occurs on Thursday, which is a second maximal strength workout because the development of strength is a major focus of this period of training. In addition, the speed and agility work has been expanded to include more exercises and to begin developing position-specific agility.

Friday is a second power workout. The power snatch and its support exercises are used. In addition, plyometrics are incorporated into this workout.

Saturday, the last workout of the week, is another conditioning workout. As with Wednesday's workout, the maximum interval training involves more time spent exercising compared with the previous period of training.

Precompetition Period

Training changes in the precompetition period because the athlete is also practicing his sport. More time has to be spent on the sport, so less time is available for other aspects of training. As a result, the training is organized differently than it was during the preparation phase. In addition, the emphasis changes during this phase. For example, more time is spent on speed and agility, but less time is spent on conditioning. Table 16.12 provides a sample microcycle from the precompetition period.

The strength training is heavier than it was in previous phases. The emphasis on Monday and Friday is on improving or maintaining maximal strength. These are also speed and agility days, but the focus is now more on position-specific speed and agility.

Table 16.11 Sample Microcycle of the Special Preparation Period

	Monday	Tuesday	Wednesday	Thursday
Strength	Back squat, 3 × 4–8 × 75–85% Romanian deadlift, 3 × 4–8 Bench press, 3 × 4–8 × 75–85% Bent-over row, 3 × 4–8 Military press, 3 × 4–8	n/a	n/a	Front squat, 3 × 4–8 × 75–85% Deadlift, 3 × 4–8 Incline press, 3 × 4–8 One-arm dumbbell row, 3 × 4–8 each arm Dumbbell military press, 3 × 4–8
Hypertrophy	n/a	n/a	n/a	n/a
Power	n/a	Power clean, hang, 3 × 4–6 × 60% Clean pull, hang, 3 × 4–6 × 60% Push jerk, 3 × 4–6 × 60% Vertical jump, 10× Box jump, 10× Standing long jump, 10× Hop, 3 × 10 yards	n/a	n/a
Speed and agility	Technique drills Stride length drills, 3 × 10 meters Standing start, 3 × 10 meters Resisted start, 3 × 5 meters	n/a	n/a	Technique drills Standing start, 3 × 40 meters Bound, 3 × 20 meters Position-specific agility drills, 15–20 minutes
Conditioning	n/a	n/a	*Bodyweight and suspension trainer circuit*, 10–15 exercises, performed for 30 seconds each with no recovery after each exercise, repeated 2–3 times	n/a

	Friday	Saturday	Sunday
Strength	n/a	n/a	n/a
Hypertrophy	n/a	n/a	n/a
Power	Power snatch, hang, 3 × 4–6 × 60% Snatch pull, 3 × 4–6 × 60% Push press, 3 × 4–6 × 60% Squat jump, 10× Jump over box, 10× Standing triple jump, 10×	n/a	n/a
Speed and agility	n/a	n/a	n/a
Conditioning	n/a	*Medicine ball and heavy ropes circuit*, 10–15 exercises, performed for 30 seconds each with no recovery after each exercise, repeated 2–3 times	n/a

Table 16.12 Sample Microcycle From the Precompetition Period

	Monday	Tuesday	Wednesday	Thursday
Strength	Back squat, 3 × 2–6 × 80–90% Deadlift, 3 × 2–6 × 80–90% Incline press, 3 × 2–6 × 80–90% Bent-over row, 3 × 2–6 Military press, 3 × 2–6	n/a		n/a
Hypertrophy	n/a	n/a	n/a	n/a
Power	n/a	n/a	Power clean, hang, 3 × 4–6 × 60% Clean pull, hang, 3 × 4–6 × 60% Push jerk, 3 × 4–6 × 60% Vertical jump, 10× Box jump, 10× Standing long jump, 10× Hop, 3 × 10 yards	n/a
Speed and agility	Technique drills Standing start, 3 × 10 meters Resisted start, 3 × 5 meters Position-specific agility drills, 15–20 minutes	n/a	Technique drills Position-specific agility drills, 45–60 minutes	n/a
Conditioning	n/a	n/a	n/a	n/a
	Friday		**Saturday**	**Sunday**
Strength	Front squat, 3 × 2–6 × 80–90% Good morning, 3 × 4–8 Dumbbell bench press, 3 × 4–8 One-arm dumbbell row, 3 × 4–8 each arm Dumbbell military press, 3 × 4–8		n/a	n/a
Hypertrophy	n/a		n/a	n/a
Power	n/a		n/a	n/a
Speed and agility	Technique drills Standing start, 3 × 40 meters Bound, 3 × 20 meters Position-specific agility drills, 15–20 minutes		n/a	n/a
Conditioning	n/a		*Bodyweight, sandbag, and suspension trainer circuit,* 10–15 exercises, performed for 30 seconds each with no recovery after each exercise, repeated 2–3 times	n/a

Tuesday, Thursday, and Sunday are recovery days. Wednesday is focused on power as well as speed and agility. The Olympic lifts and plyometrics are used to train for power. The major focus of the speed and agility component is on position-specific movements.

Saturday is a conditioning day. This day has been picked intentionally. Saturday is the day when the athlete usually competes, so a difficult conditioning session will help prepare the mind and body for this activity.

Competition Period

When an athlete is in season, training changes. During the season the athlete is competing, traveling, and practicing the sport. The athlete has to recover from these activities, all of which are more important than strength and conditioning. As a result, strength and conditioning are typically scaled back during the competition period. Coaches have to find a creative way to get more out of the athlete's available training time.

Table 16.13 provides a sample microcycle for the competition period. The assumption behind this microcycle is that the athlete is competing on Saturday. On Monday and Wednesday strength and power training are combined using something called complex training. Complex training combines heavy strength training with faster movements. So, for example, on Monday the athlete performs a set of heavy back squats and then does 10 squat jumps. This approach maintains strength and power and uses available time efficiently.

Monday and Wednesday are also speed and agility workout days. The focus is on position-specific speed and agility. Being able to move his body to perform at his best is an important focus for the athlete during the season, and the workout aligns well with what he is doing in football practices.

Friday is another speed and agility workout. This workout may be in flux depending on travel. If the team needs to spend Friday as a travel day, this workout will not occur that week. If the team is at home, this workout will take place.

Conditioning workouts do not take place during the competition period unless this is a weakness for the athlete. Between practices and games, the athlete should be getting enough to maintain his conditioning. If he is not, this work can be conducted on Tuesday or Thursday.

Table 16.13 Sample Microcycle for the Competition Period for an American Football Player

	Monday	Tuesday	Wednesday	Thursday
Strength and power	Clean pull and power clean, 3 × 4 + 3 × 70% Back squat and squat jump, 3 × 3–5 × 80–90% + 10 jumps Romanian deadlift, 3 × 6–10 Bench press and *medicine ball chest pass*, 3 × 3–5 × 80–90% + 5 throws Bent-over row and medicine ball behind-the-back toss, 3 × 6–10 + 10 throws	n/a	Snatch pull and power snatch, 3 × 4 + 3 × 70% Front squat and box jump, 3 × 3–5 × 80–90% + 5 jumps Good morning and standing long jump, 3 × 6–10 + 5 jumps Incline press and clapping push-up, 3 × 6–10 + 10 push-ups Pull-up and medicine ball front toss, 3 × max + 10 throws	n/a
Hypertrophy	n/a	n/a	n/a	n/a
Speed and agility	Technique drills Resisted starts, 3 × 5 meters Position-specific agility drills, 45–60 minutes	n/a	Technique drills Bounds, 3 × 20 meters Position-specific agility drills, 45–60 minutes	n/a
Conditioning	n/a	n/a	n/a	n/a
	Friday		**Saturday**	**Sunday**
Strength and power	n/a		n/a	n/a
Hypertrophy	n/a		n/a	n/a
Speed and agility	n/a		n/a	n/a
Conditioning	Technique drills Standing start, 3 × 40 meters Position-specific agility drills, 15–20 minutes		n/a	n/a

Transition Period

The transition period is a time of active rest and recovery. The athlete's body gets a chance to heal for the rigors of the season that just ended. Even so, we don't want athletes to get out of shape and lose everything that they have worked hard to gain during this period. One way to do this is to focus the training on maximum interval training. Table 16.14 shows an example of how this can be done. As written, each session will take about 30 to 45 minutes.

Table 16.14 Sample Transition Period Microcycle for an American Football Player

	Monday	Tuesday	Wednesday	Thursday
Strength	n/a	n/a	n/a	n/a
Hypertrophy	n/a	n/a	n/a	n/a
Power	n/a	n/a	n/a	n/a
Speed and agility	n/a	n/a	n/a	n/a
Conditioning	*Kettlebell and heavy ropes circuit,* 10–15 exercises, performed for 45 seconds each with 15 seconds of recovery, repeated 2–3 times	n/a	*Medicine ball and bodyweight exercise circuit,* 10–15 exercises performed for 45 seconds each with 15 seconds of recovery, repeated 2–3 times	n/a

	Friday	Saturday	Sunday
Strength	n/a	n/a	n/a
Hypertrophy	n/a	n/a	n/a
Power	n/a	n/a	n/a
Speed and agility	n/a	n/a	n/a
Conditioning	*Suspension trainer and sandbag circuit,* 10–15 exercises performed for 45 seconds each with 15 seconds of recovery, repeated 2–3 times	n/a	n/a

Speed

Speed is highly sought after by both athletes and coaches. The media recognizes its importance and reports about it. Speed can heavily influence an athlete's selection to a team, draft status, and earning potential.

For this book, speed refers to how quickly an athlete can run. For a track and field athlete, a sprint has three phases. Some of these phases are more relevant to sport than others are, and each phase is trained differently. These phases—acceleration, maximum velocity, and speed endurance—were briefly covered in chapter 4.

In some sports, speed is contested. In other words, the faster athlete wins the race. In almost every sport, speed is fundamental to success. Speed allows an athlete to beat the opponent to the play. It allows an athlete to move past defenders. It allows a defender to catch the person with the ball. If an athlete is fast enough, speed can compensate for mistakes that the athlete makes. For example, a fast baseball player who misjudges a ground ball may still be able to stop the ball and make the play.

HOW SPEED IS TRAINED

Speed training requires using good technique, exerting high effort, and remembering that the goal is to learn how to run fast. These requirements have implications for how speed is trained. First, you need to perform speed training at close to all-out speed. The goal is to learn how to run fast. Running slowly reinforces the ability to run slowly; it does not train you to run fast. Second, you need to recover fully after every sprint. Failing to do this results in significant fatigue, which causes you to run slowly and lose your running form. In other words, failing to recover fully teaches you to run slowly with bad technique. Finally, any exercise or tool that is used needs to focus on good running technique. Failing to observe good technique can cause injury and can cause you to run more slowly than you are capable of. With that in mind, the next part of this chapter covers the variables involved in speed training as well as the various tools that are used.

Variables

Several interrelated variables play a role in speed training, including distance, volume, intensity, rest, and recovery.

Outside track and field, few sports require an athlete to run very far in a perfectly straight line. This point must be considered because we want speed training to be applicable to the sport or situation. Recall that different distances train different phases of a sprint and different phases of a sprint require slightly different techniques. For example, sprints of 10 to 15 meters focus on pure acceleration, whereas those that are longer focus on the techniques required in maximum velocity sprinting. Therefore, training distances should be similar to the distance demands of the sport.

As with other forms of training, volume refers to the total amount of work done. With speed training in particular, more is *not* better. Too much volume leads to fatigue, poor technique, and slow running. Therefore, track and field athletes rarely go over 1,000 meters of volume in a single training session. In general, no more than 200 meters of volume are needed with speed training that is focused on acceleration or maximum velocity. Speed endurance sessions may go up to 500 or 600 meters in a session.

During a speed-training session, intensity refers to how fast you are running. Simply put, to reap any benefits, you need to run as fast as you can when conducting speed training. Keep in mind that intensity needs to be close to 100 percent for effective speed training. As a result, all speed-training sessions are performed at high intensity, which makes good technique and adequate rest all the more important.

Speed training requires high intensity, good technique, and fast running to be effective. Individually and collectively, these aspects call for full recovery between sprints. Extremely short sprints (5 to 10 meters) generally require 30 to 60 seconds of recovery, but longer sprints (60 to 100 meters) require 3 to 5 minutes. The longest sprints (500 meters or more) require up to 10 minutes of recovery.

Tools

Several tools are used for speed training. The goals of the training determine which tools are used as well as how they are used. Tools for speed training include sprints, assisted sprinting, resisted sprinting, and stride length drills.

Sprints

To become better at sprinting, you have to perform sprints. For most athletes, sprinting is a training tool that is superior to any other tool used for speed training. For sprints to be successful, the athlete has to perform them at maximum intensity, use correct technique, and get enough recovery after each sprint.

Assisted Sprinting

Assisted sprinting allows an athlete to run faster than he or she is normally capable of. Examples of this tool include being towed by something fast, running on a high-speed treadmill, and running downhill. The idea is that assisted sprinting teaches the limbs and nervous system how to run at higher speeds, which can eventually transfer to faster unassisted sprinting, resulting in a faster athlete. With assisted sprinting, technique is extremely important. Running too fast will result in poor technique and the development of bad habits, so if you cannot maintain your technique, things need to slow down!

Resisted Sprinting

Resisted sprinting is the opposite of assisted sprinting in that it makes the sprinting motion more difficult. It does this by having the athlete run against some type of external load. Examples include running with a parachute, towing something heavy, pushing a sled, running uphill, and so on. In theory, the external load requires the athlete to recruit more motor units and muscle fibers to perform the sprint. Those extra motor units and muscle fibers then cause unresisted sprinting to be faster. Too much resistance can cause poor technique, so the recommendation is that the resistance should not slow down the athlete by more than 10 percent.

Stride Length Drills

Being able to take longer strides allows you to get somewhere faster. Stride length drills focus on either taking the first few steps or running at maximum velocity. Regardless of their focus, these drills involve setting up obstacles (like miniature hurdles or a speed ladder) that dictate where you put your feet. The idea is to set the obstacles so that as your speed increases, they become farther apart, forcing you to take longer strides. This drill has to be approached carefully because strides that are too long are counterproductive. If you find yourself leaning backward when performing these drills, your strides are too long!

LIMITATIONS OF SPEED TRAINING

Like every training tool, speed training has limitations, so you need to incorporate other exercises and training approaches to overcome them. A smart metabolic conditioning program can overcome some of these limitations. The limitations of speed training are that it is typically not sport specific and that it can lead to injuries.

Speed Training Is Typically Not Sport Specific With the exception of training for track and field, speed training is rarely sport specific. Rarely in sport can athletes select their starting position and then run in a perfectly straight line without having to react to situations, opponents, and the ball. For many sports, therefore, speed training is a foundational ability unless it is performed in conjunction with sport situations.

Speed Training Can Lead to Injuries Speed training can lead to hamstring and shin splint injuries. To prevent these injuries, those who engage in this type of training must take precautions by increasing the volume slowly, selecting proper shoes, running on grass or a track, and strengthening the muscles that act on the ankle and hamstrings.

GUIDELINES FOR INTEGRATING MAXIMUM INTERVAL TRAINING

Care must be taken when integrating any kind of training with a speed-training program. If done incorrectly, it can have a negative effect on speed development and can increase injury risks. With that in mind, consider the following guidelines for integrating maximum interval training in a manner that potentially enhances a speed-training program.

Avoid Using Speed Training for Maximum Interval Training If the goal of a training program is to increase speed, then using sprints for maximum interval training will be counterproductive. If sprints are used as part of a maximum interval-training program *and* a speed development program, there are two concerns. First, the injury risks are increased because of the high volume of sprinting that will be performed. Second, the maximum interval-training part of the program may train the athlete to sprint with poor form or at less than maximal speed, which is counterproductive. Instead, bodyweight exercises, suspension training, medicine balls, heavy ropes, sandbags, kettlebells, and strongman training are appropriate.

Maximum Interval Training Should Address Injury Concerns Maximum interval training can be used to address the injury concerns associated with speed training. This can be done by employing exercises that will also strengthen the muscles that act on the shin and hamstrings. Kettlebells, sandbags, strongman training, and other implements such as weighted sleds will all be useful for this purpose. By incorporating these tools into a maximum interval-training program, conditioning is addressed in a manner that will also aid speed training.

Avoid Confusing Different Training Qualities Acceleration requires brief, all-out efforts. Maximum velocity training requires efforts that last from 4 to 15 seconds at high intensity and with full recovery. Speed endurance training may require sustained efforts that last over a minute. With this in mind, when performing maximum interval training and speed training simultaneously, maximum interval training should be employed in a manner that requires an effort level that is similar to the speed training.

SAMPLE PROGRAMS

Table 17.1 shows foundational programs using bodyweight training, suspension training, medicine balls, heavy ropes, and kettlebells. **Note: The italicized exercises are found in part II. Refer to the exercise finder for more information.** Each of these programs should be performed circuit style; you perform a set of the first exercise, then a set of the second exercise, and so on until you have run through all the exercises. Perform each exercise for 20 to 30 seconds with 10 to 15 seconds of recovery before the next exercise. Perform the circuits three times.

This training should be performed on days when no speed training is performed, so that it does not conflict with the speed training. An exception is that the foundational programs can be done on the same day that speed endurance training is being performed. Each foundational training session should focus on only one exercise mode.

The foundational programs have several goals. First, they attempt to get you more comfortable with each of the exercise modes while teaching basic techniques. Second, they develop a fitness base. Finally, these exercises target both whole-body movements and the lower body to assist with injury prevention and performance improvement.

Table 17.2 shows advanced programs using bodyweight training, suspension training, medicine balls, kettlebells and heavy ropes. These programs are also performed as circuits,

Table 17.1 Sample Foundational Speed-Training Programs

Bodyweight program	Suspension program	Medicine ball program	Heavy ropes program	Kettlebell program
Bodyweight jumping jacks	*Suspension chest press*	*Medicine ball chop*	*Heavy ropes jumping jacks*	*Kettlebell two-handed swing*
Bodyweight bear crawl	*Suspension squat*	*Medicine ball wall ball*	*Heavy ropes two-handed slam*	*Kettlebell snatch*
Bodyweight crab kick	*Suspension hip up*	*Medicine ball Bulgarian squat*	*Heavy ropes twist*	*Kettlebell goblet squat*
Bodyweight mountain climber	*Suspension reverse lunge*	*Medicine ball slam*	*Heavy ropes wave*	*Kettlebell deadlift*
Bodyweight inchworm	*Suspension row*	*Medicine ball thruster*	*Heavy ropes arm circle, clockwise and counterclockwise*	*Kettlebell clean*
Bodyweight groiner	*Suspension leg curl*	*Medicine ball seated twist*	*Heavy ropes towing*	*Kettlebell Romanian deadlift*
Bodyweight push-up	*Suspension knees to chest*	*Medicine ball touch and jump*	*Heavy ropes woodchopper*	
Bodyweight scissors	*Suspension lying leg raise*	*Medicine ball modified pike*	*Heavy ropes pulling*	
Bodyweight dip				
Bodyweight speed squat				
Bodyweight pull-up				

Table 17.2 Sample Advanced Speed-Training Programs

Program 1	Program 2	Program 3
Heavy ropes two-handed slam	*Kettlebell two-handed swing*	*Suspension squat*
Suspension squat	*Medicine ball chop*	*Kettlebell one-handed swing*
Bodyweight frog hop	*Heavy ropes one-handed slam*	*Heavy ropes twist*
Suspension reverse lunge	*Kettlebell goblet squat*	*Medicine ball thruster*
Bodyweight speed squat	*Suspension foot-in-trainer one-legged squat*	*Kettlebell deadlift*
Bodyweight squat hold	*Heavy ropes woodchopper*	*Suspension one-legged squat*
Suspension leg curl	*Kettlebell Romanian deadlift*	*Heavy ropes shuffle slam*
Kettlebell overhead squat	*Kettlebell overhead lunge*	*Medicine ball Bulgarian squat*
Suspension hip up		

but the exercises are more challenging and the volume is greater. These exercises should be performed for 45 to 60 seconds with only enough recovery to get to the next exercise. The circuits should be performed three times.

The training in the advanced programs is designed primarily to target the muscles of the lower extremity. It is not meant to be performed on the same day as speed training unless that speed training is focused on speed endurance. The advanced programs not only condition the muscles of the lower body but also serve as an excellent recovery workout from the sprint if the volume is kept high and the resistance light.

LONG-TERM PROGRAMS

When looking at how to integrate maximum interval training into a long-term speed-training program, you need to understand why speed training is organized the way that it is. The rest of this chapter presents an annual plan for a speed-training program that incorporates maximum interval training.

Training for speed has similarities to training for strength and power, but many differences are present as well. Figure 17.1 provides a sample macrocycle for a collegiate track and field athlete. The first major difference to notice is that the competition season is much longer. It begins in January with the indoor season and can extend into July with outdoor nationals. A second major difference is that speed training isn't done on a percentage basis. In other words, we're not going to be training at 75 percent of maximum velocity. For reasons explained earlier in this chapter, speed training is always performed at maximum intensity. Frequency, volume, and the training tools employed change as the athlete progresses through the macrocycle. Maximum interval training supplements the speed work to help improve the athlete's ability to be fast. With that in mind, table 17.3 highlights the goals of each period of training for an athlete focused on speed, and table 17.4 shows the volume and intensity for each period of training. Note that the distances in table 17.3 are for a 100-meter sprinter or a jumper. A 200-meter or 400-meter specialist would have different distances for the sprints.

General Preparation Period

With speed training, the general preparation period is primarily focused on the athlete's foundation. This is developed by concentrating on sprinting technique, developing speed endurance, and conditioning the muscles that are involved in sprinting. Normally, training occurs on three days a week. One session is focused on acceleration, one on maximum velocity, and one on speed endurance. Table 17.5 provides a sample week of workouts during the general preparation period.

As shown by the table, equal time is spent on acceleration, maximum velocity, and speed endurance. Although each aspect is being trained, the volume is low and the focus is on progressing the athlete to the crouch start. Plyometrics are introduced, but the volume is low. Conditioning, in the form of maximum interval training, is performed three times a

Year-long macrocycle												
Recovery phase	Preparatory phase					Competition phase						
Recovery period	General prep period		Special prep period		Precomp period	Competition period						
Aug	Sep	Oct	Nov	Dec	Jan	Feb	Mar	Apr	May	Jun	Jul
I	II	III	IV	V	VI	VII	VIII	IX	X	XI	XII

Figure 17.1 Sample macrocycle for a collegiate track and field athlete.

Table 17.3 Sample Goals for an Athlete Focused on Speed

Period	Goals	Tools
General preparation	Technical fundamentals Fitness base Improve acceleration Increase maximum velocity Injury prevention	Technique drills Conditioning Speed endurance training Short-distance sprints Work on starting technique Horizontal plyometrics 20- to 40-meter sprints A and B drills Mobility drills Maximum interval training Gradual increase in training volume
Special preparation	Technical fundamentals Maintain fitness base Increase horizontal application of force Improve acceleration Increase maximum velocity Injury prevention	Technique drills Sprints using track spikes Conditioning Speed endurance training Horizontal plyometrics Sprints up to 20 meters in length Work on starting technique 5- to 10-meter stride length drills Sprints up to 60 meters in length 20- to 60-meter stride length drills Mobility drills Maximum interval training Gradual increase in training volume
Precompetition	Technical fundamentals Maintain fitness base Race technique Improve horizontal application of force Increase acceleration Increase maximum velocity Injury prevention	Technique drills as warm-up Use of track spikes Conditioning Speed endurance training as needed Practice race pacing Horizontal plyometrics Sprints up to 20 meters in length Work on starting technique 5- to 10-meter stride length drills 5- to 10-meter resisted sprints Sprints up to 60 meters in length 20- to 80-meter stride length drills 20- to 40-meter resisted sprints 20- to 40-meter assisted sprints Mobility drills Maximum interval training Gradual increase in training volume
Competition	Technical fundamentals Peak Injury prevention	Technique drills as warm-up Use of track spikes Continued work on acceleration and maximum velocity, work on weaknesses in event Mobility drills Maximum interval training
Recovery	Conditioning	*Bodyweight exercises* *Suspension-training exercises* *Medicine ball exercises* *Sandbags* *Kettlebells* *Heavy ropes*

Table 17.4 Volume and Intensity for Each Period of Training

Period	Mode of training	Volume, intensity
General preparation	Sprints, acceleration	L, H
	Sprints, maximum velocity	L, H
	Sprints, speed endurance	M, H
	Stride length drills	n/a
	Assisted sprinting	n/a
	Resisted sprinting	n/a
	Plyometrics	L, H
	Conditioning	M, M
Special preparation	Sprints, acceleration	M, H
	Sprints, maximum velocity	M, H
	Sprints, speed endurance	L, H
	Stride length drills	L, H
	Assisted sprinting	n/a
	Resisted sprinting	L, H
	Plyometrics	M, H
	Conditioning	M, M
Precompetition	Sprints, acceleration	M, H
	Sprints, maximum velocity	H, H
	Sprints, speed endurance	L, H
	Stride length drills	L, H
	Assisted sprinting	L, H
	Resisted sprinting	L, H
	Plyometrics	L, H
	Conditioning	L, M
Competition	Sprints, acceleration	H, H
	Sprints, maximum velocity	H, H
	Sprints, speed endurance	L, H
	Stride length drills	L, H
	Assisted sprinting	L, H
	Resisted sprinting	L, H
	Plyometrics	L, H
	Conditioning	L, L
Recovery	Sprints, acceleration	n/a
	Sprints, maximum velocity	n/a
	Sprints, speed endurance	n/a
	Stride length drills	n/a
	Assisted sprinting	n/a
	Resisted sprinting	n/a
	Plyometrics	n/a
	Conditioning	H, M

week. It is designed to provide some work to the athlete's entire body while requiring a great deal of work from the lower body.

Special Preparation Period

In the special preparation period, the intensity and volume of speed training increases. During this period, acceleration is emphasized on Monday and Friday, maximum velocity on Wednesday, and speed endurance on Thursday. Maximum interval training is still being performed three times a week, now on Tuesday, Thursday, and Saturday. The complexity of the speed-training exercises are increasing with this phase; resisted sprints, stride length drills, and the use of track spikes are incorporated into the training. Table 17.6 provides a sample week of workouts during the special preparation period.

Table 17.5 Sample Week of Workouts During the General Preparation Period

	Monday	Tuesday	Wednesday
Technique	Perform 2 × 20 meters each: *Sprinting footstrike* *Sprinting lift the foot* *Sprinting swing the leg* *Sprinting put it all together*	n/a	Perform 2 × 20 meters each: *Sprinting footstrike* *Sprinting lift the foot* *Sprinting swing the leg* *Sprinting put it all together*
Acceleration	Falling starts, 3–5 × 10 meters Standing starts, 3–5 × 10 meters	n/a	n/a
Maximum velocity	n/a	n/a	Falling starts, 3–5 × 30 meters Standing starts, 3–5 × 20 meters
Speed endurance	n/a	n/a	n/a
Power	Standing long jump, 10×	n/a	Bounds, 3 × 20 meters
Conditioning	n/a	Circuit workout, perform each exercise for 45 seconds, minimize rest, repeat 3 times: *Heavy ropes two-handed slam* *Suspension squat* *Bodyweight push-up* *Bodyweight frog hop* *Suspension reverse lunge* *Bodyweight pull-up* *Bodyweight speed squats* *Bodyweight squat hold* *Kettlebell press* *Suspension leg curl* *Kettlebell overhead squat* *Suspension hip up*	n/a

	Thursday	Friday	Saturday
Technique	n/a	Perform 2 × 20 meters each: *Sprinting footstrike* *Sprinting lift the foot* *Sprinting swing the leg* *Sprinting put it all together*	n/a
Acceleration	n/a	n/a	n/a
Maximum velocity	n/a	n/a	n/a
Speed endurance	n/a	Standing start, 4 × 150 meters	n/a
Power	n/a	Hurdle hops, 3 × 20 meters	n/a
Conditioning	Circuit workout, perform each exercise for 45 seconds, minimize rest, repeat 3 times: *Kettlebell two-handed swing* *Medicine ball chop* *Suspension chest press* *Heavy ropes one-handed slam* *Kettlebell goblet squat* *Suspension row* *Suspension foot-in-trainer one-legged squat* *Suspension reverse fly* *Heavy ropes woodchopper* *Kettlebell Romanian deadlift* *Kettlebell overhead lunge*	n/a	Circuit workout, perform each exercise for 45 seconds, minimize rest, repeat 3 times: *Suspension squat* *Kettlebell one-handed swing* *Kettlebell push-up* *Heavy ropes twist* *Medicine ball thruster* *Kettlebell bent-over row* *Kettlebell deadlift* *Suspension foot-in-trainer one-legged squats* *Kettlebell press* *Heavy ropes shuffle slam* *Medicine ball Bulgarian squat*

Table 17.6 Sample Week of Workouts During the Special Preparation Period

	Monday	Tuesday	Wednesday
Technique	Perform 2 × 20 meters each: *Sprinting footstrike* *Sprinting lift the foot* *Sprinting swing the leg* *Sprinting put it all together*	n/a	Perform 3 × 20 meters each: *Sprinting footstrike* *Sprinting lift the foot* *Sprinting swing the leg* *Sprinting put it all together*
Acceleration	Stride length drills, 2 × 5 meters Falling starts, 1 × 20 meters Standing starts, 3-5 × 20 meters Crouching starts, 3-5 × 20 meters	n/a	n/a
Maximum velocity	n/a	n/a	Stride length drills, 2 × 20 meters Falling starts, 1 × 60 meters Standing starts, 1 × 60 meters Crouching starts, 1 × 60 meters Resisted sprints, 3 × 20 meters
Speed endurance	n/a	n/a	n/a
Power	Standing long jump, 10×	n/a	Bounds, 3 × 20 meters
Conditioning	n/a	Circuit workout, perform each exercise for 45 seconds, minimize rest, repeat 3 times: *Heavy ropes two-handed slam* *Suspension squat* *Bodyweight push-up* *Bodyweight frog hop* *Suspension reverse lunge* *Bodyweight pull-up* *Bodyweight speed squat* *Bodyweight squat hold* *Kettlebell press* *Suspension leg curl* *Kettlebell overhead squat* *Suspension hip up*	n/a

	Thursday	Friday	Saturday
Technique	Perform 2 × 20 meters each: *Sprinting footstrike* *Sprinting lift the foot* *Sprinting swing the leg* *Sprinting put it all together*	Perform 2 × 20 meters each: *Sprinting footstrike* *Sprinting lift the foot* *Sprinting swing the leg* *Sprinting put it all together*	n/a
Acceleration	n/a	Stride length drills, 3 × 10 meters Resisted starts, 3 × 10 meters Crouching starts, 3-5 × 10 meters	n/a
Maximum velocity	n/a	n/a	n/a
Speed endurance	Standing start, 4 × 200 meters	n/a	n/a
Power	n/a	Hurdle hops, 3 × 20 meters	n/a
Conditioning	Circuit workout, perform each exercise for 45 seconds, minimize rest, repeat 3 times: *Kettlebell two-handed swing* *Medicine ball chop* *Suspension chest press* *Heavy ropes one-handed slam* *Kettlebell goblet squat* *Suspension row* *Suspension foot-in-trainer one-legged squat* *Suspension reverse fly* *Heavy ropes woodchopper* *Kettlebell Romanian deadlift* *Kettlebell overhead lunge*	n/a	Circuit workout, perform each exercise for 45 seconds, minimize rest, repeat 3 times: *Suspension squat* *Kettlebell one-handed swing* *Kettlebell push-up* *Heavy ropes twist* *Medicine ball thruster* *Kettlebell bent-over row* *Kettlebell deadlift* *Suspension foot-in-trainer one-legged squat* *Kettlebell press* *Heavy ropes shuffle slam* *Medicine ball Bulgarian squat*

Precompetition Period

In the precompetition period, athletes perform two acceleration sessions and two maximum velocity sessions each week. Speed endurance is not done unless it is a weakness. The volume is higher on the speed workouts on Monday and Wednesday, lower on Friday and Saturday. The complexity of the exercises and the distances are increased. In addition, stride length drills, resisted sprints, and track spikes are used. Because of the expanded focus on speed work, maximum interval training is reduced to two days per week.

During this period, athletes may enter some competitions that will occur primarily on weekends. When that happens, the training schedule needs to be adjusted accordingly to either reduce the number of training sessions or reorganize the day on which they occur. Table 17.7 provides a sample week of workouts during the precompetition period. Note that during the week sampled no competitions occur.

Competition Period

The competition period for any type of athlete presents programming challenges. Table 17.8 provides a sample week of workouts for a speed athlete during the competition period. The workouts in the table assume that Friday is a travel day and that meets occur on Saturday and Sunday. If that is not the case, training will have to be adjusted accordingly.

Conditioning is cut back to one session per week, on Wednesday. The kettlebells are emphasized to maintain muscle mass, strength, and power during the competition period. The Monday session emphasizes maximum velocity, Tuesday is a low-volume acceleration workout, and Thursday is another maximum velocity session (with lower volume than Monday).

Transition Period

During the transition period, the intent is to give the speed athlete a chance to recover from the season and get away from organized speed training for a few weeks. Maximum interval training is an ideal training tool to keep the athlete in shape while getting away from speed training. Table 17.9 provides a sample week of workouts during the transition period.

In this example, the athlete is training on Monday, Wednesday, and Friday. Monday, the heaviest training session of the week, involves kettlebells and medicine balls. Wednesday involves heavy ropes and suspension training. Friday is a day involving short sprints for conditioning combined with bodyweight training. For each of these circuits, the intent is to perform the exercise for 30 seconds, get 10 to 15 seconds of recovery, and then perform the next exercise. The circuits should be repeated three times.

Table 17.7   Sample Week of Workouts During the Precompetition Period

	Monday	Tuesday	Wednesday
Technique	Perform 3 × 20 meters each: *Sprinting footstrike* *Sprinting lift the foot* *Sprinting swing the leg* *Sprinting put it all together*	n/a	Perform 3 × 20 meters each: *Sprinting footstrike* *Sprinting lift the foot* *Sprinting swing the leg* *Sprinting put it all together*
Acceleration	Stride length drills, 3 × 5 meters Crouching starts, 5 × 20 meters Resisted starts, 3 × 10 meters	n/a	n/a
Maximum velocity	n/a	n/a	Stride length drills, 3 × 40 meters Crouching starts, 3 × 60 meters Resisted sprints, 3 × 20 meters
Speed endurance	n/a	n/a	n/a
Power	Standing long jump, 10×	n/a	Bounds, 3 × 40 meters
Conditioning	n/a	Circuit workout, perform each exercise for 45 seconds, minimize rest, repeat three times: *Heavy ropes two-handed slam* *Suspension squat* *Bodyweight push-up* *Bodyweight frog hop* *Suspension reverse lunge* *Bodyweight pull-up* *Bodyweight speed squat* *Bodyweight squat hold* *Kettlebell press* *Suspension leg curl* *Kettlebell overhead squat* *Suspension hip up*	n/a

	Thursday	Friday	Saturday
Technique	n/a	Perform 3 × 20 meters each: *Sprinting footstrike* *Sprinting lift the foot* *Sprinting swing the leg* *Sprinting put it all together*	Perform 3 × 20 meters each: *Sprinting footstrike* *Sprinting lift the foot* *Sprinting swing the leg* *Sprinting put it all together*
Acceleration	n/a	Crouching starts, 5 × 20 meters	n/a
Maximum velocity	n/a	n/a	Crouching starts, 5 × 40 meters
Speed endurance	n/a	n/a	n/a
Power	n/a	Hurdle hops, 3 × 20 meters	Bounds, 3 × 20 meters
Conditioning	Circuit workout, perform each exercise for 45 seconds, minimize rest, repeat 3 times: *Kettlebell two-handed swing* *Medicine ball chop* *Suspension chest press* *Heavy ropes one-handed slam* *Kettlebell goblet squat* *Suspension row* *Suspension foot-in-trainer one-legged squat* *Suspension reverse fly* *Heavy ropes woodchopper* *Kettlebell Romanian deadlift* *Kettlebell overhead lunge*	n/a	n/a

Table 17.8 Sample Week of Workouts During the Competition Period

	Monday	Tuesday	Wednesday
Technique	Perform 3 × 20 meters each: *Sprinting footstrike* *Sprinting lift the foot* *Sprinting swing the leg* *Sprinting put it all together*	Perform 15–20 minutes of mobility drills	n/a
Acceleration		Crouching starts, 5 × 20 meters	n/a
Maximum velocity	Stride length drills, 3 × 40 meters Crouching starts, 3 × 60 meters Resisted sprints, 3 × 20 meters	n/a	n/a
Speed endurance	n/a	n/a	n/a
Power	Bounds, 3 × 40 meters	n/a	n/a
Conditioning	n/a	n/a	Circuit workout, perform each exercise for 45 seconds, minimize rest, repeat 3 times: *Kettlebell two-handed swing* *Medicine ball chop* *Suspension chest press* *Heavy ropes one-handed slam* *Kettlebell goblet squat* *Suspension row* *Suspension foot-in-trainer one-legged squat* *Suspension reverse fly* *Heavy ropes woodchopper* *Kettlebell Romanian deadlift* *Kettlebell overhead lunge*

	Thursday	Friday	Saturday	Sunday
Technique	Perform 3 × 20 meters each: *Sprinting footstrike* *Sprinting lift the foot* *Sprinting swing the leg* *Sprinting put it all together*	n/a	n/a	n/a
Acceleration	n/a	n/a	n/a	n/a
Maximum velocity	Crouching starts, 5 × 40 meters	n/a	n/a	n/a
Speed endurance	n/a	n/a	n/a	n/a
Power	Hurdle hops, 3 × 20 meters	n/a	n/a	n/a
Conditioning	n/a	n/a	n/a	n/a

Table 17.9 Sample Week of Workouts During the Transition Period

	Monday	Wednesday	Friday
Conditioning	Kettlebell two-hand swing Medicine ball chop Kettlebell snatch (right hand) Medicine ball thruster Kettlebell snatch (left hand) Medicine ball Bulgarian squat Kettlebell goblet squat Medicine ball modified pike Kettlebell deadlift Medicine ball seated twist Kettlebell push-up Medicine ball wall ball Kettlebell row Medicine ball seated twist Kettlebell press	Heavy ropes two-handed slam Suspension squat Heavy ropes one-handed slam (right hand) Suspension reverse lunge Heavy ropes one-handed slam (left hand) Suspension leg curl Heavy ropes woodchopper Suspension chest press Heavy ropes twist Suspension row Heavy ropes arm circle, clockwise and counterclockwise Suspension reverse fly Heavy ropes jumping jacks	Bodyweight jumping jacks Sprint 10 meters Bodyweight bear crawl Sprint 10 meters Bodyweight crab kick Sprint 10 meters Bodyweight mountain climber Sprint 10 meters Bodyweight inchworm Sprint 10 meters Bodyweight groiner Sprint 10 meters Bodyweight push-up Sprint 10 meters Bodyweight speed squat Sprint 10 meters Bodyweight walking lunge Sprint 10 meters

CHAPTER 18

Endurance

Endurance is defined as the ability to sustain activity for an extended time. Although this concept seems simple, different types of endurance may be more or less important depending on the nature of the sport or activity being performed.

For example, when people think of endurance they tend to picture long-duration, steady-state bouts of exercise using repetitive movements, performed predominately in a linear fashion, such as swimming, rowing, jogging, and cycling—the classic examples of aerobic endurance activities. These types of activities require the aerobic energy system, and to some extent the glycolytic energy system, to provide ATP to sustain activity.

But endurance is also essential for high-level performance in field-based and court-based sports. For example, basketball, soccer, and lacrosse players need to have good aerobic endurance so that they can last the entire duration of a game. But unlike traditional aerobic endurance events, these sports require athletes to perform quick and explosive changes of direction and repeated intermittent speed efforts. Athletes use a blend of the aerobic and anaerobic energy systems to produce ATP.

Understanding the differences between these kinds of endurance is essential because longer-duration aerobic endurance training might actually hinder performance in activities that require repeated sprint efforts. Conversely, a program that focuses exclusively on repeat sprint efforts or anaerobic endurance would not optimize performance in a longer-duration endurance event such as a full or half marathon. How we train each of these forms of endurance is significantly different.

HOW ENDURANCE IS TRAINED

Aerobic endurance is critical for sports that require athletes to sustain an activity for a long duration, such as triathlons, marathons, cycling contests, and various types of adventure races. The main goal of these types of events, other than enjoyment, is to cover the given distance in the shortest time possible. Because of the distances that must be covered, participants must work at low intensity to persist. Otherwise, fatigue significantly hinders performance.

Aerobic power is generally measured by determining maximal oxygen uptake, or $\dot{V}O_2$max. After a person reaches a certain level, however, improvements in $\dot{V}O_2$max become more marginal. In fact, the ability to maintain activity at a high percentage of $\dot{V}O_2$max may be a better predictor of performance than aerobic capacity alone. Specifically, people who can maintain exercise at a higher percentage of their $\dot{V}O_2$max without accumulating a large amount of lactic acid have a distinct advantage over their competitors. To improve this ability, people must train at or near their maximal lactate steady state, or the exercise intensity at which maximal lactate production is equal to maximal lactate clearance. This training can be done by using some of the methods that we will discuss in this section. In addition to $\dot{V}O_2$max, movement economy is a critical factor for endurance performance. People who have better technique and form waste less energy during training and events. Similar to the novice weight lifter, a person who begins and then regularly performs a specific type of endurance activity becomes more efficient at the movements required to execute the task.

For instance, when testing for $\dot{V}O_2$max, runners would likely achieve a higher score using an assessment that emphasizes running. Conversely, if asked to perform a maximal aerobic test on an indoor rowing machine, runners would likely struggle to reach their true aerobic capacity because they would probably waste a lot of energy trying to gain proficiency in executing a foreign movement. Instead, they would achieve their $\dot{V}O_2$peak, which is simply the highest $\dot{V}O_2$ that they are able to achieve on a given test. This further explains why sport specificity is important for reaching peak performance. In essence, a person who has a goal of participating in a specific endurance event such as a half marathon (13.1 miles, or 21 km) would need to run at a distance and intensity similar to the event on a consistent basis. Furthermore, other forms of endurance and resistance training and maximal interval training may be effectively used to complement aerobic endurance performance. But performing resistance training or maximal interval training (MIT) alone and expecting to run a full marathon would likely produce a poor performance.

Conversely, when seeking to improve anaerobic endurance for intermittent sports, the focus of training tends to favor developing speed endurance, at or above the lactate threshold, rather than steady-state endurance. This is generally done by performing repeated short (3- to 10-second) sprints with brief recovery (10 to 60 seconds) between bouts (Bishop, Girard, and Mendez-Villanueva 2011; Dawson 2012; Girard, Mendez-Villanueva, and Bishop 2011). This form of training is aimed at improving the athlete's ability to sustain her or his average maximal speed over a match or improve average peak power and work capacity over the duration of a game. In addition to repeat sprint ability (RSA) training, the use of conditioning games is popular among coaches and athletes. The aim of these games is to help athletes play their way into shape by using activities that are contextually appropriate to game scenarios.

Repeat sprint ability becomes critically important during the latter stages of a match or competition. As fatigue sets in over the course of the game, a player's physical ability diminishes. RSA training can help improve the ability to sustain and reproduce maximal speed efforts and recover more quickly between sprints. Fatigue may also hinder the movement mechanics necessary to execute skill-related tasks because fatigued muscles do not produce force as effectively. Additionally, a player's perceptual skills, decision-making ability, and focus tend to diminish as fatigue takes hold.

Variables

Given the demands of endurance training, creating a careful balance among training variables is essential. In general, as the intensity and duration of the activity increase, the amount of rest required increases. Highly trained athletes require less rest to recover between training bouts than those who are less trained. In general, two to five endurance-training sessions per week are adequate for most people. More than five training sessions per week may increase the risk of repetitive injuries, so the decision to add more training sessions should be evaluated based on the needs of the person and adjusted with caution. Obviously, as the number of training sessions increases, the intensity of those sessions should decrease, and vice versa. Generally, those who are engaged in more speed endurance training versus aerobic endurance training would perform fewer sessions to allow adequate recovery between high-intensity work bouts.

Intensity, or how hard an athlete is working, is quantified and monitored in many endurance endeavors by using the target heart method (THR) and by estimating or tracking heart rate during training. To calculate THR, we must first determine the theoretical maximum heart rate (MHR). This number can be easily found by subtracting the age of the athlete from 220. For instance, a 30-year-old athlete has a theoretical maximum heart rate of approximately 190 beats per minute (bpm). If this athlete wants to train at 80 to 85 percent of his or her estimated maximal heart rate, he or she would perform the following equation:

Target heart rate at 80 percent of estimated maximal heart rate of 190 beats per minute

$$THR = 190 \times .80$$

$$THR = 152 \text{ bpm}$$

Target heart rate at 85 percent of estimated maximal heart rate of 190 beats per minute

$$THR = 190 \times .85$$

$$THR = 161.5 \text{ bpm}$$

Setting a heart rate range for training is useful because the athlete can then push a bit harder at times and back off slightly at other times during a session while still remaining in the target range. Heart rate during activity can be monitored by taking a 10-second pulse at the carotid or radial artery and multiplying the count by 6 to get the estimated beats per minute. For example, if the 10-second pulse is 27, we would solve the following simple equation:

10-second heart rate = 27 beats per minute

$$60 \text{ sec HR} = 27 \times 6$$

$$60 \text{ sec HR} = 162 \text{ bpm}$$

This number would coincide with a heart rate just above 85 percent of the MHR in the previous example.

Many athletes prefer to streamline the process of tracking their intensity through the use of heart rate monitors. These monitors provide the user with an instantaneous reading of HR, making it easy to maintain the desired intensity throughout the duration of the activity. A more crude, but effective, method for determining exercise intensity is to rate the perceived exertion level during a training bout on a scale of 1 to 10, with 1 being not difficult at all and 10 being extremely difficult. For example, a rating of 8 would reflect an intensity of about 80 percent of the athlete's perceived maximal effort. Although this method is a bit less precise, it helps athletes gauge training intensity and may be more practical in settings in which monitoring equipment cannot be used or it is difficult for the player to stop to get a pulse, such as when performing conditioning games.

Globally speaking, duration and intensity for endurance activities are inversely related, meaning that the longer the training session is, the lower the intensity must be to sustain the activity. For example, exercise performed at between 85 and 93 percent of target heart rate generally coincides with an intensity at or near the maximal lactate steady state. Subsequently, when exercise is performed at this intensity, the work bouts will be relatively short; after 20 to 30 minutes, the accumulation of lactic acid will make it increasingly difficult for the athlete to continue. Exercise performed at lower intensity (70 to 75 percent) can be sustained for longer periods, often up to several hours, depending on the person's fitness.

The intensity selected depends largely on the particular energy system we wish to develop. Lower intensity, below 85 percent of THR, tends to favor aerobic endurance adaptations, whereas submaximal intensity between 85 and 93 percent begins to challenge the glycolytic energy system to a greater extent and helps improve the ability to sustain exercise at a higher training threshold.

Tools

A variety of methods can be used to improve endurance performance. Many of these methods focus on using intensity at or near the maximal lactate steady state to improve the ability to work at a higher percentage of the $\dot{V}O_2$max. For many team sports, however, the ability to repeat short bursts of explosive, high-intensity sprints may be more critical than being able to sustain steady-state activity for a long time. This section explains several techniques for improving endurance in both areas.

Long, Slow Distance Training

Long, slow distance (LSD) training is used primarily to improve aerobic capacity. This form of training is performed at low to moderate intensity (between approximately 70 and 85 percent of THR) for a long duration (greater than 30 minutes). Although the term *long, slow distance* may be a bit of a misnomer because the person is still usually trying to cover the distance in a relatively short time, the name emphasizes the relationship between intensity and duration. To sustain activity for a longer period, a lower intensity must be employed. Training modalities generally use the larger muscle groups of the legs and hips and are performed using repetitive movements for greater than 15 to 20 minutes at submaximal intensity (70 to 85 percent). Some options include running outdoors or on a treadmill; using a step trainer, elliptical trainer, or rower; lap swimming; spinning; and road or mountain biking. As previously discussed, however, you should select the most sport-specific activity for the bulk of your training and do another form of aerobic training periodically as a method of reducing repetitive motion stress on the body. That approach helps reduce the risk of injury or overtraining.

For improving speed endurance or RSA, short bouts of high-intensity (90 to 100 percent) effort over relatively short periods (less than 10 seconds) with a rest of 10 to 60 seconds between repetitions and a rest of 2 to 3 minutes between sets should be used. Although the majority of training should focus on activities similar to the sport (usually running), other methods of training such as games that use a blend of high, low, and moderate intensity can also be used when performing team conditioning. These games are excellent for disguising work as play and for providing a break from traditional training methods aimed at performing specific distances, times, and work-to-rest ratios.

Interval Training

Interval training consists of performing short or moderately long work bouts at a relatively high intensity interspersed with periods of reduced intensity or complete rest within a single training session. This method of training is often used to improve speed endurance and $\dot{V}O_2$max and to enhance aerobic metabolism by improving the ability to buffer lactic acid build-up. Long work intervals can be performed for approximately 2 to 3 minutes at an intensity of around 80 to 90 percent of maximal effort or for shorter work bouts (15 seconds to 2 minutes) at 85 to 100 percent of maximal effort.

As the intensity and duration of the interval increase, so does the time needed for the person to recover from the bouts. Generally, for longer intervals performed at 80 to 90 percent of maximal effort, a 1:0.5 to 1:2 work-to-rest ratio is used. For shorter work bouts performed at 85 to 100 percent effort, a 1:2 to 1:5 work-to-rest ratio should be allowed. This form of training can be performed on one or two days per week.

Fartlek Training

Fartlek is a Swedish word that means "speed play." This type of training combines random higher-intensity intervals with continuous training based on how the person feels during a training session. Fartlek training does not rely on the use of specific durations or intensities; instead, the athlete varies the intensity over the course of the training session. If the person feels as if she or he can go at a higher intensity, the person simply adjusts the speed or cadence to a faster pace. When the person feels that she or he can no longer sustain the pace, the person simply reduces the intensity to recover. This unstructured form of interval training can be especially useful for beginners because it allows them the freedom to adjust the training session based on their current level of fitness. In addition, it reduces the boredom and monotony often associated with LSD or steady-state training.

LIMITATIONS OF ENDURANCE TRAINING

Endurance training, especially aerobic endurance training, is typically associated with a high incidence of repetitive stress injuries based on the long duration and repetitive nature of these activities. Additionally, these activities are performed predominately in one primary plane of movement. Consequently, some muscles and muscle groups receive a larger volume of training than others, which may further predispose a person to risk of muscular imbalances, injury, and poor movement efficiency. For example, because they sit in a crunched positon with the shoulders rounded for extended periods, cyclists are predisposed to injury of the muscles of the lower and upper back. Repeatedly maintaining the crouched position can create tightness in the anterior muscles (e.g., chest, hip flexors, quads), causing them to shorten over time. These changes also tend to weaken the muscles. This tightness and shortening can affect the muscles of the posterior chain (e.g., upper and lower back, glutes) and can lead to tight hamstrings, IT band syndrome, and reduced mobility. Subsequently, these imbalances lead to poor posture and greater stress on the body both while training and while at rest. Unfortunately, in many cases these issues set the stage for chronic pain and overuse injuries.

Another concern with endurance training is selecting the correct mix of training. Performing strictly aerobic endurance training with athletes who require speed and power may cause the intermediate muscle fibers to take on more slow-twitch fiber characteristics, which can hinder force production and reduce speed and explosive power, especially under fatigue.

GUIDELINES FOR INTEGRATING
MAXIMUM INTERVAL TRAINING

When integrating MIT into an endurance-training program, several factors should be considered.

■ MIT should be used to complement endurance training, not detract from it. If the primary goal of the training program is to improve endurance performance, MIT should be performed *after* the endurance-training session. Otherwise, fatigue may interfere with the ability to perform the specific endurance activity that the athlete is trying to improve. For example, performing MIT before running may hinder the ability to complete the run in the desired time because of cumulative fatigue.

■ MIT should be used to help strengthen the smaller stabilizer muscles surrounding the joints of the upper and lower body that tend to fatigue with aerobic training. This training will lead to a more balanced body that can better tolerate the stresses created during aerobic training over long periods or distances.

■ MIT can be effective when used as a form of cross-training, especially for runners. Running tends to pound on the joints more than other forms of endurance training do.

MIT is an excellent tool for reducing the risk of repetitive joint trauma and for maintaining aerobic and anaerobic fitness while recovering from minor injuries.

■ MIT can also be used to improve anaerobic endurance and help athletes exert consistent force as the body fatigues. The effect is similar to traveling farther on a tankful of fuel in your automobile. Such training can also help endurance athletes produce more force while pedaling, executing a foot strike, or pulling with the arms when swimming or rowing, thus leading to greater economy of movement.

SAMPLE PROGRAMS

Two sample endurance-training programs are presented in this section. The first shows how MIT can be used to complement a training program focused on improving performance in an aerobic endurance event such as the half marathon, whereas the second shows how MIT can be used for an intermittent-type sport such as soccer. These samples are used for illustrative purposes only; the basic concepts can be applied to similar sports or activities.

Table 18.1 shows a few foundational programs that use bodyweight exercises, suspension training, and kettlebell work. **Note: The italicized exercises are found in part II. Refer to the exercise finder for more information.** Each of these programs has been designed to follow a circuit format. Each exercise should be performed for 12 to 15 repetitions, with a 10- to 20-second rest period between exercises. Each exercise in the circuit should be performed in the sequence displayed and repeated three times.

Within each program, specific emphasis is placed on improving strength in the upper back, mobility of the hips, dynamic stability of the lumbar spine, and flexibility of the hamstrings. Addressing these areas is critical to preventing injuries in endurance athletes. Because these workouts are performed in the initial stages of the aerobic endurance-training program, the intensity is relatively low and the volume is relatively high. As the training program progresses and the volume of aerobic endurance work increases, the intensity of the MIT sessions increases and the volume decreases. This adjustment is made to account for the greater amount of time dedicated to performing increasingly longer training distances as the competition approaches.

At the beginning of the training program, when the distances and times required for the endurance-training sessions are low, MIT sessions can be performed on the same days as the endurance activity. But as the time dedicated to endurance training increases, the preferable approach is to conduct these sessions on nonendurance training days or on days when training time and distance are limited. If both training sessions are performed on the same day, the MIT session should always follow endurance training. Training in this sequence ensures that the fatigue caused from the MIT session does not interfere with the main training priority, which is improving endurance performance.

Table 18.2 shows advanced programs using body weight, kettlebells, a suspension trainer, and sandbags as resistance. As with the foundational program, these exercises are performed in a circuit manner, although the intensity is much greater and the volume of training is lower. This reduction in volume in the MIT sessions allows for better recovery as the duration of endurance-training sessions continues to increase.

Similar to the foundational programs, each of these programs is performed as a circuit for two or three sets of 8 to 10 repetitions, with little to no rest between exercises. Each exercise in the circuit should be performed in the sequence displayed and repeated two or three times.

LONG-TERM PROGRAMS

Two sample endurance-training program designs are presented in this section. The first is a distance-running program for a recreational runner, and the second program outlines a

Table 18.1 Sample Foundational MIT Workouts for Endurance Athletes

Sample session 1	Sample session 2	Sample session 3
Medicine ball Bulgarian squat *Suspension row* *Bodyweight push-up* *Kettlebell one-handed swing* Circuit workout. Perform each exercise for three sets of 12 to 15 reps with little to no rest between sets.	*Kettlebell goblet squat* *Bodyweight inchworm* *Bodyweight groiner* *Bodyweight pull-up* *Sandbag overhead press* Circuit workout. Perform each exercise for three sets of 12 to 15 reps with little to no rest between sets.	*Bodyweight lateral squat* *Kettlebell Romanian deadlift* Modified chin-up *Bodyweight dip* *Bodyweight plank (30 sec)* Circuit workout. Perform each exercise for three sets of 12 to 15 reps with little to no rest between sets.

Table 18.2 Advanced MIT Workouts for Endurance Athletes

Sample session 1	Sample session 2	Sample session 3
Suspension row *Bodyweight push-up* *Kettlebell one-handed swing* *Medicine ball alphabet* Circuit workout. Perform each exercise for two or three sets of 8 to 10 reps with little to no rest between sets.	*Medicine ball multiplanar squat* *Bodyweight inchworm* *Kettlebell Romanian deadlift* *Bodyweight groiner* *Bodyweight pull-up* *Bodyweight dip* Circuit workout. Perform each exercise for two or three sets of 8 to 10 reps with little to no rest between sets.	*Medicine ball Bulgarian squat* *Kettlebell Romanian deadlift* *Kettlebell bent-over row* *Kettlebell press* Side plank (60 sec) Circuit workout. Perform each exercise for two or three sets of 8 to 10 reps with little to no rest between sets.

training program for a soccer athlete. The first program emphasizes aerobic endurance (half marathon), whereas the second addresses the endurance requirements of an intermittent sport.

Traditional Endurance Example: Half Marathon

It is beyond the scope of this book to delve into every specific competitive endurance event, but a training program for a representative event, the half marathon, is presented in table 18.3. This program is designed for recreational runners who are running between 5 and 12 miles (between 12 and 19 km) per week. The goal of this training program is to develop a good foundation of fitness and help reduce injures commonly seen from performing repetitive movement as distance progressively increases. This program is different from most half-marathon programs because it emphasizes performing quality runs rather than just accumulating distance. In fact, the program requires only two or three days of running per week. Within this program, both strength training and maximal interval training play essential roles in terms of cross-training and prehabilitation.

General Preparation Period

During the general preparation period (weeks 1 through 4) the main goals are to develop a good base of cardiorespiratory fitness and prepare the body for the rigors of the more intense training periods to follow. In the first three weeks there are only two running days. The training session between those days is a maximum interval-training session. This workout helps reduce muscle soreness and focuses on improving overall muscular fitness and balance. With distance running, people may experience repetitive stress injuries as their distance and volume of training increase. Improving specific muscle qualities, such as endurance and general strength, during this phase may help alleviate some of those issues. In addition, better muscular endurance will help reduce compensations and poor technique that result from fatigue as duration increases. Furthermore, with greater strength of the stabilizer muscles and supporting structures, the person is able to put more force in the ground with each step, resulting in greater stride length with each step. This improvement is critical because speed is a product of both stride length and frequency.

The foundational MIT sessions should be emphasized during this stage. Initially, while the running volume is low, the runner should focus on performing one MIT session per week and two resistance-training sessions per week. For each exercise, performing two or three sets of 12 repetitions is recommended during this phase. MIT sessions in the general preparation phase should be performed either on days between runs or on days when shorter runs are performed (never on the day when the long run is performed). Table 18.4 presents a sample two-week resistance-training program for the general preparation phase. The goal of this program is to develop a good foundation of general fitness to accommodate the higher levels of stress that will be placed on the body throughout the training schedule.

Special Preparation Period

During this phase (weeks 5 through 19) the number of running session increases from two to three per week. Additionally, the duration of each run is progressively increased to start building the person's tolerance and stamina for longer training sessions. At week 12, interval and fartlek training is incorporated into the training program on the short-run days to work on speed endurance. By this point, a descent aerobic base should have been established, allowing the person to work at a higher percentage of his or her $\dot{V}O_2$max for longer periods. These intervals should last between 30 to 60 seconds depending on the intensity selected.

Table 18.3 Sample Half-Marathon Training Program

Week		Activity	Intensity	Target distance or time
1	Day 1	Run	70–80%	1.5 miles (2.4 km)
	Day 2	MIT (perform sample session 1, table 18.1)	70–80%	20 min
	Day 3	Run	60–70%	3 miles (4.8 km)
2	Day 1	Run	70–80%	1.5 miles (2.4 km)
	Day 2	MIT (perform sample session 2, table 18.1)	80–90%	20 min
	Day 3	Run	60–70%	3 miles (4.8 km)
3	Day 1	Run	70–75%	2 miles (3.2 km)
	Day 2	MIT (perform sample session 3, table 18.1)	80–90%	20–25 min
	Day 3	Run	60–70%	3.5 miles (5.6 km)
4	Day 1	Run	75–85%	1 mile (1.6 km)
	Day 2	MIT (perform sample session 1, table 18.1)	60–70%	20 min
	Day 3	Run	60–65%	3 miles (4.8 km)
5	Day 1	Run	70–80%	3.25 miles (5.2 km)
	Day 2	Run MIT (perform sample session 1, table 18.2)	80–85%	1 mile (1.6 km) or 20 min
	Day 3	Run	60–70%	4 miles (6.4 km)
6	Day 1	Run	70–80%	3.5 miles (5.6 km)
	Day 2	Run MIT (perform sample session 2, table 18.2)	80–85%	1.5 miles (2.4 km) or 20–25 min
	Day 3	Run	60–70%	4.5 miles (7.2 km)
7	Day 1	Run	70–80%	3.5 miles (5.6 km)
	Day 2	Run	80–85%	2 miles (3.2 km) or 15–20 min
	Day 3	Run	60–70%	5 miles (8 km)

Week		Activity	Intensity	Target distance or time
8	Day 1	Run MIT (perform sample session 3, table 18.2)	70–80%	2.5 miles (4 km)
	Day 2	Run	70–80%	3.5 miles (5.6 km) or 10 min
	Day 3	Run	70–80%	4.5 miles (7.2 km)
9	Day 1	Run MIT (perform sample session 2, table 18.2)	60–70%	3 miles (4.8 km)
	Day 2	Run	75–80%	3.5 miles (5.6 km)
	Day 3	Run	60–65%	6 miles (9.7 km)
10	Day 1	Run MIT (perform sample session 2, table 18.2)	60–70%	2.5 miles (4 km)
	Day 2	Run	75–80%	3.5 miles (5.6 km)
	Day 3	Run	60–65%	6.5 miles (10.5 km)
11	Day 1	Run MIT (perform sample session 3, table 18.2)	70–80%	3 miles (4.8 km)
	Day 2	Run	75–80%	3.5 miles (5.6 km)
	Day 3	Run	60–65%	6.5 miles (10.5 km)
12	Day 1	Run (interval or fartlek) MIT (perform sample session 1, table 18.2)	70–80% Intervals (80–90%)	3 miles (4.8 km)
	Day 2	Run	70–80%	4 miles (6.4 km)
	Day 3	Run	60–65%	6.5 miles (10.5 km)
13	Day 1	Run (interval or fartlek) MIT (perform sample session 2, table 18.2)	70–80% Intervals (80–90%)	3 miles (4.8 km)
	Day 2	Run	75–80%	4 miles (6.4 km)
	Day 3	Run	60–65%	7 miles (11.3 km)
14	Day 1	Run (interval or fartlek)	75–80% Intervals (80–90%)	3 miles (4.8 km)
	Day 2	Run MIT (perform sample session 3, table 18.2)	75–80%	3 miles (4.8 km)
	Day 3	Run	60–65%	7.5 miles (12.1 km)
15	Day 1	Run (interval or fartlek) MIT (perform sample session 3, table 18.2)	70–80% Intervals (80–90%)	3 miles (4.8 km)
	Day 2	Run MIT (perform sample session 1, table 18.2)	70–80 %	4 miles (6.4 km)
	Day 3	Run	70–80%	8 miles (12.9 km)
16	Day 1	Run MIT (perform sample session 1, table 18.2)	65–70%	4 miles (6.4 km)
	Day 2	Run (interval or fartlek)	75–80% Intervals (80–90%)	4 miles (6.4 km)
	Day 3	Run	65–75%	9 miles (14.5 km)

(continued)

Table 18.3 *(continued)*

Week		Activity	Intensity	Target distance or time
17	Day 1	Run	65–75%	5 miles (8 km)
	Day 2	Run (interval or fartlek)	75–80% Intervals (80–90%)	3 miles (4.8 km)
	Day 3	Run	65–75%	9.5 miles (15.3 km)
18	Day 1	Run	70–80%	4 miles (6.4 km)
	Day 2	Run (interval or fartlek)	75–80% Intervals (80–90%)	4 miles (6.4 km)
	Day 3	Run	65–75%	8 miles (12.9 km)
19	Day 1	Run	70–80%	4 miles (6.4 km)
	Day 2	Run	70–80 %	4 miles (6.4 km)
	Day 3	Run	65–75%	10.5 miles (16.9 km)
20	Day 1	Run (interval or fartlek)	80–85% Intervals (80–90%)	4 miles (6.4 km)
	Day 2	Run	75–80%	6 miles (9.7 km)
	Day 3	Run	70–80%	6 miles (9.7 km)
21	Day 1	Run	75–85%	4 miles (6.4 km)
	Day 2	Run	80–85%	2 miles (3.2 km)
	Day 3	Run	Competition	

Table 18.4 Sample Two-Week Resistance-Training Program (General Preparation Period)

WEEK 1	
Day 1	**Day 2**
Barbell back squat 2 × 10–12 Barbell bench press 2 × 10–12 Lat pull-down 2 × 10–12 Barbell Romanian deadlift 2 × 10–12 Hanging leg raise 2 × 10 Weighted back extension 2 × 10	Bulgarian squat 2 × 10–12 Dumbbell overhead press 2 × 10–12 Seated row 2 × 10–12 Single-leg dumbbell Romanian deadlifts 2 × 10–12 Glute–ham raise 2 × 10–12

WEEK 2	
Day 1	**Day 2**
Bulgarian squat 2 × 10–12 Dumbbell overhead press 2 × 10–12 Seated row 2 × 10–12 Single-leg dumbbell Romanian deadlift 2 × 10–12 Glute–ham raise 2 × 10–12	Lunge 2 × 10–12 Dumbbell bench press 2 × 10–12 Lat pull down 2 × 10–12 Dumbbell Romanian deadlifts 2 × 10–12 Hanging leg raise 2 × 10 Weighted back extension 2 × 10

Intense intervals should be about 30 seconds long, whereas less intense intervals should be between 30 and 60 seconds long.

The MIT training sessions displayed in table 18.2 can be used in this stage. MIT training during this stage should be performed twice a week at moderately high intensity for two or three sets of 8 to 12 reps. Ideally, these sessions would be spaced a minimum of 72 hours apart to distribute the sessions evenly over the course of the week so that there are never more than three days of rest between MIT sessions. One MIT session per week can be performed on a run day (preferably on the day when the shortest run is scheduled, but never on a long-run day). Resistance training should be performed twice per week depending on how well the person is recovering from training runs. Table 18.5 presents a sample one-week resistance-training program for weeks 5 through 16. Again, a minimum of 48 hours should be allowed between resistance training and MIT sessions. Additionally, on weeks 8, 12, and 16, the number of resistance training session should be cut back to one to aid recovery.

For weeks 17 through 19, the intensity of training during resistance-training sessions increases while the overall volume of training decreases. This plan allows the athlete to maintain the strength developed through the other training cycles while accounting for the increased volume of run training. Resistance training should be performed twice a week at a moderately high intensity for two sets of 6 to 10 reps. During this period, MIT sessions are cut out of the training program (with the exception of interval and fartlek runs). Table 18.6 presents a sample one-week training program for weeks 17 through 19.

Precompetition Period

For weeks 20 through 21 the focus shifts to maintaining intensity while decreasing run duration to allow the athlete to recover from the rigors of training and peak for competition. During this stage MIT training should not be performed. Rather, the resistance-training sessions outlined in weeks 17 through 19 should be performed for one or two sets per training session with a resistance that is challenging at 6 to 10 reps. This plan will help the athlete maintain strength while tapering the volume of endurance training in preparation for competition.

Competition Period

For the purpose of this program the competition period is short. In fact, it is the day of the event only. In the few weeks leading up to the competition, intensity should have remained relatively high while the overall volume of training decreased. This approach allows the runner to maintain the fitness developed through the training program and recover so that she or he can peak on the day of the event.

Recovery Period

When the competition ends, the recovery period begins. This stage may last from two to four weeks depending on the person's training goals and next competition. During this phase

Table 18.5 Sample Two-Week Resistance-Training Program (Special Preparation Period)

Day 1	Day 2
Lateral lunge 2 × 8-10	Bulgarian squat (or lunge) 2 × 8-10
Incline dumbbell bench press 2 × 8-10	Dumbbell push press 2 × 8-10
Chin-up 2 × 8-10	Chin-up 2 × 10-12
Dumbbell Romanian deadlift 2 × 8-10	Single leg dumbbell Romanian deadlift 2 × 10-12
Plank 2 × 30-60 sec.	Side plank 2 × 30-60 sec.
Weighted back extension 2 × 10	

Table 18.6 Sample One-Week Resistance-Training Program (Special Preparation Period)

Day 1	Day 2
Horizontal leg press 2 × 6	Step-up 2 × 8
Barbell incline press 2 × 6–8	Dumbbell push jerk 2 × 6
Chin-up 2 × 8–10	Seated row 2 × 8
Dumbbell Romanian deadlift 2 × 8	Single-leg dumbbell Romanian deadlifts 2× 10
Plank 2 × 30–60 sec.	Side plank 2 × 30–60 sec.
Weighted back extension 2 × 10	

MIT is the ideal method of training because it maintains a sufficient level of cardiorespiratory fitness and muscular strength and endurance. Additionally, MIT can be used to focus on other muscle groups and movement patterns to reduce the stress placed on the muscles used for distance running. During this stage the runner should return to the foundational MIT workouts covered in table 18.1. These workouts help the runner recover from the long training cycle leading up to the race and, by incorporating different MIT programs, may help reduce boredom and maintain enthusiasm for training. Any cardiorespiratory endurance performed during this stage should be something other than running. Using an alternative form of training will help the body recover from the previous training program and the competition and will reduce the injury risk.

Intermittent Endurance Example: Soccer

Soccer requires a high level of technical skill, good eye–foot coordination, and good understanding of game strategy. With the exception of the goalkeeper, there are no specialists on the field, so all players must be able to play both offense and defense simultaneously. Players must be able to accelerate in any direction to defend against an opponent or create space as an attacker. Subsequently, players have to be able to transition quickly from lower-intensity activities (e.g., walking, jogging, or striding) to higher-intensity activities (e.g., sprints, cuts, changes of direction, jumping) during a 90-minute match. Soccer requires efficiency in both the aerobic and anaerobic energy systems to maintain speed and power while minimizing the effects of fatigue as the match progresses.

Because of the metabolic demands of this sport, approaching training from an aerobic conditioning standpoint will leave players ill prepared for competition. Because soccer players use all three energy systems, all three must be addressed in the conditioning program. Table 18.7 is a 52-week conditioning program for a Division II women's collegiate soccer team. This program was developed to encompass all three energy systems, establish an appropriate base of aerobic fitness, and improve anaerobic and speed endurance. Initially, a general conditioning approach is used to enhance the appropriate physiological attributes critical for high-level soccer performance. As the program progresses from the off-season to in-season, the conditioning methods become increasingly more sport specific to maximize the transfer of training effects from practice situations to match scenarios.

Table 18.8 shows a few foundational programs using bodyweight training, medicine balls, and suspension training. These exercises are performed in a circuit. Players should perform each exercise for 20 to 30 seconds, rest for 10 to 15 seconds, and then move to the next exercise in the series. Each circuit should be performed three times.

Within each of these programs, specific emphasis is placed on improving stability and mobility. These attributes are the cornerstones of efficient human movement and are essential for injury reduction. Additionally, these exercises improve muscular endurance and lactate tolerance, which builds a foundation for more intense sprint intervals and heavier resistance-training sessions that will follow in subsequent training stages.

Table 18.9 displays advanced programs using bodyweight and suspension-training exercises. The focus of these sessions is to improve and maintain stability and mobility while challenging anaerobic endurance. These programs can be used in both the special preparation period and during the in-season portion of this training program. Each exercise in these circuits should be performed for 20 to 30 seconds with 10 to 15 seconds of rest between exercises. Each circuit should be repeated two to three times.

Table 18.7 52-Week Conditioning Program for a Women's College Soccer Team

<table>
<tr><td colspan="4" align="center">GENERAL PREPARATION PERIOD</td></tr>
<tr><td></td><td>Day 1</td><td>Day 2</td><td>Day 3</td></tr>
<tr><td>1</td><td>Endurance 2 miles (3.2 km), fartlek</td><td>Endurance 2 miles (3.2 km), fartlek</td><td>MIT circuits (perform sample session 1, table 18.8)</td></tr>
<tr><td>2</td><td>Endurance 2 miles (3.2 km), interval</td><td>Endurance 2 miles (3.2 km), interval</td><td>MIT circuits (perform sample session 2, table 18.8)</td></tr>
<tr><td>3</td><td>Endurance 2 miles (3.2 km), fartlek</td><td>Endurance 2 miles (3.2 km), interval</td><td>MIT circuits (perform sample session 3, table 18.8)</td></tr>
<tr><td>4</td><td colspan="3">Recovery week—active rest</td></tr>
<tr><td colspan="4" align="center">SPECIAL PREPARATION PERIOD</td></tr>
<tr><td>5</td><td>Acceleration, interval</td><td>Acceleration, sprint training</td><td>Endurance 2 miles (3.2 km), interval</td></tr>
<tr><td>6</td><td>Acceleration, interval</td><td>Acceleration, sprint training</td><td>Endurance 2.25 miles (3.6 km), interval</td></tr>
<tr><td>7</td><td>Acceleration, interval</td><td>Acceleration, sprint training</td><td>Endurance 2.5 miles (4 km), interval</td></tr>
<tr><td>8</td><td>MIT circuits (perform sample session 1, table 18.8)</td><td>MIT circuits (perform sample session 2, table 18.8)</td><td>Endurance 2 miles (3.2 km), interval</td></tr>
<tr><td>9</td><td>Acceleration, interval</td><td>Acceleration, sprint training</td><td>Endurance 2.25 miles (3.6 km), interval</td></tr>
<tr><td>10</td><td>Acceleration, interval</td><td>Acceleration, sprint training</td><td>Endurance 2.5 miles (4 km), interval</td></tr>
<tr><td>11</td><td>Acceleration, interval</td><td>Acceleration, sprint training</td><td>Endurance 2.5 miles (4 km), interval</td></tr>
<tr><td>12</td><td>MIT circuits (perform sample session 1, table 18.9)</td><td>MIT circuits (perform sample session 2, table 18.9)</td><td>Endurance 2.5 miles (4 km), interval</td></tr>
<tr><td>13</td><td>Acceleration, interval</td><td>Acceleration, sprint training</td><td>Acceleration, interval</td></tr>
<tr><td>14</td><td>Acceleration, sprint training</td><td>Acceleration, interval</td><td>Acceleration, sprint training</td></tr>
<tr><td>15</td><td>Acceleration, interval</td><td>Acceleration, sprint training</td><td>Acceleration, interval</td></tr>
<tr><td>16</td><td>MIT circuits (perform sample session 3, table 18.9)</td><td>MIT circuits (perform sample session 1, table 18.8)</td><td>Recovery—active rest</td></tr>
<tr><td>17</td><td>Acceleration, interval</td><td>Acceleration, sprint training</td><td>Acceleration, interval</td></tr>
<tr><td>18</td><td>Acceleration, sprint training</td><td>Acceleration, interval</td><td>Acceleration, sprint training</td></tr>
<tr><td>19</td><td>Acceleration, interval</td><td>Acceleration, sprint training</td><td>Acceleration, interval</td></tr>
<tr><td>20</td><td>MIT circuits (perform sample session 2, table 18.8)</td><td>MIT circuits (perform sample session 2, table 18.8)</td><td>Recovery—active rest</td></tr>
<tr><td>21</td><td>Acceleration, sprint training</td><td>Acceleration, interval</td><td>Acceleration, sprint training</td></tr>
<tr><td>22</td><td>Acceleration, interval</td><td>Acceleration, sprint training</td><td>Acceleration, interval</td></tr>
<tr><td>23</td><td>Acceleration, sprint training</td><td>Acceleration, interval</td><td>Endurance 2 miles (3.2 km), fartlek</td></tr>
<tr><td>24</td><td>Endurance 2 miles (3.2 km), fartlek</td><td>Acceleration, interval</td><td>Endurance 2 miles (3.2 km), Fartlek</td></tr>
<tr><td>25</td><td>Endurance 2 miles (3.2 km), interval</td><td>Acceleration, sprint training</td><td>Endurance 2 miles (3.2 km), interval</td></tr>
<tr><td>26</td><td>Acceleration, interval</td><td>Acceleration, sprint training</td><td>Acceleration, interval</td></tr>
<tr><td>27</td><td>Acceleration, sprint training</td><td>Acceleration, interval</td><td>Acceleration, sprint training</td></tr>
<tr><td>28</td><td>Acceleration, interval</td><td>Acceleration, sprint training</td><td>Acceleration, interval</td></tr>
<tr><td>29</td><td>Acceleration, interval</td><td>Acceleration, sprint training</td><td>Acceleration, interval</td></tr>
<tr><td>30</td><td>Acceleration, sprint training</td><td>Acceleration, interval</td><td>Acceleration, sprint training</td></tr>
<tr><td>31</td><td>Acceleration, interval</td><td>Acceleration, sprint training</td><td>Acceleration, interval</td></tr>
<tr><td>32</td><td>MIT circuits (perform sample session 1, table 18.9)</td><td>MIT circuits (perform sample session 2, table 18.9)</td><td>Recovery—active rest</td></tr>
</table>

(continued)

Table 18.7 *(continued)*

	Day 1	Day 2	Day 3	
PRECOMPETITION PERIOD				
33	Scrimmages	Scrimmages	Scrimmages	
34	Scrimmages	Scrimmages	Scrimmages	
COMPETITION PERIOD				
35	SSG	Acceleration, SSG	Games	Games
36	SSG	Acceleration, SSG	Games	Games
37	SSG	Acceleration, SSG	Games	Games
38	SSG	Acceleration, SSG	Games	Games
40	SSG	Acceleration, SSG	Games	Games
41	SSG	Acceleration, SSG	Games	Games
42	SSG	Acceleration, SSG	Games	Games
43	SSG	Acceleration, SSG	Games	Games
44	SSG	Acceleration, SSG	Games	Games
45	SSG	Acceleration, SSG	Games	Games
46	SSG	Acceleration, SSG	Games	Games
47	SSG	Acceleration, SSG	Games	Games
48		Playoffs, championship		
49				
RECOVERY				
50		Active rest		
51		Active rest		
52		Active rest		

SSG = small-sided games.

Table 18.8 Foundational MIT Workouts for Intermittent Endurance Athletes

Sample session 1 Suspension training	Sample session 2 Medicine balls	Sample session 3 Body weight
Suspension squat *Suspension push-up* *Suspension reverse lunge* *Suspension row* *Suspension biceps curl* *Suspension triceps extension* *Suspension reverse fly* Circuit workout. Perform each for 30 seconds and rest for 15 seconds between exercises. Rest for 1 minute between circuits and repeat.	*Medicine ball chop* *Medicine ball lift* *Medicine ball thruster* *Medicine ball slam* *Medicine ball multiplanar squat* *Medicine ball modified pike, right leg elevated* *Medicine ball modified pike, Left leg elevated* *Medicine ball bomb toss to sprint* Circuit workout. Perform each for 20 seconds and rest for 10 seconds between exercises. Rest for 1 minute between circuits and repeat.	*Bodyweight groiner* *Bodyweight frog hop* *Bodyweight inchworm* *Bodyweight bear crawl* *Bodyweight walking plank* *Bodyweight jumping jacks* *Bodyweight scissors* Circuit workout. Perform each for 30 seconds and rest for 15 seconds between exercises. Rest for 1 minute between circuits and repeat.

Table 18.9   Advanced MIT Workouts for Intermittent Endurance Athletes

Sample session 1 Suspension training	Sample session 2 Medicine balls	Sample session 3 Bodyweight
Suspension hip up *Suspension leg curl* *Suspension lying leg raise* *Suspension pike* *Suspension clock* Circuit workout. Perform each for 30 seconds and rest for 15 seconds between exercises. Rest for 1 minute between circuits and repeat.	*Medicine ball chop* *Medicine ball lift* *Medicine ball thruster* *Medicine ball slam* *Medicine ball bomb toss to sprint* Circuit workout. Perform each for 20 seconds and rest for 10 seconds between exercises. Rest for 1 minute between circuits and repeat.	*Bodyweight jumping jacks* *Bodyweight 180-degree squat turn* *Bodyweight speed squat* *Bodyweight inchworm* *Bodyweight hockey lunges* *Bodyweight scissors* Circuit workout. Perform each for 30 seconds and rest for 15 seconds between exercises. Rest for 1 minute between circuits and repeat.

Quickness and Agility

In one sense, quickness and agility can be thought of as the ability to react to a stimulus, select the appropriate movement pattern, and execute it quickly and correctly. For an athlete, quickness and agility are the ability to combine strength, power, speed, conditioning, mobility, and sport skills and put them to use during sport-specific situations. In many ways, this is the most direct application of strength and conditioning to sport.

HOW AGILITY IS TRAINED

Agility is difficult to train. It involves specific skills, performed in a specific situation, that occur in a random and chaotic setting. To coach and train agility requires knowledge of the event we are trying to perform, its movement patterns, its skills, and its offenses and defenses. This task can be daunting to many people. Typically, agility training involves several steps. First, the important skills for the event are identified and trained in isolation. Next, some of these skills are combined to increase the complexity of the drill. Finally, the athlete is asked to react to situations and cues and to select the appropriate movement patterns, just like in real life.

Variables

Quickness and agility training involves many of the same variables as other modes of training: volume, intensity, training frequency, rest, and recovery. Volume can be expressed in terms of distance or repetitions. Intensity is usually measured by the stopwatch. Agility can be trained daily, but this should be done in a way that supports the rest of the athlete's training. Finally, the athlete must have enough time between sets and repetitions to recover.

In terms of the training variables, two considerations are important. First, because agility involves sudden, explosive changes of directions, a tired athlete may perform the movements incorrectly, which could lead to injury. The wise approach is to keep the training volume low and to allow full recovery. Second, the intensity is usually high on these drills, especially as the complexity increases. The athlete should walk through the drill the first time to get comfortable with what is going on.

Tools

Several classifications of tools are commonly used in agility training. These include fundamental skills, combination drills, and reactive drills. These classifications also represent a progression; typically, athletes begin with fundamental skills, move to combination drills, and then do reactive drills.

Fundamental Skills

These skills are movements performed in the sport. Skills common to many sports include starting, stopping, backpedaling, shuffling, turning, running a curve, and changing direction suddenly. These skills are normally trained in isolation as an athlete is mastering them. In the long term they can serve as excellent warm-up drills after the athlete has mastered them. These skills are often trained for specific distances (for example, backpedalling for 10 meters).

Combination Drills

The challenge with performing fundamental skills is that these movements are not used in real life. For example, a basketball player is never going to be shuffling to the left for 10 yards during a game. Combination drills combine several fundamental skills and therefore come closer to resembling real-life situations. They allow the athlete to continue to master the individual skills while learning how to move effortlessly between skills. Eventually, these drills may even incorporate the ball or a defender to make them more sport specific.

For example, a basketball player might be asked shuffle to the right, turn around, sprint five yards, and then reestablish a defensive stance. This example simulates covering an opposing player who has the ball, having to run down the opponent after a breakaway, and getting between the opponent and the basket. In that example, the athlete is working on shuffling, turning, starting, stopping, and sprinting, all in a basketball-specific context.

Reactive Drills

Reactive drills closely simulate an athlete's reality. They require the athlete to react successfully to a situation, a defender, or a coach. These drills require the athlete to process the situation, select the appropriate movement patterns, and execute those movement patterns correctly—and do all those things quickly. Reactive drills are the most advanced agility drills. They are safe and effective only after the athlete has mastered the previous two types of agility tools.

The drill described in the combination section can be modified by having the athlete defend a live player who has the ball. The player with the ball is instructed to try to break away from the defender and sprint down the court for a layup. The athlete defending the ball handler is instructed to stay between the ball and the basket, attempting to prevent a breakout and layup.

LIMITATIONS OF AGILITY TRAINING

This chapter presents agility training in conjunction with maximum interval training only. It is rarely performed this way in practice. Normally, athletes perform agility training in conjunction with speed training, plyometrics, and strength training.

Agility Training Eventually Must Be Sport Specific or Situation Specific

Fundamental skills and combination drills are easy to program and coach. The challenge is that although they provide a foundation, they don't do a good job of preparing athletes for the speed, chaos, and unpredictability of a game. Therefore, agility training has to become sport specific and situation specific at some point. Meeting this condition is a challenge because to program athletes in this manner, you have to understand the movement patterns and situations inherent to that sport.

Agility Training Can Cause Injuries

By definition, agility training involves sudden and explosive changes in direction. These movement patterns can cause hamstring strains, groin strains, ankle sprains, and knee ligament injuries. To help reduce the risk of these injuries, several factors must be kept in mind when employing agility training.

- Athletes must be grounded in proper techniques.
- Avoid extreme fatigue; overtired athletes will have sloppy technique.
- Athletes need a strength-training foundation to develop their joints and muscles.

Agility Training Must Be Integrated With Other Training Modes

Normally, quickness and agility training is a portion of an athlete's training; rarely do athletes perform only quickness and agility training. Agility training is normally done along with speed training, strength training, plyometrics, sport practices, and games. Typically, agility training is linked with either practices or speed training.

If agility training is linked with practice, then the two activities should emphasize similar things. For example, if practice emphasizes short offensive or defensive situations, then the agility training should do the same. On the other hand, if practice focuses on longer scrimmages or small-sided games, then the agility training can feature longer and more complex drills.

If agility training is linked with speed training, then the focus of the speed training should help to influence the kind of agility training that is being performed. If speed training is focused on acceleration, then agility drills should be shorter, generally in the 5- to 6-second range. If speed training is focused on maximum velocity, then agility drills can be longer, more complex, and last up to 20 seconds. If speed training is focused on speed endurance, then the agility drills may last longer than 20 seconds.

GUIDELINES FOR INTEGRATING MAXIMUM INTERVAL TRAINING

Quickness and agility training should be conducted on the days that speed training is conducted. Remember that quickness and agility training is rarely a stand-alone training modality. It is part of a larger, more comprehensive training program that may include practices, competitions, strength training, speed training, plyometrics, and conditioning. With this in mind, maximum interval training should be integrated into a larger training program in a way that ensures that it supports the bigger picture of training. The long-term programs take this comprehensive approach to show how real-world agility is integrated and then to show how maximum interval training is integrated.

SAMPLE PROGRAMS

Most forms of conditioning can be performed in conjunction with a quickness and agility program. Table 19.1 shows sample foundational programs that could be used with a quickness and agility program. **Note: The italicized exercises are found in part II. Refer to the exercise finder for more information.** With the exception of the sprint program, these programs are circuits of 30 seconds of exercise and 10 to 15 seconds of recovery. Each circuit is repeated three times. The sprint program is a stepwise program (from table 4.1), so the first number in parenthesis after each distance is the time that you have to perform the sprint and the second number is how much rest you have before the next sprint. If you complete the sprint in less than the allotted time, you have more time to rest!

Table 19.2 shows sample advanced programs that could be used in conjunction with a quickness and agility workout. These longer circuits integrate multiple modes of exercise and sprinting. Exercises might be performed for 30 to 60 seconds, followed by a sprint. Recovery between exercises is minimal, just enough to position or adjust equipment.

Table 19.1 Sample Foundational Programs to Use With Quickness and Agility Training

Bodyweight program	Suspension program	Stepwise sprint program	Medicine ball program	Heavy ropes program	Kettlebell program
Bodyweight jumping jacks Bodyweight bear crawl Bodyweight crab kick Bodyweight mountain climber Bodyweight inchworm Bodyweight groiner Bodyweight push-up Bodyweight scissors Bodyweight dip Bodyweight squat hold Bodyweight pull-up	Suspension chest press Suspension squat Suspension hip up Suspension reverse lunge Suspension row Suspension leg curl Suspension knees to chest Suspension lying leg raise	1 × 20 meters (10 sec, 20 sec) 1 × 40 meters (15 sec, 30 sec) 1 × 60 meters (20 sec, 40 sec) 1 × 80 meters (25 sec, 50 sec) 1 × 100 meters (30 sec, 60 sec) 1 × 80 meters (25 sec, 50 sec) 1 × 60 meters (20 sec, 40 sec) 1 × 40 meters (15 sec, 30 sec) 1 × 20 meters	Medicine ball chop Medicine ball wall ball Medicine ball Bulgarian squat Medicine ball slam Medicine ball thruster Medicine ball seated twist Medicine ball touch and jump Medicine ball modified pike	Heavy ropes jumping jacks Heavy ropes two-handed slam Heavy ropes twist Heavy ropes wave Heavy ropes arm circle, clockwise then counterclockwise Heavy ropes towing Heavy ropes woodchopper Heavy ropes pulling	Kettlebell two-handed swing Kettlebell snatch Kettlebell goblet squat Kettlebell deadlift Kettlebell clean Kettlebell Romanian deadlift

Table 19.2 Sample Advanced Programs to Use With Quickness and Agility Training

Program 1	Program 2	Program 3
Heavy ropes two-handed slam Sprint 10 meters Suspension squat Sprint 10 meters Bodyweight frog hop Sprint 10 meters Suspension reverse lunge Sprint 10 meters Bodyweight speed squat Sprint 10 meters Bodyweight squat hold Sprint 10 meters Suspension leg curl Sprint 10 meters Kettlebell overhead squat Sprint 10 meters Suspension hip up	Kettlebell two-handed swing Sprint 5 meters Medicine ball chop Sprint 5 meters Heavy ropes one-handed slam Sprint 5 meters Kettlebell goblet squat Sprint 5 meters Suspension suspended foot squat Sprint 5 meters Heavy ropes woodchopper Sprint 5 meters Kettlebell Romanian deadlift Kettlebell overhead lunge	Suspension squat Sprint 5 meters Kettlebell one-handed swing Sprint 10 meters Heavy ropes twist Sprint 20 meters Medicine ball thruster Sprint 20 meters Kettlebell deadlift Sprint 10 meters Suspension one-legged squat Sprint 5 meters Heavy ropes shuffle slam Medicine ball Bulgarian squat

LONG-TERM PROGRAMS

For the long-term programming of quickness and agility training, we'll use the example of a collegiate basketball player. Our long-term example takes the approach that the athlete is focusing only on quickness and agility training. Keep in mind that in reality an athlete is training with every training mode.

Figure 19.1 shows the 2014 macrocycle for the collegiate basketball player. The preparatory phase lasts five months, from May through September. The competition phase lasts from October through March. April is the recovery phase.

An athlete who is training primarily for quickness and agility needs maximum interval training to do a number of things. It needs to help the athlete prevent injuries, particularly hamstring, groin, and shin injuries. It needs to help the athlete develop the strength

Year-long macrocycle												
Competition phase							Recovery phase	Preparatory phase				
Precomp period	Competition period						Recovery period	General preparation period			Special preparation period	
Oct	Nov	Dec	Jan	Feb		Mar	April	May	Jun	July	Aug	Sep
I	II	III	IV	V	VI	VII	VIII	IX	X	XI	XII	XIII

Figure 19.1 Sample macrocycle for a collegiate basketball player.

and power foundation required to be successful with agility. This means that kettlebells, sandbags, bodyweight training, suspension training, and implements like those covered in chapter 10 form the foundation of maximum interval training. In addition, using speed training as part of maximum interval training will help enhance the athlete's agility.

Table 19.3 provides the goals and tools to be used in each period of training for agility and maximum interval training. Agility is divided into the fundamental skills, combination drills, and reactive drills mentioned earlier. The table shows that the complexity of the agility training and basketball training increases as the athlete progresses through the

Table 19.3 Goals and Tools for Each Period of the Cycle

Period	Goals	Tools
General preparation	Fitness base Injury prevention Fundamental skills Basketball skills	*Maximum interval training using kettlebells, heavy ropes, sprinting, bodyweight exercises, suspension training, alternative training devices, and sandbags* *Maximum interval training using kettlebells, bodyweight exercises, suspension training, alternative training devices, and sandbags* Drills focused on shuffling, backpedaling, starting, stopping, zigzags, and running curves Ballhandling, defending against the ball, passing, pass denial, shooting
Special preparation	Fitness base Injury prevention Fundamental skills Combination drills Basketball skills	*Maximum interval training using kettlebells, heavy ropes, sprinting, bodyweight exercises, suspension training, alternative training devices, and sandbags* *Maximum interval training using kettlebells, bodyweight exercises, suspension training, alternative training devices, and sandbags* Drills focused on jab step, V cuts, shuffling, backpedaling, starting, stopping, zigzags, and running curves Stop the breakthrough, weave, down and back, figure 8, and breakout and shoot Ballhandling with one ball and two, defending against the ball, passing, pass denial, shooting, rebounding, basic team offense and defense
Precompetition	Fitness base Injury prevention Fundamental skills Combination drills Reactive drills Basketball skills	Small-sided games, *maximum interval training using kettlebells, heavy ropes, sprinting, bodyweight exercises, suspension training, alternative training devices, and sandbags* *Maximum interval training using kettlebells, bodyweight exercises, suspension training, alternative training devices, and sandbags* Drills focused on jab step, V cuts, shuffling, backpedaling, starting, stopping, zigzags, and running curves Stop the breakthrough, weave, down and back, figure 8, breakout and shoot, jab step drill Deny the red zone, box out, get open Ballhandling with one ball and two, defending against the ball, passing, pass denial, shooting, rebounding, basic team offense and defense

Period	Goals	Tools
Competition	Fitness base Injury prevention Fundamental skills Combination drills Reactive drills Basketball skills	Small-sided games, *maximum interval training using kettlebells, heavy ropes, sprinting, bodyweight exercises, suspension training, alternative training devices, and sandbags* *Maximum interval training using kettlebells, bodyweight exercises, suspension training, alternative training devices, and sandbags* Drills focused on jab step, V cuts, shuffling, backpedaling, starting, stopping, zigzags, and running curves Stop the breakthrough, weave, down and back, figure 8, breakout and shoot, jab step drill Deny the red zone, box out, get open Ballhandling with one ball and two, defending against the ball, passing, pass denial, shooting, rebounding, team offense and team defense
Recovery	Conditioning	*Kettlebells* *Heavy ropes* *Suspension training* *Bodyweight exercises* *Sandbags* *Alternative training devices* *Sprinting*

macrocycle. In addition, both maximum interval training and, eventually, small-sided games (i.e., scrimmages with fewer than five players on each side) are used for conditioning when the precompetition period begins. Table 19.4 shows an overview of how the volume and intensity for the various modes of training will change during each period of the macrocycle.

General Preparation Period

Table 19.5 shows a sample microcycle from the general preparation period. The agility training is focused on starting, accelerating, stopping, shuffling, backpedaling, turning, and zigzags. The agility drills are meant to sync up with what the athlete is training in terms of basketball skills. So, for example, on Monday the focus is on ballhandling and defense. As a result, the agility training is focused on shuffling, starting, accelerating for short distances, and backpedaling. Three short agility-training sessions occur each week. Keep in mind that an athlete may also be strength training and performing plyometrics.

Maximum interval training is performed three times a week, on days when the athlete is not performing agility training. This schedule is also meant to sync up with the basketball training that is being done. In this microcycle the focus is on kettlebells, medicine balls, suspension training, heavy ropes, and bodyweight training. The circuit workouts focus on addressing most of the muscles and joints of the body. Besides providing a fitness base, the workouts help condition the muscles that are prone to injury from agility training.

Special Preparation Period

Table 19.6 shows a sample microcycle from the special preparation period. The fundamental skills now essentially become warm-ups, which is why the volume of those exercises is reduced. The athlete is beginning to shift to more complicated agility movements and the practice of basketball skills. In this period, a number of sport-specific combination drills are included.

Table 19.4 Volume and Intensity for Each Period of the Macrocycle

Period	Mode of training	Volume, intensity
General preparation	Fundamental skills	M, M
	Combination drills	n/a
	Reactive drills	n/a
	Basketball skills	L, L
	Conditioning	M, M
Special preparation	Fundamental skills	L, L
	Combination drills	M, M
	Reactive drills	n/a
	Basketball skills	M, M
	Conditioning	M, M
Precompetition	Fundamental skills	L, L
	Combination drills	L, M
	Reactive drills	L, H
	Basketball skills	H, H
	Conditioning	L, L
Competition	Fundamental skills	L, L
	Combination drills	L, M
	Reactive drills	M, H
	Basketball skills	H, H
	Conditioning	L, L
Recovery	Fundamental skills	n/a
	Combination drills	n/a
	Reactive drills	n/a
	Basketball skills	n/a
	Conditioning	M, M

Precompetition Period

During the precompetition period, team practices ramp up. The emphasis on basketball increases, which has ripple effects on the rest of the training program. Agility becomes more specific, so reactive drills are introduced. Small-sided games are added to serve as a bridge between conditioning and basketball practice. In the precompetition period, exhibition games may be scheduled, so travel may be required. As a result, training modes like maximum interval training are reduced. A sample microcycle from this period is found in table 19.7.

Competition Period

Because of competition and travel, the hope is to get in two training days per week during the competition period (table 19.8). A basketball athlete may practice basketball more than this, but the goal is to get in at least two agility sessions each week. During this period, everything is as basketball-specific as possible. Most of the fundamental skills, combination drills, and reactive drills are done with the ball when appropriate.

Recovery Period

The recovery period for this athlete focuses on three maximum interval-training sessions per week. The sessions described in table 19.9 are appropriate for basketball players. These sessions allow the athletes to maintain their fitness while giving them a break from the rigors of basketball-specific training.

Table 19.5 Sample Week of Workouts During the General Preparation Period

	Monday	Tuesday	Wednesday
Fundamental skills	Falling starts, 3–5 × 10 meters Shuffle right and left, 3 × 5 meters each way Backpedal, 3 × 5 meters	n/a	Standing starts, 3–5 × 20 meters Sprint 5 meters, stop, sprint 5 more, 3× L drill, 3–5×
Combination drills	n/a	n/a	n/a
Reactive drills	n/a	n/a	n/a
Basketball skills	Ballhandling Defense	n/a	Ballhandling Passing and pass denial
Conditioning	n/a	Circuit workout, perform each exercise for 45 seconds, minimize rest, repeat 3 times: *Kettlebell two-handed swing* *Medicine ball chop* *Suspension chest press* *Heavy ropes one-handed slam* *Kettlebell goblet squat* *Suspension row* *Suspension foot-in-trainer one-legged squat* *Suspension reverse fly* *Heavy ropes woodchopper* *Kettlebell Romanian deadlift* *Kettlebell overhead lunge*	n/a

	Thursday	Friday	Saturday
Fundamental skills	n/a	Standing starts, 3–5 × 5 meters Suicides, 5× whole court Zigzag drill, 3–5×	n/a
Combination drills	n/a	n/a	n/a
Reactive drills	n/a	n/a	n/a
Basketball skills	Shooting	Ballhandling (one and two balls)	Shooting
Conditioning	Circuit workout, perform each exercise for 45 seconds, minimize rest, repeat 3 times: *Heavy ropes two-handed slam* *Suspension squat* *Bodyweight push-up* *Bodyweight frog hop* *Suspension reverse lunge* *Bodyweight pull-up* *Speed squat* *Bodyweight squat hold* *Kettlebell press* *Suspension leg curl* *Kettlebell overhead squat* *Suspension hip up*	n/a	Circuit workout, perform each exercise for 45 seconds, minimize rest, repeat 3 times: *Suspension squat* *Kettlebell one-handed swing* *Kettlebell push-up* *Heavy ropes twist* *Medicine ball thruster* *Kettlebell bent-over row* *Kettlebell deadlift* *Suspension one-legged squat* *Kettlebell press* *Heavy ropes shuffle slam* *Medicine ball Bulgarian squat*

Table 19.6 Sample Week of Workouts During the Special Preparation Period

	Monday	Tuesday	Wednesday
Fundamental skills	Falling starts, 3–5 × 10 meters Shuffle right and left, 1 × 5 meters each way Backpedal, 1 × 5 meters	n/a	Standing starts, 3–5 × 20 meters Sprint 5 meters, stop, sprint 5 more, 1× L drill, 15×
Combination drills	Stop the breakthrough, 5× Figure 8, 5×	n/a	Weave, 5× Breakout and shoot, 5×
Reactive drills	n/a	n/a	n/a
Basketball skills	Ballhandling (one and two balls) Defense Team offense and defense	Shooting Rebounding	Ballhandling (one and two balls) Passing and pass denial Team offense and defense
Conditioning	n/a	Circuit workout, perform each exercise for 45 seconds, minimize rest, repeat 3 times: *Heavy ropes two-handed slam* *Suspension squat* *Bodyweight push-up* *Bodyweight frog hop* *Suspension reverse lunge* *Bodyweight pull-up* *Bodyweight speed squat* *Bodyweight squat hold* *Kettlebell press* *Suspension leg curl* *Kettlebell overhead squat* *Suspension hip up*	n/a

	Thursday	Friday	Saturday
Fundamental skills	n/a	Standing starts, 3–5 × 5 meters Suicides, 5× whole court Zigzag drill, 15×	n/a
Combination drills	n/a	Weave, 5×	n/a
Reactive drills	n/a	n/a	n/a
Basketball skills	Shooting Rebounding	Ballhandling (one and two balls) Team offense and defense	Shooting
Conditioning	Circuit workout, perform each exercise for 45 seconds, minimize rest, repeat 3 times: *Kettlebell two-handed swing* *Medicine ball chop* *Suspension chest press* *Heavy ropes one-handed slam* *Kettlebell goblet squat* *Suspension row* *Suspension foot-in-trainer one-legged squat* *Suspension reverse fly* *Heavy ropes woodchopper*	n/a	Circuit workout, perform each exercise for 45 seconds, minimize rest, repeat 3 times: *Suspension squat* *Kettlebell one-handed swing* *Kettlebell push-up* *Heavy ropes twist* *Medicine ball thruster* *Kettlebell row* *Kettlebell deadlift* *Suspension one-legged squat* *Kettlebell press* *Heavy ropes shuffle slam*

Table 19.7 Sample Week of Workouts During the Precompetition Period

	Monday	Tuesday	Wednesday
Fundamental skills	Falling starts, 3–5 × 10 meters Shuffle right and left, 1 × 5 meters each way Backpedal, 1 × 5 meters	n/a	Standing starts, 3–5 × 20 meters Sprint 5 meters, stop, sprint 5 more, 1× L drill, 15×
Combination drills	Stop the breakthrough, 3× Figure 8, 3×	n/a	Weave, 3× Breakout and shoot, 3×
Reactive drills	Deny the red zone drill, 5×	Box out drill, 5×	Get open drill, 5×
Basketball skills	Ballhandling (one and two balls) Defense Team offense and defense	Shooting Rebounding Team offense and defense Small-sided games	Ballhandling (one and two balls) Passing and pass denial Team offense and defense
Conditioning	n/a	Circuit workout, perform each exercise for 45 seconds, minimize rest, repeat 3 times: *Heavy ropes two-handed slam* *Bodyweight suspension squat* *Bodyweight push-up* *Bodyweight frog hop* *Suspension reverse lunge* *Bodyweight pull-up* *Bodyweight speed squat* *Bodyweight squat hold* *Kettlebell press* *Suspension leg curl* *Kettlebell overhead squat* *Suspension hip up*	n/a

	Thursday	Friday	Saturday
Fundamental skills	n/a	Standing starts, 3–5 × 5 meters Suicides, 5× whole court Zigzag drill, 15×	n/a
Combination drills	n/a	Weave, 3×	n/a
Reactive drills	Box out drill, 5×	n/a	n/a
Basketball skills	Shooting Rebounding Team offense and defense Small-sided games	Ballhandling (one and two balls) Team offense and defense	Shooting
Conditioning	Circuit workout, perform each exercise for 45 seconds, minimize rest, repeat 3 times: *Kettlebell two-handed swing* *Medicine ball chop* *Suspension chest press* *Heavy ropes one-handed slam* *Kettlebell goblet squat* *Suspension row* *Suspension foot-in-trainer one-legged squat* *Suspension reverse fly* *Heavy ropes woodchopper* *Kettlebell Romanian deadlift* *Kettlebell overhead lunge*	n/a	n/a

Table 19.8 Sample Week of Workouts During the Competition Period

	Day 1	Day 2
Fundamental skills	Falling starts, 3–5 × 10 meters Shuffle right and left, 1 × 5 meters each way Backpedal, 1 × 5 meters	Standing starts, 3–5 × 20 meters Sprint 5 meters, stop, sprint 5 more, 1× L drill, 15×
Combination drills	Stop the breakthrough, 3× Figure 8, 3×	Weave, 3× Breakout and shoot, 3×
Reactive drills	Deny the red zone drill, 5× Box out drill, 5×	Get open drill, 5× Jab step drill, 5×
Basketball skills	Ballhandling (one and two balls) Defense Team offense and defense Small-sided games	Ballhandling (one and two balls) Passing and pass denial Team offense and defense Small-sided games
Conditioning	n/a	Circuit workout, perform each exercise for 45 seconds, minimize rest, repeat 3 times: *Kettlebell two-handed swing* *Medicine ball chop* *Suspension chest press* *Heavy ropes one-handed slam* *Kettlebell goblet squat* *Suspension row* *Suspension foot-in-trainer one-legged squat* *Suspension reverse fly* *Heavy ropes woodchopper* *Kettlebell Romanian deadlift* *Kettlebell overhead lunge*

Table 19.9 Sample Week of Workouts During the Recovery Period

	Monday	Wednesday	Friday
Conditioning	*Kettlebell one-handed swing* *Heavy ropes two-handed slam* *Kettlebell snatch (right hand)* *Bodyweight jumping jacks* *Kettlebell snatch (left hand)* *Medicine ball Bulgarian squat* *Kettlebell goblet squat* *Medicine ball modified pike* *Kettlebell deadlift* *Medicine ball seated twist* *Bodyweight push-up* *Medicine ball wall ball* *Kettlebell bent-over row* *Medicine ball seated twists* *Kettlebell press*	*Kettlebell two-handed swing* *Suspension squat* *Kettlebell clean (right hand)* *Suspension reverse lunge* *Kettlebell clean (left hand)* *Bodyweight inchworm* *Heavy ropes woodchopper* *Suspension chest press* *Heavy ropes twist* *Suspension bent-over row* *Heavy ropes arm circle* *Suspension reverse fly* *Heavy ropes jumping jacks*	*Bodyweight jumping jacks* *Sprint 10 meters* *Bodyweight bear crawl* *Sprint 10 meters* *Bodyweight crab kick* *Sprint 10 meters* *Bodyweight mountain climber* *Sprint 10 meters* *Bodyweight inchworm* *Sprint 10 meters* *Bodyweight groiner* *Sprint 10 meters* *Bodyweight push-up* *Sprint 10 meters* *Bodyweight speed squat* *Sprint 10 meters* *Bodyweight lunge* *Sprint 10 meters*

CHAPTER 20

Tactical Training

Tactical athletes are those whose primary job responsibility is to protect the safety of their country and community in time of need, such as military soldiers, law enforcement officers, firefighters, and rescue personnel. Based on many of the job tasks that they must perform, tactical athletes work in some of the most physically demanding occupations outside professional athletics. Consequently, maintaining and attaining optimal levels of physical conditioning is necessary. If these people fail to do so, the stakes can be much greater than losing a game or championship. Fitness may literally mean the difference between life and death.

As explained in chapter 11, the first step in designing any strength and conditioning program is to perform a needs or goals analysis. This analysis should include the primary energy systems used and the biomechanical needs of specific job tasks. In addition, creating an injury profile that includes common occupational injuries seen on the job and an individual injury profile is helpful in developing a safe and effective prehabilitation program to improve occupational resilience.

Although a good deal of overlap is seen within the tactical professions, some subtle differences are present in job tasks. Tables 20.1 through 20.5 list job tasks based on some of the categories of tactical athletes. Within each of these categories you will see the primary energy systems used and a list of movements that may be required to execute each task. Although this list does not describe all the possible movement combinations required to perform a task, it provides a good general template to start breaking down movements.

DEVELOPING OPERATIONAL FITNESS

Many similarities are found between the programs of occupational athletes and those of sport athletes. In this section we discuss how to maximize fitness for operational readiness. The training program presented here has been designed in a general manner, so it will require some modifications to suit the specific circumstances, job requirements, injury profile, and training experience of the individual.

Building a Foundation for Efficient Movement and Conditioning

One of the critical aspects of training the tactical athlete is optimizing movement performance. Therefore, the emphasis of training these people should be to develop efficient movement patterns. This should be done by first emphasizing fundamental movement skills in an unloaded (without resistance) environment and then progressing to loaded activities (with resistance) as skill and proficiency are demonstrated.

People often falsely assume that because tactical athletes perform highly demanding physical tasks on a daily basis, they are ready to engage in an aggressive training program from day one. In fact, remedial training to address flaws in movement proficiency should be addressed first within the training program. Many people in this population have movement limitations created by poor mobility and stability. These issues may lead to muscle imbalances

Table 20.1 Essential Job Tasks for Law Enforcement Officers

	Primary energy system	Muscle quality	Movement patterns
Sustained pursuit	Glycolytic	Strength, power, endurance	Sprint mechanics
Sprints	ATP–PCr	Strength, power	Sprint mechanics
Dodging	ATP–PCr, glycolytic	Strength, power, endurance	Sprint mechanics, agility
Lifting and carrying	ATP–PCr, glycolytic	Strength, power, endurance	Squat, lunge, push, pull
Dragging and pulling	ATP–PCr, glycolytic	Strength, power, endurance	Squat, lunge, pull
Pushing	ATP–PCr, glycolytic	Strength, power, endurance	Squat, lunge
Jumping and vaulting	ATP–PCr	Strength, power	Squat, lunge, drop landing
Crawling	ATP–PCr	Strength, power, endurance	Core training, coordinating limbs in an oppositional movement pattern
Use of force for less than 2 minutes	ATP–PCr, glycolytic	Strength, power, endurance	Squat, lunge, push, pull
Use of force for more than 2 minutes	ATP–PCr, glycolytic, and oxidative		Squat, lunge, push, pull

Adapted from R. Hoffman and T.R. Collingwood, 2005, *Fit for duty*, 2nd ed. (Champaign, IL: Human Kinetics), 8-9.

Table 20.2 Essential Job Functions for Special Weapons and Tactics Officers

Crawling
Jumping over, off, or across obstacles
Maintaining balance while traversing a narrow object or wall
Maintaining a tactical position for an extended period and remaining alert
Climbing fences, walls, elevator shafts, multiple flights of stairs, ladders, fire escapes, ropes, poles, and trees to gain an objective or tactical position
Lifting and carrying necessary equipment—rams, breeching tools, ladders, and shields—over rough terrain
Lifting; dragging wounded officers or citizens to safety
Running to escape an area of danger or to cross an open area
Running to pursue a suspect or rescue a hostage
Functioning on roof tops, ledges, and high positions
Functioning in crawl spaces, tunnels, vents, shafts, and other tight spaces
Low and high crawling to objectives

Source: National Tactical Officers Association.

that create postural issues, which in turn can cause improper movement mechanics. This problem may not only hinder performance but also increase injury risk. For example, police officers must spend long periods sitting in their cars while on patrol. The result may be a shortening of the hip flexor muscles and a rounding of the shoulders because of increased tightness in the anterior muscles surrounding the shoulder girdle (pectorals) and progressive elongation of the muscles on the posterior side of the shoulder girdle (rhomboids). These physical changes may increase the risk that officers will experience shoulder and back

Table 20.3 Firefighter Job Tasks

Structural firefighters	Wildland firefighters
Vertical climb	Hiking
Hose hoist	Load carriage
Ladder carry and raise	Lift and lower heavy objects
Forcible entry	Digging and clearing
Hose advance	Tree cutting
Crawl and search	Hose advance
Casualty evacuation	Casualty evacuation
Salvage	
Overhaul	

Source: National Strength and Conditioning Association.

Table 20.4 General Occupational Tasks for Military Soldiers

Climbing
Casualty carrying
Lifting heavy and light objects
Sprinting to cover or to overtake a hostile position
High and low crawling
Digging
Foot marching
Load carrying loads over short and long distances
Running
Throwing

Adapted from S.E. Sauers and D.E. Scofield, 2014, "Strength and conditioning strategies for females in the military," *Strength and Conditioning Journal* 36(3): 1-17.

Table 20.5 Military Urban Operation Skills

Crossing open areas
Moving parallel to buildings
Moving past windows
Moving around corners
Crossing a wall
Using of doorways
Moving between positions

Adapted from J.J. Knapik, W. Rieger, F. Palkoska, S. Van Camp, and S. Darakjy, 2009, "United States Army Physical Readiness Training: Rationale and evaluation of the physical training doctrine," *Journal of Strength and Conditioning Research* 23(3): 1353-1362.

problems. Additionally, duty belts worn by officers can cause increased anterior tilt of the pelvis, which is often associated with lower back pain and injury. These postural issues are further accentuated when a person is required to perform movement tasks under load (carrying equipment, wearing protective clothing, and so on). Therefore, tactical athletes must learn to control and redirect the forces and stressors placed on their bodies so that they can perform well and be more resistant to injury.

During this foundation-building phase, performing training activities that require the use of low loads, high repetitions, and longer work durations is the emphasis. This form of training tends to favor the development of muscular endurance, aerobic fitness, and technique development. Doing repetitions in a slow, controlled manner and performing isometric holds emphasizes the development of the stabilizing structures of the joints and trunk. Bodyweight exercise, suspension training, light resistance tubing, and light medicine ball work is recommended during this phase.

Additionally, improving mobility should be addressed during this stage. Repetitive motions, previous injuries, and improper movement mechanics may lead to restricted mobility in certain joints, which in turn may cause movement restrictions and lead to compensatory movement patterns that may hinder performance and increase injury risk.

Table 20.6 provides a sample dynamic warm-up. This warm-up focuses on a series of exercises aimed at improving fundamental movement skills, motor control and stability of the trunk, and mobility of the joints. Basic form running drills can also be used as part of the warm-up to help develop good movement mechanics for accelerations and sprints. **Note: The italicized exercises are found in part II. Refer to the exercise finder for more information.**

Table 20.7 provides a sample introductory resistance-training program that can be used during the foundation-building phase. It emphasizes the use of supersets, alternating between agonist and antagonist muscle groups, to improve the time efficiency of the workout and maintain high metabolic demand. Mostly bodyweight and suspension exercises have been selected in this phase to emphasize proper technique before adding additional weight. Each exercise should be performed in sequential order for the recommended number of repetitions before the second set is performed.

Aerobic energy system development should also be emphasized in this stage by including activities that can be sustained for longer than three minutes. Improving aerobic capacity helps establish a base of fitness for more intense and specific energy system training in the future. Improved aerobic capacity may also assist in occupational tasks such as foot marches, load carriage over long distances, searches, casualty evacuations, and hiking. But the tactical athlete does not need to perform traditional aerobic training that focuses on repetitive, long-duration, steady-state activities. Rather, a series of drills and exercise can be sequenced in a manner to emphasize various movement patterns at low training loads that emphasize this energy system. A sample weeklong aerobic training program is shown in table 20.8. This program should be performed immediately after the resistance-training session.

For the beginner, this portion of the foundation-building phase should be performed for approximately 6 to 12 weeks. For those who are more advanced and have resistance-training experience, this portion of the program may last between 2 and 6 weeks.

Table 20.6 Sample Dynamic Warm-Up

Exercise	Repetitions or distance
Bodyweight jumping jacks	× 20 reps
Bodyweight bear crawl	× 20 yards
Bodyweight inchworm	× 10 yards
Arm swing drill	× 20 reps
Jog	× 40 yards
Bodyweight groiner	× 10 reps each leg
Bodyweight frog hop	× 10 reps
Bodyweight speed squat	× 10 reps
Bodyweight push-up	× 10 reps
Bodyweight lateral squat	× 10 reps (5 each side)

Perform this series of exercises one or two times with minimal or no rest between exercises.

Table 20.7 Sample Introductory Resistance-Training Program for a Tactical Athlete

Monday		Wednesday		Friday	
Exercise	**Sets × reps**	**Exercise**	**Sets × reps**	**Exercise**	**Sets × reps**
Bodyweight push-up	2–4 × 15–20	*Bodyweight elevated push-up*	2–4 × 10–12	*Suspension push-up*	2–4 × 12–15
Suspension row	2–4 × 15–20	*Suspension one-armed row*	2–4 × 10–12	*Suspension row*	2–4 × 12–15
Bodyweight walking lunge	2–4 × 15–20 per leg	Medicine ball Bulgarian squat	2–4 × 10–12	*Suspension reverse lunge*	2–4 × 12–15
Suspension lying leg raise	2–4 × 15–20	*Suspension knees to chest*	2–4 × 10–12	*Suspension hip up*	2–4 × 12–15

Note: When performing suspension exercises the feet should be adjusted in relation to the anchor point to increase or decrease the intensity of the movement so that only the desired number of repetitions can performed.
Rest: less than 30 seconds between exercises
Beginners should perform two or three times, whereas advanced people can perform three or four times.

Table 20.8 Sample Aerobic Training Program

Monday	Wednesday	Friday
Rower for 5 minutes Stairmaster for 5 minutes Jog for 5 minutes	Spin bike or rower: Sprint 30 seconds at 70% effort. Recover for 30 seconds at 50% effort. Repeat for 15 minutes	Walk or jog 1.5–2 miles (2.4–3.2 km)
Note: Attempt to cover as much distance as possible in the time allotted.	**Note:** On a subjective rating scale of 1–10, 70% effort would equate to a 7 whereas a 5 would equate to 50% effort.	**Note:** Attempt to cover the distance in as little time as possible.

Building Fitness

After completing the first phase of this program, the tactical athlete will have a solid foundation of mobility, stability, and aerobic fitness that will support fitness training. At this point the athlete can begin to focus on improving muscular size and strength. These muscle qualities will set the stage for more explosive forms of training aimed at increasing power and speed of movement. Table 20.9 presents a sample four-week resistance-training program for this stage. Notice that each day has a few training options (e.g., dumbbells or barbells). Periodically selecting different modalities forces the muscles to work slightly differently to accommodate the different stressors placed on the body. For instance, when using dumbbells rather than a barbell, greater stabilization is required because dumbbells allow more freedom of movement at the joint. Therefore, most people are able to lift heavier weights with barbells. But to address the ability to produce force as well as to stabilize, both modalities should be incorporated in a training program. Switching between the use of barbells and dumbbells every other workout or every third workout not only helps reduce staleness and training monotony but also promotes gains. The fourth week in this fitness development portion of the program is an unloading week to allow the athlete to recover from the rigors of exercising before repeating this training block.

During this stage, improving metabolic capacity also becomes a priority. Performing conditioning that begins to emphasize both the aerobic and glycolytic energy systems is appropriate. Training the glycolytic energy system means performing activities at an intensity that can be sustained for at least 30 seconds but no more than 2 minutes. This type of conditioning is beneficial for improving performance in activities of moderate duration and

Table 20.9 Sample Four-Week Resistance-Training Program for Building Fitness

WEEK 1

Monday		Wednesday		Friday	
Exercise	Sets × reps	Exercise	Sets × reps	Exercise	Sets × reps
Barbell bench press	3–4 × 10–12	Overhead dumbbell press	3–4 × 8–10	Incline dumbbell press	2–4 × 12–15
Barbell bent-over row	3–4 × 10–12	Single-arm rows	3–4 × 8–10	Bodyweight pull-up	3–4 × 10–15
Barbell deadlift	3–4 × 10–12	Bulgarian squat with dumbbells	3–4 × 8–10	Lateral lunge with dumbbells	3–4 × 12–15 per leg
Barbell Romanian deadlift	3–4 × 10–12	Dumbbell Romanian deadlift	3–4 × 8–10	Suspension leg curl	3–4 × 12–15
Hanging leg raise	3–4 × 10–12	Hanging oblique crunch	3–4 × 10–12	Back hyperextension	3–4 × 12–15

WEEK 2

Monday		Wednesday		Friday	
Exercise	Sets × reps	Exercise	Sets × reps	Exercise	Sets × reps
Dumbbell bench press	3–4 × 10–12	Overhead barbell press	3–4 × 8–10	Incline barbell press	2–4 × 12–15
Lat pull-down	3–4 × 10–12	Bent-over barbell row	3–4 × 8–10	Bodyweight pull-up	3–4 × 10–15
Barbell squat	3–4 × 10–12	Lateral squat with dumbbells	3–4 × 8–10 per leg	Walking lunge with dumbbells	3–4 × 12–15 per leg
Barbell Romanian deadlift	3–4 × 10–12	Single-leg Romanian deadlift	3–4 × 8–10 per leg	Suspension leg curl	3–4 × 12–15
Hanging leg raise	3–4 × 10–12	Back hyperextension (holding weight plate or medicine ball)	3–4 × 10–12	Hanging oblique crunch	3–4 × 12–15

WEEK 3:
Repeat week 1 and adjust training loads accordingly to stay within the desired repetition ranges.

WEEK 4:
Unloading week

Monday		Wednesday		Friday	
Exercise	Sets × reps	Exercise	Sets × reps	Exercise	Sets × reps
Bodyweight push-up	3 × 15–20	Bodyweight elevated push-up	3 × 10–12	Suspension push-up	3 × 12–15
Suspension row	3 × 15–20	Suspension single-arm row	3 × 10–12	Suspension row	3 × 12–15
Bodyweight walking lunge	3 × 15–20 per leg	Medicine ball Bulgarian squat	3 × 10–12	Suspension reverse lunge	3 × 12–15
Suspension lying leg raise	3 × 15–20	Suspension knee to chest	3 × 10–12	Suspension hip up	2–4 × 12–15

Note: When performing suspension exercises the feet should be adjusted in relation to the anchor point to increase or decrease the intensity of the movement so that only the desired number of repetitions can performed.

Rest: 60 to 90 seconds between exercises.

Sets: Beginners should perform three sets, whereas advanced athletes can perform three or four sets.

After completing this cycle, repeat the training cycle in the following order: week 2, 3, 1, and 4.

intensity, such as sustained pursuits, vertical climbing, and use-of-force situations lasting less than 2 minutes. Table 20.10 details a weeklong sample maximal interval-training program emphasizing both the aerobic and glycolytic energy systems.

The beginner should perform this program for approximately 8 to 12 weeks. An experienced lifter may perform this portion of the program for 4 to 8 weeks.

Training for Power, Speed, and Strength

Power and speed training is performed at the peak of the training cycle. These attributes represent the optimal expression of velocity and strength. During this stage emphasis is on maintaining and improving strength while shifting to higher-velocity movements that emphasize the ATP–PCr energy system. Therefore, heavy resistance training at slow velocity is used to improve strength, whereas moderate to light loads are integrated at higher velocity to improve power and speed of movement. Additionally, plyometric and speed training are performed at this stage. Before performing plyometric training, the athlete must build a good foundation of strength to control the rapid eccentric loading of the muscle tissues while decelerating.

Table 20.11 shows a sample plyometric and speed-training program that can be performed before the strength-training session (table 20.12). Note that because power, speed, and resistance training are all being performed on the same day, the volume of training is relatively low.

Periodization

The program, discussed up to this point, has focused on a linear periodization program, meaning that every phase of the training program builds on the previous phase. During each

Table 20.10 Sample Maximal Interval-Training Program for Building Fitness

Monday	Wednesday	Friday
Weighted sled push, 30 sec	*Heavy boxing bag jab, 30 sec, rest 30 sec*	*Water-filled stability ball carry, 20 yards, jog up and back 20 yards, water-filled stability ball carry 20 yards back to start*
Weighted sled pull, 30 sec	*Heavy boxing bag cross, 30 sec, rest 30 sec*	*Heavy boxing bag walking lunge, 10 yards and back*
Jog 30 sec	*Heavy boxing bag, hook 30 sec, rest 30 sec*	*Bodyweight bear crawl, 20 yards up and back*
Rest 1 min		
Repeat 6× (total time 15 min)	Repeat 6× (total time 18 min)	Repeat as many times as possible for 12 min

Table 20.11 Sample Plyometric and Speed Program

Monday	Wednesday	Friday
Box jumps 3 × 10 Rest 2–3 min between sets	Depth jumps 3 × 4–6 Rest 2–3 min between sets	6 in. cone hops 3 × 10 Rest 1–2 min between sets
Speed work: acceleration 　10 yards × 4 　15 yards × 4 　20 yards × 4 Rest 2 min between sets 180 total yards	Speed work: acceleration 　10 yards × 4 　15 yards × 2 Rest 2 min between sets Agility: 　5-10-5 (pro-agility) × 4 Rest 2–3 min between sets 130 total yards	Speed work: acceleration from a prone position 　0 yards × 2 　15 yards × 4 Rest 1–2 min between sets Agility: 　T-test × 2 Rest 2 min between sets 160 total yards

Table 20.12 Sample Strength-Training Program

WEEK 1

Monday		Wednesday		Friday	
Exercise	**Sets × reps**	**Exercise**	**Sets × reps**	**Exercise**	**Sets × reps**
Barbell bench press	3 × 4–6	Overhead dumbbell press	3 × 8	Incline dumbbell press	3 × 6–8
Barbell bent-over row	3 × 8	Single-arm row	3 × 6–8	Seated row	3 × 6–8
Bulgarian squat with dumbbells	3 × 6–8	Barbell deadlift	3 × 4–6	Lateral lunge with dumbbells	3 × 8 per leg
Barbell Romanian deadlift	3 × 8	Dumbbell Romanian deadlifts	3–4 × 8–10	Crunch	3 × 12–20
Hanging leg raise	3 × 10–12	Hanging oblique crunch	3 × 10–12	Back hyperextension	3 × 12–20

WEEK 2

Monday		Wednesday		Friday	
Exercise	**Sets × reps**	**Exercise**	**Sets × reps**	**Exercise**	**Sets × reps**
Dumbbell bench press	2–3 × 6–8	Overhead barbell press	2–3 × 4–6	Incline barbell press	2–3 × 8
Lat pull-down	2–3 × 8	Bent-over barbell row	3–4 sets 8–10	Bodyweight pull-up	2–3 × 10–15
Barbell squats	2–3 × 4–6	Lateral squat with dumbbells	3–4 sets 8–10 per leg	Barbell deadlift	2–3 × 6–8
Barbell Romanian deadlift	2–3 × 8–10	Single-leg Romanian deadlift	2–3 sets 10–12 per leg	Suspension leg curl	2–3 × 12–15
Crunch	2–3 × 15–20			Suspension hip up	3–4 × 15–20

phase, the athlete will likely become proficient at performing the specific attributes that are emphasized. At the initiation of a training program for the tactical athlete, it is appropriate to follow this basic model to establish a good training base. A traditional linear periodization model is frequently used in sports that require an athlete to peak at a certain time of year or for a specific competition. Thus, this model may work well for the tactical athlete in developing a base of fitness for academy training, training for a personal fitness test (PFT), or training for a scheduled deployment.

Although linear periodization has a place in the training of the tactical athlete, it is not always appropriate. In the tactical population, every day may be game day. Periodizing a training program isn't possible in all instances for members of these groups. A firefighter cannot predict when a fire will happen, a police officer does not know when a suspect will resist arrest or flee, and a soldier may not know when a deployment will begin. Therefore, after a base of fitness has been developed through a more conventional linear periodization model, more advanced models may be used. Nonlinear periodization programs are useful in simultaneously attempting to maintain and improve muscular strength, power,

Table 20.13 Sample One-Week Nonlinear Program

Monday		Wednesday		Friday	
Dynamic warm-up Light speed work and plyometrics		Dynamic warm-up Maximum-effort speed work and high-intensity plyometrics		Dynamic warm-up	
RESISTANCE TRAINING					
Exercise	**Sets × reps**	**Exercise**	**Sets × reps**	**Exercise**	**Sets × reps**
Barbell squat	3 × 10–12	Deadlift	3 × 4–6	*Suspension training, bodyweight circuit*	
Dumbbell incline press	3 × 10–12	Bench press	3 × 4–6		
Bodyweight pull-up	3 × 10–12	Single-arm row	3 × 6		

Back hyperextension	3 × 10–12	Barbell Romanian deadlift	3 × 6–8	Conditioning:
				    Rower × 5 min
				    Stairmaster × 5 min
				    Bike × 5 min
				Cover as much distance as possible in time allotted	

Suspension pike	3 × 10–12	Conditioning: None or light walking (50–60%) for recovery			
Conditioning: *Medicine ball circuit, 10–15 min*					

and endurance while enhancing each of the three energy systems. The benefit of this model is that people maintain a relatively high level of operational readiness at all times. Table 20.13 outlines a sample one-week nonlinear program that emphasizes both strength training and conditioning.

GUIDELINES FOR INTEGRATING MAXIMUM INTERVAL TRAINING INTO A TACTICAL TRAINING PROGRAM

Maximal interval training should be used in this population as part of a comprehensive training program, not as a stand-alone method of training. Maximum interval training should be incorporated with other forms of strength, power, and speed training to enhance metabolic capacity and reduce potential risks of injury by improving mobility and stability. Maximum interval training can be used to address many of the issues discussed earlier with typical injuries and imbalances created by occupational movements. For example, by performing mobility training within the context of a maximal interval-training session, the tactical athlete may be able to improve movement limitations created by repetitive motion or lack of motion, such as sitting in a patrol car for extended periods. It can also be used to train basic movement patterns, such as hip hinging, squatting and lunging, pushing, pulling, and rotating, that may be necessary to execute job tasks safely and effectively, all while improving metabolic efficiency.

Developing a training program for the tactical athlete is a complicated process that requires a detailed needs analysis that emphasizes specific movements, skills, energy systems, and the underpinning physiological attributes needed to enhance each of those components. A structured program designed to develop these attributes should be the primary focus at the onset of the training. Linear periodization models tend to work well in accomplishing these goals. After a good base of movement, conditioning, and fitness has been established, more advanced methods of periodization, specifically nonlinear models, can be used to maintain operational fitness levels and to continue making consistent improvement.

CHAPTER 21

Total-Body Conditioning

Not everyone is interested in training for strength, speed, agility, tactical fitness, or endurance. Each of these approaches to training will appeal to a specific population, but any approach can be problematic for those who don't fit into a particular category. Some people just enjoy training, are interested in being more fit, are interested in looking better, and prefer the maximum interval approach to training. This chapter includes principles, tools, and programs for people who want to use maximum interval training as the mainstay in their fitness regimen.

HOW TOTAL-BODY CONDITIONING IS TRAINED

Using maximum interval training as the training approach has several benefits. Maximum interval training has built-in variety in terms of exercises, training tools, and training variables that just isn't available to people who are training for something specific. For example, an athlete who is training to increase strength will focus primarily on free weights and get some help from kettlebells. Any other training tool will be used in a purely supplementary role. An athlete who trains for strength will focus primarily on heavy weights, low volume, and lots of recovery. On the other hand, someone who uses maximum interval training as the primary training approach can use any type of exercise, apply any training tool, and manipulate training variables with great variety.

Tools

Every training tool covered in this book can be used for total-body conditioning, offering a huge advantage to those who use maximum interval training as their training approach. Depending on goals, kettlebells, body weight, suspension trainers, heavy ropes, sandbags, sprinting, medicine balls, and other training implements can be used. This variety keeps the body adapting and results in a more fit and well-rounded person compared with those who rely on a single training tool.

Variables

Maximum interval training used as total-body conditioning can be used to increase muscle mass, increase strength, improve power, improve agility and quickness, increase speed, and improve endurance. But this approach is not going to be more effective than more traditional approaches to developing these qualities (i.e., the approaches described in chapters 16 through 20). If your goal is to maximize the development of one of those qualities (for example, maximal strength), then you should follow the training approaches detailed in the previous chapters. If, however, your goal is all-around development, then you can use maximal interval training to help develop those qualities. Table 21.1 provides examples of how to program the training variables to achieve various goals. Note that if you are not

Table 21.1 Guidelines for Adjusting Variables to Meet Other Goals

Goal	Volume	Intensity
Increase muscle mass	8–15 reps per set	60–80% of maximum
Increase strength	1–8 reps per set	>80% of maximum
Improve power (weight room)	1–6 reps per set	50–70% of maximum
Improve power (plyometrics)	50–100 foot contacts per workout	100%
Increase endurance	>15 reps per set	<60% of maximum
Improve speed (acceleration)	Up to 20-meter sprints; no more than 200 meters per session	100%
Improve speed (maximal speed)	40- to 60-meter sprints; no more than 200–400 meters per session	100%
Improve speed (speed endurance)	Up to 150-meter sprints; no more than 300–600 meters per session	100%

focused on performance, you don't have to train for any of these goals. You can feel free to change the volume, intensity, and so on.

Training Approaches

You can use maximum interval training in several ways to develop a total-body conditioning routine. These programs all present unique challenges to your body, and some lend themselves better to specific goals. These various approaches provide you with variety to keep your workouts interesting and challenging.

Total-Body Circuit Training

Total-body circuit training is an approach that trains almost every muscle of the body. Up to this point in the book, it represents the majority of the maximum interval training that has been used. Table 21.2 provides a sample of this approach. This method is a good way to increase endurance and integrate sprinting into total-body conditioning. **Note: The italicized exercises are found in part II. Refer to the exercise finder for more information.**

Table 21.2 Sample Total-Body Workout Circuit

Kettlebell two-handed swing
Kettlebell goblet squat
Heavy rope slams
Bodyweight lunge
Kettlebell Romanian deadlift
Bodyweight push-up
Kettlebell one-handed swing (right hand)
Bodyweight pull-up
Kettlebell one-handed swing (left hand)

Table 21.3 Sample Alternating Upper-Body and Lower-Body Workout

Sandbag front squat
Bodyweight push-up
Bodyweight reverse lunge
Bodyweight pull-up
Sandbag Romanian deadlift
Suspension reverse fly
Suspension leg curls
Suspension biceps curl
Suspension hip up
Suspension triceps extension

Alternating Upper-Body and Lower-Body Training

This method still uses a circuit approach to training, but it uses only exercises that can be identified as upper body or lower body in emphasis. In this training approach, upper body and lower body exercises are alternated. Table 21.3 provides a sample of this approach. This type of training would be best used for increasing muscle mass or increasing strength.

Head to Feet Training

Head to feet training is a type of circuit training in which you begin with the exercises at the top of your body and progressively move down. As with a typical circuit, you perform the exercises in order, one set of each exercise. After you complete the circuit, you repeat it as many times as necessary. Table 21.4 provides a sample of this approach. This approach to training is best for increasing endurance, increasing muscle mass, or increasing strength. The set approach is a different concept from those that have been explored previously. With the set approach, you perform all the sets of a given exercise before moving on to the next exercise. Between these sets, you do some type of sprint or cardiovascular exercise while you "rest." Table 21.5 provides a sample of a workout using the set approach. This type of training is best for increasing power, increasing strength, and increasing muscle mass. It is also a way to improve speed because sprinting can be incorporated into the program.

Table 21.4 Sample Head to Feet Circuit Training Program

Suspension chest press
Bodyweight pull-up
Sandbag overhead press
Suspension reverse fly
Suspension triceps extension
Suspension biceps curl
Kettlebell goblet squat
Sandbag split squat
Kettlebell Romanian deadlifts

Table 21.5 Sample Head to Feet Set Program

Kettlebell two-handed swing
Kettlebell snatch
Sandbag front squat
Suspension reverse lunge
Kettlebell Romanian deadlift
Suspension push-up
Kettlebell bent-over row
Sandbag overhead press
Suspension reverse fly
Perform 8 to 12 repetitions of each exercise. After a set of 8 to 12 reps, sprint 20 meters. Walk back and then immediately perform the next set. Perform three sets of each exercise.

GUIDELINES FOR TOTAL-BODY CONDITIONING

No approach to training is perfect, and this caution is certainly true when using maximum interval training as your workout program. This section gives you some things to keep in mind when putting together your program. By understanding these limitations, you will be able to overcome them and keep your workouts effective.

Total-Body Conditioning Must Follow the Principles of Exercise A frequent mistake made when using maximum interval training as the primary method of working out is failing to observe the principles of exercise. Recall that chapter 14 listed the following principles of exercise: specificity, overload, progression, muscle balance, and individualization. All these principles need to be applied to a maximum interval-training program.

Total-Body Conditioning Must Be Organized Carefully Total-body conditioning needs to be organized so that it is easy to move between exercises and tools with a minimal break in the activity. For example, let's say that a workout includes the following exercises: kettlebell two-handed swing, medicine ball chest pass, 20-meter sprint, suspension chest press, and suspension knees to chest. The kettlebell exercise is performed in one place; in other words, you don't change your location while you perform it. But after tossing the medicine ball, you have to go get it to continue performing the repetitions. If you keep moving away from your starting point with each rep, you could get pretty far away. Then you have to perform the sprint, perform the chest press, and then take time to adjust the suspension trainer to perform the knees to chest exercise. All this could result in too much downtime to have an effective workout.

A better approach would be to organize the training session as follows. First, perform the kettlebell two-handed swing. Second, perform the medicine ball chest pass, but after the first toss, toss it back to the start line for the second toss. Continue tossing it back and forth, first away from the start line and then back toward the start line. Make the last toss toward the start line. Third, sprint the 20 meters. Fourth, after the sprint perform push-ups instead of the chest press. No equipment is necessary, so you can perform the exercise anywhere. Fifth, sprint back to the suspension trainer and perform the knees to chest exercise. These modifications are an example of how to organize training to maximize what you have access to while minimizing things that waste your time.

LONG-TERM PROGRAMS

The long-term program presented in this chapter is meant to keep you interested, give you lots of variety, increase your fitness level, and force your body to adapt to the training. The long-term program consists of several mesocycles, each of which builds on the one that came before. After you have completed all the steps, you should start the whole program over again. The mesocycles are called Get in Shape, Build Those Muscles, Use Those Muscles, and Train Like an Athlete.

Get in Shape

The Get in Shape mesocycle lasts four weeks. It involves training three times a week, ideally with a day off after each training session. The training revolves around total-body circuit training with sprints, total-body exercises (like heavy ropes slams), and cardiovascular exercises mixed in between the circuits. This fast, high-volume training is designed to burn a lot of calories and improve your endurance. This training also lays the foundation for the future steps.

Table 21.6 shows a week of workouts for this part of training. Note that each workout is a little different in terms of the exercises, the amount of time spent performing each exercise, and the activity to be performed during "recovery." All the workouts are designed so that minimal changes to equipment are required. The first day involves heavy ropes and body-weight exercises, so all the exercises can be performed in the same location. The second day involves alternating between suspension-training exercises and medicine ball exercises. The third day involves alternating between sandbags and kettlebells.

Build Those Muscles

This four-week mesocycle builds on the fitness base developed in the previous mesocycle. The training is a little heavier. It incorporates both a circuit approach and a set approach, and it uses a combination of total-body exercises and core exercises as recovery tools. This mesocycle develops the ligaments, tendons, and bones, so it helps prevent future injuries from training in the next two cycles.

Table 21.7 shows a week of workouts for this part of training. The first thing to notice is that training occurs on four days each week with one day off. Days 1 and 4 are focused on lower-body training, and days 2 and 5 are focused on upper-body training. Days 4 and 5 use a set format. For each of these exercises, three sets should be performed.

Use Those Muscles

This mesocycle takes the fitness base developed in the first mesocycle and the muscle and soft-tissue development from the second and trains you how to apply those improvements.

Table 21.6 Sample Week of Workouts for Get in Shape Cycle

	Day 1	Day 2	Day 3
Work intervals	Perform each exercise for 30 seconds.	Perform each exercise for 45 seconds.	Perform each exercise for 60 seconds.
Rest intervals	Sprint 20 to 40 meters after each exercise, walk back, and then perform the next exercise.	After each exercise, perform 30 seconds of *kettlebell two-handed swings*. Select a weight that you can handle with good form for 30 seconds of swinging.	After each exercise, perform 30 seconds of *heavy ropes slams*.
Total-body circuits	*Heavy ropes jumping jacks* *Bodyweight bear crawl* *Heavy ropes slams* *Bodyweight inchworm* *Heavy ropes wave* *Bodyweight crab kick* *Heavy ropes woodchopper* *Bodyweight groiner* *Heavy ropes oblique woodchopper* *Bodyweight pull-up* *Heavy ropes arm circle, clockwise and counterclockwise* *Bodyweight push-up*	*Medicine ball chop* *Suspension chest press* *Medicine ball thruster* *Suspension row* *Medicine ball touch and jump* *Suspension biceps curl* *Medicine ball chop with knee punch* *Suspension triceps extension* *Medicine ball rotational slam* *Suspension squat* *Medicine ball off-centered plyo push-up* *Suspension leg curl*	*Kettlebell two-handed swing* *Sandbag front squat* *Kettlebell deadlift* *Sandbag Romanian deadlift* *Kettlebell push-up* *Sandbag bent-over row* *Kettlebell one-handed swing (right hand)* *Sandbag Y press* *Kettlebell one-handed swing (left hand)* *Sandbag upright row*

Table 21.7 Sample Week of Workouts for Build Those Muscles Cycle

	Day 1	Day 2	Day 3	Day 4	Day 5
Work intervals	Select a resistance that you can use for 12 to 15 reps or 45 seconds. This day uses a circuit format.	Select a resistance that you can use for 12 to 15 reps or 45 seconds. This day uses a circuit format.	Off	Select a resistance that you can use for 8 to 12 reps or 30 seconds. This day uses a set approach.	Select a resistance that you can use for 8 to 12 reps or 30 seconds. This day uses a set approach.
Rest intervals	Perform *heavy ropes slams* for 20 seconds after each exercise.	Perform *kettlebell two-handed swings* for 20 seconds after each exercise.	Off	Perform *medicine ball modified pikes* for 30 seconds after each exercise.	Perform *medicine ball seated twists* for 30 second after each exercise.
Circuits	*Medicine ball multiplanar squat* *Suspension squats* *Medicine ball Bulgarian squat* *Suspension reverse lunge* *Medicine ball Bulgarian squat* *Suspension hip up* *Suspension leg curl*	*Medicine ball chest pass* *Suspension chest press* *Medicine ball off-centered plyo push-up* *Suspension row* *Medicine ball thruster* *Suspension reverse fly* *Medicine ball alphabet* *Suspension biceps curl* *Suspension triceps extension*	Off	*Kettlebell goblet squat* *Sandbag front squat* *Sandbag deadlift* *Kettlebell overhead lunge* *Sandbag overhead press* *Sandbag split squat* *Kettlebell Romanian deadlift*	*Kettlebell push-up* *Sandbag push-up to overhead press* *Kettlebell bent-over row* *Kettlebell prone row* *Kettlebell press* *Sandbag Y press* *Sandbag upright row*

Table 21.8 Sample Week of Workouts for Use Those Muscles Cycle

	Day 1	Day 2	Day 3
Work intervals	Select a resistance that you can use for 4 to 8 reps or 30 seconds. Use a set approach on this day.	Select a resistance that you can use for 8 to 12 reps or 45 seconds. Use a set approach on this day.	Select a resistance that you can use for 12 to 20 reps or 60 seconds. Use a set approach on this day.
Rest intervals	Perform *medicine ball pikes* for 30 seconds after each set.	Perform *suspension knees to chest* for 30 seconds after each set.	Perform *medicine ball seated twists* for 30 seconds after each set.
Circuits	*Kettlebell two-handed swing* *Kettlebell one-handed swing (right hand)* *Medicine ball thrusters* *Kettlebell one-handed swing (left hand)* *Medicine ball slams* *Kettlebell overhead squat (right hand)* *Medicine ball chops with knee punch* *Kettlebell overhead squat (left hand)* *Medicine ball rotational slams*	*Kettlebell one-handed swing (right hand)* *Heavy ropes slam* *Kettlebell one-handed swing (left hand)* *Heavy ropes wave* *Kettlebell one-handed clean (right hand)* *Heavy ropes one-handed slam (right hand)* *Kettlebell one-handed clean (left hand)* *Heavy ropes one-handed slam (left hand)*	*Sandbag swing and lift* *Sandbag deadlift* *Kettlebell one-hand jerk (right hand)* *Sandbag push-up to overhead press* *Kettlebell one-hand jerk (left hand)* *Kettlebell windmills (right hand)* *Sandbag overhead squats* *Kettlebell windmills (left hand)*

This mesocycle focuses more on developing strength and power, and it places greater emphasis on total-body movements than the previous two mesocycles did. Weights are heavier, volume is lower, and the set approach receives greater emphasis.

Table 21.8 shows a sample week of workouts from this mesocycle. Note that the workouts occur on only three days a week. The workouts are total body and heavier in nature, so a day off should be scheduled after each workout for recovery. A set approach is used for each workout. Three sets of each exercise should be performed.

Train Like An Athlete

This mesocycle builds on everything you have developed to this point. It trains everything, but it requires you to have developed a fitness base, strength, and power. In addition, you need to have spent time injury proofing your joints. It also assumes that you have had a chance to develop your technique on the exercises.

Table 21.9 shows a sample week of workouts from this mesocycle. The training is organized around four days of training per week, with a day off between the second and fourth days. The first day involves heavier training, and the second day is more total-body training in nature. Both the first and second days are meant to use circuit approaches. Note that there are no rest periods between exercises. The fourth day is focused on a stepwise sprinting workout. During the time between sprints, you should be performing the designated bodyweight exercise as your recovery. The last day uses a set approach and focuses on a combination of agility drills and medicine ball exercises. With the exception of the T-test and the L drill, the agility drills are to be performed for 10 meters each. During the rest periods after each set, you should perform medicine ball exercises for 30 seconds. Ideally, you should perform three sets of each agility exercise.

Using maximum interval training as your workout approach offers the potential for a great deal of variety. The workouts covered in this chapter provide exposure to many exercises and training tools. These workouts will help you develop comprehensive, well-rounded fitness.

Table 21.9 Sample Week of Workouts for Train Like an Athlete Cycle

	Day 1	Day 2	Day 3	Day 4	Day 5
Work intervals	Select a resistance that allows you to perform 4 to 8 repetitions or 30 seconds of work.	Select a resistance that allows you to perform 4 to 8 repetitions or 30 seconds of work.	Day off	This is a stepwise sprinting workout. The sprints are alternated with bodyweight exercises.	This is an agility workout. Perform each drill for 10 meters or for the prescribed drill. Between drills, perform medicine ball exercises for 30 seconds. Note that a set approach is used on this day.
Rest intervals	No rest, circuit approach.	No rest, circuit approach.	Day off	Perform bodyweight exercises for the rest periods after each sprint.	Perform medicine ball drills for 30 seconds after each set.
Circuit	*Heavy ropes two-handed slam* *Sandbag front squat* *Heavy ropes slam* *Kettlebell overhead squat* *Heavy ropes slam* *Kettlebell Romanian deadlift* *Heavy ropes slam* *Kettlebell push-up* *Heavy ropes slam* *Sandbag bent-over row* *Heavy ropes slam* *Kettlebell press*	*Kettlebell two-handed swing* *Sandbag clean* *Kettlebell two-handed clean* *Sandbag jerk* *Kettlebell windmill (right hand)* *Sandbag high pull* *Kettlebell windmill (left hand)* *Kettlebell get-up (right hand)* *Kettlebell get-up (left hand)*	Day off	1 × 20 meters (10 sec, 20 sec) *Bodyweight speed squat* 1 × 40 meters (15 sec, 30 sec) *Bodyweight reverse lunge* 1 × 60 meters (20 sec, 40 sec) *Bodyweight crab kick* 1 × 80 meters (25 sec, 50 sec) *Bodyweight bear crawl* 1 × 100 meters (30 sec, 60 sec) *Bodyweight push-up* 1 × 80 meters (25 sec, 50 sec) *Bodyweight mountain climber* 1 × 60 meters (20 sec, 40 sec) *Bodyweight thruster* 1 × 40 meters (15 sec, 30 sec) 1 × 20 meters	Backpedal *Medicine ball thruster* Shuffle right *Medicine ball slam* Shuffle left *Medicine ball chop with knee punch* T-test *Medicine ball modified pike* L drill *Medicine ball seated twist*

References

Chapter 1

Baechle, T.R., and R.W. Earle., eds. 2008. *Essentials of Strength Training and Conditioning.* Champaign, IL: Human Kinetics.

Brewer, C. 2008. *Strength and Conditioning for Sport: A Practical Guide for Coaches.* Headingley, United Kingdom: Sports Coach UK.

Boutcher, S.H. 2011. "High-Intensity Intermittent Exercise and Fat Loss." *Journal of Obesity.* doi:10.1155/2011/868305.

Gibala, M.J., and S.L. McGee. 2008. "Metabolic Adaptations to Short-Term High-Intensity Interval Training: A Little Pain for a Lot of Gain?" *Exercise and Sport Sciences Reviews* 36 (2): 58–63.

Talanian, J.L., S.D. Galloway, G.J. Heigenhauser, A. Bonen, and L.L. Spriet. 2007. "Two Weeks of High-Intensity Aerobic Interval Training Increases the Capacity for Fat Oxidation During Exercise in Women." *Journal of Applied Physiology* 102 (4): 1439–47.

Tremblay, A., J.A. Simoneau, and O. Bouchard. 1994. "Impact of Exercise Intensity on Body Fatness and Skeletal Muscle Metabolism." *Metabolism* 43: 814–818.

Chapter 2

Bergeron, M.F., M. Hargreaves, E.M. Haymes, G.W. Mack, and W.O. Roberts. 2007. "Exercise and Fluid Replacement." *Medicine and Science in Sports and Exercise* 39 (2): 377–390.

Chapter 5

Chandler, J.T. and B. Reuter. 1994. "An Inexpensive Medicine Ball for Strength, Conditioning, and Rehabilitation Programs." *Strength and Conditioning Journal* 16 (4): 45–47.

Thomas, Ed. 2002. "The Medicine Ball—Pro Salute Animae." *TaeKwon Do Times*, November, 44–50.

Chapter 11

Harman, E. 2008. "Principles of Test Selection and Administration." In *Essentials of Strength Training and Conditioning*, edited by T.R. Baechle, R.W. Earle. Champaign, IL: Human Kinetics.

Murray B. 2007. "Hydration and Physical Performance." *Journal of the American College of Nutrition* 26: 542s–548s,

Research CIfA. 2002. *Common Questions Regarding Physical Fitness Tests, Standards, and Programs for Public Safety.*

Spivey 2010.

Chapter 12

Harman E., and J. Garhammer. 2008. "Administration, Scoring and Interpretation of Selected Tests." In *Essentials of Strength Training and Conditioning*, edited by T.R. Baechle and R.W. Earle, 237–246. Champaign, IL: Human Kinetics.

Jones, J. 2012. "Testing Agility and Quickness." In *Developing Agility and Quickness*, edited by J. Dawes and M. Roozen. Champaign, IL: Human Kinetics.

Kritz, M., J. Cronin, and P. Hume. 2009a. "The Bodyweight Squat: A Movement Screen for the Squat Pattern." *Strength and Conditioning Journal* 31: 76–85.

Kritz, M., J. Cronin, and P. Hume. 2009b. "Using the Bodyweight Forward Lunge to Screen an Athlete's Lunge Pattern." *Strength and Conditioning Journal* 31: 15–24.

Reiman, M.P., and R.C. Manske. 2009. *Functional Testing in Human Performance*. Champaign, IL: Human Kinetics.

Chapter 13

Dimkpa, U. 2009. "Post-Exercise Heart Rate Recovery: An Index of Cardiovascular Fitness." *Journal of Exercise Physiology* (online) 12: 10–22.

Fletcher, G.F., V.F. Froelicher, L.H. Hartley, W.L. Haskell, and M.L. Pollock. 1990. "Exercise Standards. A Statement for Health Professionals From the American Heart Association." *Circulation* 82: 2286–2322.

McGuigan, M.R., T.L.A. Doyle, M. Newton, D.J. Edwards, S. Nimphius, and R.U. Newton. 2006. "Eccentric Utilization Ratio: Effect of Sport and Phase of Training." *Journal of Strength and Conditioning Research* 20: 992–995.

Reiman, M.P., and R.C. Manske. 2009. *Functional Testing in Human Performance*. Champaign, IL.: Human Kinetics.

Sayers, S.P., D.V. Harackiewicz, E.A. Harman, P.N. Frykman, and M.T. Rosenstein. 1999. "Cross-Validation of Three Jump Power Equations." *Medicine and Science in Sports and Exercise* 31: 572–577.

Turner, A.N., and P.F. Stewart. 2013. "Repeat Sprint Ability." *Strength and Conditioning Journal* 35: 37–41.

Chapter 18

Bishop, D., O. Girard, and A. Mendez-Villanueva. 2011. "Repeated-Sprint Ability—Part II: Recommendations for Training." *Sports Medicine* 41 (9): 741–756. doi: 10.2165/11590560-000000000-00000

Dawson, B. 2012. "Repeated-Sprint Ability: Where Are We?" *International Journal of Sports Physiology and Performance* 7 (3): 285–289.

Girard, O., A. Mendez-Villanueva, and D. Bishop. 2011. "Repeated-Sprint Ability—Part I: Factors Contributing to Fatigue." *Sports Medicine* 41 (8): 673–694. doi: 10.2165/11590550-000000000-00000

Chapter 20

Knapik, J.J., W. Rieger, F. Palkoska, S. Van Camp, and S. Darakjy. 2009. "United States Army Physical Readiness Training: Rationale and Evaluation of the Physical Training Doctrine." *Journal of Strength and Conditioning Research* 23: 1353–1362.

National Strength and Conditioning Association. 2014. *Need Analysis for the Tactical Officer*. Presented at NSCA Facilitators Course, Colorado Springs, CO.

National Tactical Officers Association. 2008. *SWAT Standards for Law Enforcement Agencies*.

Cooper Institute for Aerobic Research. *Frequently Asked Questions Regarding Fitness Standards in Law Enforcement*. Dallas TX: Cooper Institute of Aerobic Research.

Sauers, S.E., and Scofield, D.E. 2014. "Strength and Conditioning Strategies for Females in the Military." *Strength and Conditioning Journal* 36: 1–7.

About the Authors

John Cissik is the president and owner of Human Performance Services, LLC (HPS), which helps athletics professionals solve their strength and conditioning needs. He coaches youth baseball, basketball, and Special Olympics sports and runs fitness classes for children with special needs. He has written 10 books and more than 70 articles on strength and speed training that have been featured in *Muscle & Fitness*, *Iron Man*, and track and field and coaching publications. He is also the author of Human Kinetics' *Speed for Sports Performance* DVD series. Cissik specializes in education, strength training for baseball, basketball, track and field, and speed and agility training. He has worked with athletes from high school to Olympic levels. John is certified by the National Strength and Conditioning Association as a strength and conditioning specialist and personal trainer and by the National Academy of Sports Medicine as a personal trainer and corrective exercise specialist. He has held level I and level II certifications from USA Track and Field and was certified with the former U.S. Weightlifting Federation.

Jay Dawes is an assistant professor in the department of health sciences at the University of Colorado at Colorado Springs. Before joining UCCS, Dawes was an assistant professor of kinesiology at Texas A&M at Corpus Christi and the director of education for the National Strength and Conditioning Association. Jay has worked as a strength and performance coach, personal trainer, educator, and postrehabilitation specialist for more than 15 years. A frequent presenter both nationally and internationally on topics related to health, fitness, and human performance, Dawes received his PhD from Oklahoma State University in the School of Applied Health and Educational Psychology with an emphasis in health and human performance. He is certified by the National Strength and Conditioning Association as a strength and conditioning specialist and personal trainer, by the American College of Sports Medicine as a health fitness specialist, and by USA Weightlifting as a club coach. He became a fellow of the NSCA in 2009.

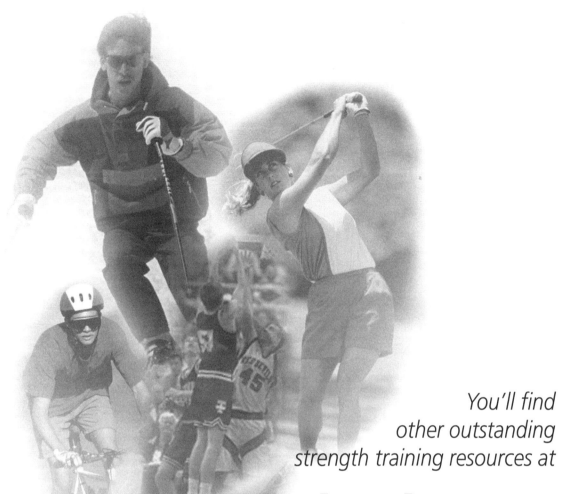

*You'll find
other outstanding
strength training resources at*

www.HumanKinetics.com

In the U.S. call

1-800-747-4457

Australia	08 8372 0999
Canada	1-800-465-7301
Europe	+44 (0) 113 255 5665
New Zealand	0800 222 062

HUMAN KINETICS
The Premier Publisher for Sports & Fitness
P.O. Box 5076 • Champaign, IL 61825-5076 USA